34.95

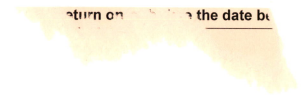

Scientific Errors and Controversies in the U.S. HIV/AIDS Epidemic

Scientific Errors and Controversies in the U.S. HIV/AIDS Epidemic

How They Slowed Advances and Were Resolved

SCOTT D. HOLMBERG, M.D.

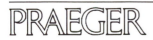
PRAEGER

Westport, Connecticut
London

Library of Congress Cataloging-in-Publication Data

Holmberg, Scott D., 1950–
Scientific errors and controversies in the U.S. HIV/AIDS epidemic : how they slowed advances and were resolved / Scott D. Holmberg.
    p. cm.
  Includes bibliographical references and index.
  ISBN: 978–0–313–34717–7 (alk. paper)
    1. AIDS (Disease)–Research–United States–History.   2. HIV infections–Research–United States–History.   3. AIDS (Disease)–United States–Epidemiology.   4. HIV infections–United States–Epidemiology.   5. Errors, Scientific.   6. Medical errors.
    [DNLM: 1. HIV Infections–epidemiology.   2. HIV Infections–history.
3. Epidemiologic Methods.   4. Medical Errors–prevention & control. WC 503
H747s 2007]   I. Title.
  RA643.83.H65   2008
  614.5′99392–dc22   2007035419

British Library Cataloguing in Publication Data is available.

Library of Congress Catalog Card Number: 2007035419
ISBN: 978–0–313–34717–7

First published in 2008

Praeger Publishers, 88 Post Road West, Westport, CT 06881
An imprint of Greenwood Publishing Group, Inc.
www.praeger.com

Printed in the United States of America

The paper used in this book complies with the Permanent Paper Standard issued by the National Information Standards Organization (Z39.48–1984).

10 9 8 7 6 5 4 3 2 1

Contents

Preface

As the first section of this book indicates, all scientific advance and understanding comes from teamwork, and I have been especially lucky with my teammates. Over almost 20 years in CDC's Division of HIV/AIDS Prevention, many intramural and extramural colleagues and I have continually compared notes and sometimes groused about the role of ideologic scientific prejudice (I don't have a better term) in skewing data and opinions about HIV epidemiology and treatment. Sometimes, my colleagues and I felt we were spending half our time "undoing" clearly wrong science, especially wrong research promulgated by prominent figures or published in prestigious journals.

It would be impossible to cite and adequately thank them all, but the collaborators with whom I have worked especially closely in recent years on large cohort studies include: at CDC, Anne Moorman, Alan Greenberg (now at George Washington University), Martha Rogers (now at The Carter Center, Atlanta), Dawn Smith, Tony Tong, and John Brooks; Frank Palella, Northwestern University, Chicago; Ken Lichtenstein, University of Colorado Health Center, Denver; and Ellen Tedaldi, Temple University, Philadelphia. Going back further in time, several professional friends have been consistently supportive, collegial, and insightful over the years, and many other HIV/AIDS scientists, clinicians, and patients will recognize their names: Ken Mayer, Brown University AIDS Program; Sten Vermund, Vanderbilt University, Nashville; and Susan Buchbinder, San Francisco Department of Public Health.

Recent and proximate contributors of insights, quotes, data, and suggestions for this book include: Harold W. Jaffe, St. Cross College and Department of Public Health, University of Oxford, England; Charles A. Schable, Scientific Technologies Corporation, Tucson; Paul O'Malley, San Francisco Public Health Foundation; Roger Dodd, American Red Cross Holland Laboratory, Rockville, MD; James Richardson, Cerner Corporation, McLean, VA; Mary E. Chamberland, Division of Viral and Rickettsial Diseases, CDC, Atlanta; Ken A. Lichtenstein; Ruth L. Berkelman, Emory University, Atlanta; and Richard Jefferys, Treatment Action Group, New York. Special mention should also go to my freelance-writing friend, Mark Pendergrast, for some experienced authorial and publishing suggestions.

In addition to these colleagues, this is a good opportunity to thank again my very patient and supportive immediate supervisors over the years, Harold Jaffe, Martha Rogers, and Alan Greenberg. Finally, but not least, I wish to thank my most important teammates for their support of not only this book, but my life, namely my wife Maureen and my son Matthew.

CHAPTER ONE

Background

This is a book about errors: not only about how scientific errors developed, got propagated, and sometimes still persist in the field of HIV/AIDS, but also about how errors got corrected and controversies resolved. All scientific endeavors are distracted by many detours and dead ends, controversies and resolutions, and this is certainly the case with our understanding the U.S. HIV/AIDS epidemic over the past 25 years.

About Teamwork

Contrary to some popular opinion, almost all of what we now accept as true was not the result of a lone scientist toiling at his bench long into the night, holding a pastel-colored, smoking test tube in the air, and shouting "Eureka." HIV/AIDS science is not only done at bench tops, but also in hospitals and clinics, in communities, in computers, and in reference (not just research) laboratories. Advances almost always result from a team effort of various combinations of clinicians, statisticians, laboratorians, epidemiologists, supervisors, computer programmers, and, lest we forget, a host of usually unrecognized support personnel such as data managers, writer-editors, nurses, lab technicians, and on and on. Thus, almost no major article on HIV/AIDS hosts fewer than several coauthors, and the best efforts of medical journal editorial staff some years ago, now largely abandoned, to prune nonessential authors from the masthead have been met with resistance. Most coauthors have had an essential, even if small, part in the team effort of putting together any scientific analysis and peer-reviewed journal publication about HIV. Also, for many aspiring scientists, recognition as a coauthor on an important paper may be far more important in the long run than their immediate paycheck.

Teamwork has many virtues: an important one is that collaborators can review each other's work to minimize the chances that the wrong data or conclusions will be broadcast. However, this presumes that no one or two researchers can enforce their own biases and that several on the team have the insight and courage to correct or at least bring up problems with the data or its analysis.

Research teams are motivated at least in part to report the next scientific breakthrough and to be both first and correct. Indeed, the impatience to be first to report something often breeds carelessness and biased analyses. This intense competitiveness sometimes dismays nonscientists: why must motivations be so nonaltruistic; why can't government agencies and academic and research centers play with one another nicely; or, why must different organizations set up separate, competing studies? In fact, scientists and their organizations more often cooperate than compete with one another, but competition is vital to progress in the area of HIV/AIDS. As described in this book, no one study ever completely answers a question: the first study of an issue can be wrong in part or in full, and, even if it isn't, it must be verified by the findings of others independently.

Also, to be a true breakthrough, not only must the analysis or report be reproducible, but people also need to pay attention to it. A letter to an obscure regional or specialist journal does not count; an original article that is cited hundreds of times—that is, referenced by others in their articles as determined, for example, in the *Science Citation Index*—can easily result in tenure, invitations to speak to other doctors and scientists, the esteem of those colleagues, and a personal sense of accomplishment. As important for many, research lab or clinical funding is ever harder to obtain and increasingly contingent on good results. Many assistants and colleagues may lose their positions and salaries if funding dries up: this puts tremendous pressure to find something to justify the underwriting of the endeavor. Money, too, in the form of honoraria for speaking or a position as a "clinical investigator" funded by a pharmaceutical company provides motivation for many.

Still, for the vast majority of doctors, scientists, and epidemiologists with whom I have worked for over 20 years within and outside the Centers for Disease Control (CDC), most in the Division of HIV/AIDS Prevention (1986–2005), it seems unlikely that any one of them would purposely propagate a scientific error. Most scientists do science because, as for mountain climbers, the mountain beckons. Unlike mountain climbers, however, they can ascribe their motivations to a greater social good and so hide the fact that they do science because it is really interesting. As Harold Jaffe commented at the time of his retirement in 2004 as Director for CDC's National Center for HIV, STD and TB Prevention: "So what were the first few years of the AIDS epidemic really like at CDC? Although it seems almost sacrilegious to say so, it was actually fun. You couldn't look in the back of the book to find the answer. Each phone call could turn into a new lead . . ." For "each phone call," one could insert "the next set of experiments" or "the next data run," and for "AIDS" one can substitute almost any other disease: the idea remains the same.

Sources of Error and Epidemiologic Thinking

We often read about fraud as the source of bad science. Fraud by scientists certainly exists, and indeed, the claims of Robert Gallo to discovery of the HIV virus (HTLV-III) have been criticized as "fraudulent" (see Chapter 2). However, it is somewhat difficult to believe that someone who is smart enough to consciously manufacture fraudulent data would actually do so. The rewards for being correct are too great and the loss of esteem by one's fellows is too onerous for most scientists to set out to report something that one knows is false, as virtually all fraudulent science of any import is eventually discovered.

However, much, much more common and much harder to eventually ferret out are "cherry-picking" information or analyses, nibbling at the edges of truth, or squinting and seeing data in a prejudicial light. These are all common and usually done semiconsciously. The result is a litter of discarded theories and opinions that this book will admittedly select in a biased manner to point out how errors occurred in HIV/AIDS science and how they eventually garner credence and later rejection. While there have been many successes, the errors and failures are usually more instructive.

Much of what will be described here relates to epidemiology, technically the study of epidemics, be they HIV/AIDS, cancer, obesity, injury, or any medical condition. Some readers will find the following brief description didactic and well below their level of knowledge; they may also well resent the simplistic way I have chosen to explain epidemiologic thinking, or perhaps take issue with it, so perhaps they will spare themselves reading the next few pages. However, for those who do not often think about such topics, epidemiology is a science of comparison, as it is for most biologic and medical science. Typically, against a comparison (control) group without disease or condition "y," is the risk factor "x" more likely found in a (case) group of people of interest who do have condition y? In a retrospective study early in the epidemic, for example, did gay men with HIV infection have more sex partners, or riskier sex practices, than a comparison group of HIV-uninfected gay men?

If an association is indeed found between condition y (in this simple case, HIV/AIDS) and risk factor x (in this case, sex activity), it is expressed statistically two ways. First, the differences are usually expressed as a relative risk or relative hazard (RR or RH, usually when comparing two cohorts or large groups, especially if time-dependent statistics are used), or an odds ratio (OR, as in comparing smaller numbers of "case-persons" and their matched "control-persons"). We might say, "In our study, HIV-infected gay men had three times the number of lifetime sex partners (RR or OR=3.0) than gay men in our study who were not HIV-infected." This is a really simple and basic example, and almost all studies—especially modern studies of complicated drug regimens—are far more complex, looking at several factors and their relationship to each other and the outcome variable of interest. Still, the basic "building block" is the same—a comparison, a measure of the *strength of association*, of two groups of people. (In addition to clinical and epidemiologic studies, much lab work also rests on comparison.)

The other statistic universally used is the p-value, the probability that the association found could have occurred by chance, a fluke, of the natural variation in both y and x. The statistically "significant" p-value was set at 0.05 many years ago by one of the earliest statisticians and remains the standard today. That is, scientists will always look to see whether p is less than 0.05, indicating that there is less than a 5 percent probability that the association of x with y occurred by chance.

This would all be straightforward, if there weren't so many hidden statistical and other land mines. First, no matter how high the OR or RR and no matter how low the p-value, it is not possible to prove that x actually led to y. This relates to our basic problem with demonstrating causation. Fortunately, most scientists end up having a jovial disregard for this philosophical point: if, in our simple example, the gay men who have HIV infection have 50-fold the number of sex partners over the past 5 years compared to gay men without infection, and the p-value for the association is 10^{-8}, that is certainly good enough for anyone's purposes. The authors of a paper describing such an association will usually slip into talking about how having many sex partners predisposes or leads to getting HIV infection, when, technically, they should only talk about the "association." (However, I am unaware that anyone has been sued for letting the language of causation slip into a report.) This theoretical nit-picking leads, though, to an important practical problem when critics focus on the lack of absolute proof of causation rather than a mountain of evidence that such causation does indeed occur, as, for instance, the claim that HIV does not cause AIDS.[1]

Second, and more important, is the problem of "confounding," simply put, the observed and measured variable x may actually be a marker of or otherwise closely associated with another variable–let's call it x_n–that may reflect the true association with condition y. Thus, variable x_n may "confound" (obscure) the real association of x with y. For instance, if a study reports that HIV-infected people (x) are twice as likely to develop, say, cardiovascular disease (y) than non-HIV-infected people, is this because the HIV-infected people are twice as likely to be long-term cigarette smokers (x_1); or more than twice as likely to be men (x_2), who also have a higher incidence of cardiovascular disease; or simply older (x_3), another risk factor for this disease? In fact, over 60 percent of HIV-infected people are current or past cigarette smokers, and, until recently, 80 percent or more of HIV-infected people and AIDS cases were men. Do high rates of cigarette-smoking or male gender confound the association between HIV infection and cardiovascular disease? Unless the study has selected participants ahead of time to be equally distributed in their amount and duration of smoking history and gender, or, more usually, "controlled" after the fact by stratification or regression analysis for cigarette smoking and gender, we call the association of HIV and cardiovascular disease potentially "confounded."

A fundamental property of epidemiologic thinking is to immediately start thinking of potential confounders the moment an association is described. To take another example from the HIV/AIDS epidemic, poverty or race is often associated with HIV infection in many studies, but the real association may be between number and types of sex activity–for example, more so for indigent, drug-using women who may exchange sex for money or drugs–and HIV infection. Most good studies spend a lot of time trying to "control" for confounding variables such as this either ahead of time by matching cases and controls, or by later stratification or other analytic means. Some of the studies referenced in this book were ultimately found to be wrong because a critical risk factor was not measured or measured poorly, and it confounded the reported association, such as the association between protease inhibitor drugs and HIV-associated lipodystrophy (Chapter 8).

Another common problem is what we call a "bias of ascertainment." For example, if one is only investigating hospitalized AIDS patients, one might conclude that the time between HIV infection and death is comparatively short; however, if the time of HIV infection were known for such patients it may turn out that the incubation period between HIV infection and developing AIDS is actually rather long, as, indeed, it is–that is, about 8–11 years in the absence of treatment, longer if modern therapies are included. In this crude and obvious example, the problem here is that we are "ascertaining" our HIV patients late in their HIV infection. The problem may be quite subtle when, as we shall see, some investigators reported that women had shorter incubation periods to AIDS or survival before dying than men,[2] when the women were probably "ascertained" later in their disease course.

In an egregious instance of how the data itself can be badly biased, Robert Redfield and other military investigators reported in 1985 that 10 (28%) of male uniformed personnel who were interviewed by them reported "no identified risk" other than heterosexual contact.[3] This report was widely taken and cited as evidence of female-to-male transmission in the United States, although by 1985 it was evident that many African heterosexual men had acquired AIDS and such transmission was certainly occurring outside Africa. These investigators from the Uniformed Services were certainly correct on the larger issue: heterosexual contact was then and remains the major mode of transmission in almost the whole world outside some developed nations. Twenty years later heterosexual spread in the South is currently increasing as a mode of transmission at an alarming rate. However, their basis for drawing the principle was suspect, and a letter from officials at the New York City Department of Health questioned the "epidemiologic reasoning" as "Certainly, discharge from military service for [admitting to investigators] homosexuality and/or intravenous (IV) drug use would dissuade self-reporting of these behaviors."[4] The response from the original report authors (the military investigators) missed the point: "We are unaware of any evidence to support the often-repeated statement that soldiers are more likely than civilians to lie to their personal physicians."[5] Perhaps soldiers are no more likely than civilians to lie, but a follow-up study of 26 no-identified-risk AIDS cases in active-duty military—including some of those same interviewees described in the original report![4]—showed that 20 (77%) reported to civilian investigators behaviors defined as HIV risk factors, usually homosexual activity.[6] So, to avoid discharge from the service, some of these soldiers, anyway, had lied.

There is the problem with interpretation of statistics, even by otherwise sophisticated researchers. p-values can be accepted in a facile and mechanical fashion to misinterpret the results of a published study, when more nuanced or fuller interpretation is required. The tyranny of the p-value has been commented on by many thinkers[7] because, interpreted alone, it presents a double-edged problem. If one looks at large groups of people—say, thousands—small differences may be "statistically significant" with a p-value much less than 0.05. However, what is the practical difference if your risk of acquiring condition y is only increased a percentage or two by factor x? That percentage or two of additional risk may be cost-beneficial in terms of population health if factor x is easily eliminated or controlled. However, for the purposes of a doctor counseling a patient, it probably makes no real difference: there is so much more that needs to be done in the 10–15 minutes the typical HIV clinician now has with his or her HIV patient.

Another overinterpretation of p-values relates to looking at the association of several variables to the outcome y. If one analyzes several factors for their independent association with condition y, the chance that one of these analyses will have a p-value less than 0.05 rapidly increases. For example, if we look at 10 potential risk factors for HIV infection, even if they are not associated in reality, we have about a 40 percent chance of finding one association with a p-value less than 0.05.

p-values also have the opposite problem: that is, if the numbers of people being compared is small, the RR or OR may be large, but the p-value may not be under 0.05. This book will point to some examples where a p-value of, say, between 0.05 and 0.10, led the authors, the reviewers, or the readers to conclude that "no association exists," when, more properly, the association actually does exist and the p-value is pretty low, but it simply does not fit the criterion that we all arbitrarily accept. We may say such a study is "underpowered" because, while the association may be strong, the numbers of people or events compared are relatively small or rare and the p-value, reflecting variation in the factors and outcome being compared, is higher than 0.05.

One underlying problem is that many, if not most, medical personnel have had brief education in statistics and epidemiology, and this is usually the tedious memorization of a set of statistical equations, rather than a true understanding of epidemiologic and critical thinking and the use of statistics to support it. They may be unduly impressed with statistical esoterica such as complicated tests unknown to any outside the biostatistical community, by the size of the study, or by mountains of p-values, risk ratios and confidence limits, β-coefficients, etc. Nonetheless, a spate of statistics may hide many methodologic weaknesses such as biases and confounding.

Thus, the way most AIDS researchers report and read analyses requires examining both the strength of the association, reflected in the RR or OR, and also the likelihood that the association is true and not an artifact of variability in the factors examined, as expressed in a low p-value. Experience teaches that any report with a risk or odds ratio less than 2.0, or especially less than 1.5, needs to be interpreted with an open mind, as too many unmeasured confounders may be operating. This requires assessing not only how well an original report "fits" what is known, but also considering ways in which the analysis may have ultimately been confounded by unsuspected, unmeasured or poorly measured variables.

In addition to the "strength of association," another consideration that may determine the credibility of a report includes whether, within limits, there is a "dose-response." For example, increasing the dosage of a drug– above a threshold of efficacy and below toxic dosage (within a "therapeutic index")–should be associated with better outcomes; similarly, increasing the frequency, or amount of a risk factor for disease should increase the likelihood (or amount) of the disease. This is not always possible to demonstrate, for example with all-or-none type outcomes or within narrow therapeutic indices. Still, when a research team can demonstrate a dose-response, this lends credence to their conclusion.

Much more tricky is the question of "biologic plausibility." It is always good to be able to point to some biologic mechanism that makes sense of the association–for example, the toxic or adverse effects of a drug or a disease process has a recognized biologic basis. Thus, if certain antiretroviral drugs increase serum cholesterol levels, it is biologically plausible that over time they may have negative consequences for cardiovascular health (Chapter 8). However, many times a given phenomenon–say, lipodystrophy, the fat wasting or accumulation (maldistribution) seen in many HIV patients treated with protease inhibitor (PI) and nucleoside reverse transcriptase inhibitor (NRTI) drugs after 1996–has no clear biologic mechanism. It is possible to conjecture many different pathways for the unexpected outcome, and, indeed, there are: all of these may seem plausible. Biologic plausibility can be postulated for almost any observed phenomenon, and this limits its helpfulness in evaluating many reports.

Simple "error" has always been a major problem in HIV/AIDS research, especially with new laboratory tests or statistical modeling exercises that are well beyond the expertise of the reader. We are often impressed by what we cannot do ourselves, and this may obscure real problems with a study or its analysis. For example, early in the use of polymerase chain reaction (PCR) to test for the presence or number of copies of HIV genomes, some prominent studies reported startling findings that both misled many in the AIDS community and, on retrospect, resulted from laboratory error, contamination, or poor technique in the hands of novices (Chapter 4).

Somewhat different problems pertain to modeling as the mathematics can be obtuse and the result predetermined by the assumptions put into the model. Readers of articles in general scientific, medical, or public health literature will not be able to understand the calculus, other than in a general way, involved in most mathematical models. Reminiscent of the Wizard of Oz's warning "Ignore that man behind the curtain," many of the assumptions upon which models rest are large, based on scant data and not always clear or even presented to the reader. A measurement used in many stochastic models of HIV is "R-naught" (R_o), the basic reproductive rate, that is, how many others will be infected from a given infected individual. If R_o is greater than 1, the epidemic will propagate; if R_o is less than 1, the epidemic will abate of its own accord. However, to determine this value, one needs to know properties of the agent that are almost never available. We know, for example, that different people with HIV infection are more or less likely to transmit HIV (their infectiousness) and their strains of HIV may have different likelihood of transmission (viral infectivity) over the long course of HIV infection (see Chapter 4).

And then there is a basic error rate to human endeavors, no matter how careful one is. Blood bankers, an extremely nervous group of professionals, must worry about clerical errors all the time,[8, 9] as such errors may now be much more likely than the extremely low likelihood of transmission by blood transfusion screened as "negative" for HIV infection.[10]

Error frequently occurs as well in data management both before and after data entry into the computer. Clerical errors and misassignment of values and incorrect programming of data can easily occur. This author has had the experience of finding completely different results once computer-programming errors were corrected (fortunately, before journal submission).

Finally, the biggest problem, in the writer's opinion, is only indirectly but powerfully related to the conduct of studies, the selection of factors to be analyzed, or the statistical test that is applied to the data. This is called personal bias or, if you will, wishful thinking. Many studies have been undertaken and reported by investigators, and then read by reviewers and editorialists, with a real bias to find or not find a particular association. A treasured teacher, colleague, leader in the field, or journal article has told one that something is so, and thus, a certain attitude is taken. Or, conversely, perhaps one is by nature an iconoclast, ready to disbelieve. In any case, most good scientists believe that personal bias is, like error, fundamentally human and unavoidable, and the best scientists spend their professional lives trying to recognize bias not only in others but also especially in themselves.

In HIV/AIDS science, there are certainly what we may call "alpha-scientists" who, when they start in a certain direction, will pull any number of "beta-scientists" along with them. This problem is inextricably related to the personal popularity of the scientist. Presently, more researchers are more likely to believe Dr. Anthony Fauci (former Director, National Institute of Allergic and Infectious Disease, NIH) than Dr. Robert Gallo (former Director, National Cancer Institute's Laboratory of Tumor Cell Biology). Most people have great difficulty separating the message from the messenger, but this sifting is essential to good science. This is particularly the problem, as seen in later Chapters, when the messenger is exceptionally popular or revered, yet just plain wrong.

Personal bias may be detected in a scientific report or article when one or more of the following conditions pertain: the association has not been completely corrected for potential confounding—for example, factor x is probably associated with something else the investigator(s) did not or could not examine; the strength of the association (RR or OR), no matter what the *p*-value, is low; or the report focuses on a weak association that does not fit the main thesis—for example, some secondary factor (such as lack of drug toxicity) is reported, as the main variable of interest (drug's efficacy) did not turn out to be statistically associated.

HIV/AIDS science has often gone awry, taking time as other, independent researchers try to find out whether a new and surprising finding is indeed correct. Incidentally, these efforts that result in confirmation or refutation of a report usually circulate only in the HIV/AIDS scientific community and a small subset of the general AIDS community concerned with a particular issue, and may not make it into the general public media. Ultimately, though, most people now understand that HIV causes AIDS, that HIV is not spread by toilet seats, and that HIV-infected people can now be treated moderately successfully. However, the public ultimately comes to these pieces of knowledge based on personal experience, news reports, or how many people they respect say these things are so, rather than on a careful reading of the scientific literature (which, one supposes, gets back to the problem with bias).

Interpreting the Relative Value of Studies

Generally, when an original report comes out in the medical/scientific literature, other scientists tend to credit the analysis to a large extent on the basis of the type of methodology that is used: certain studies have more credence than others. The simplest kind of report is the case report or case series. These are essentially anecdotes that may reflect something new or unusual that is happening, or may be flukes. The first report of an unusual infection in five gay men in California in CDC's *Morbidity and Mortality Weekly Report* (*MMWR*) in 1981 was the harbinger of hundreds of thousands of U.S. AIDS cases. Was this cluster of *Pneumocystis carinii* infection in gay men simply a coincidence, an artifact of some common exposure?

In 1981 no one could know, but clearly these few cases represented an "outbreak" by the definition of an occurrence of a disease or condition significantly out of proportion to its baseline occurrence (endemicity) in the population. Case reports or case series are often the way a new disease or syndrome, their successful treatment, or adverse reactions to treatment are first reported. These simple reports are invaluable; they also have many problems. For example, many reserchers have examined and reported unusual cancer clusters, investigations of which have largely been abandoned as these appear to be random geographical groupings of cancer cases. Early on, there were some thoughts that AIDS clusters were similar to these cancer clusters—that is, case reports and small case series (clusters) may be the report of a coincidence or a rare oddity, so they must be read with an open mind. Thus, while it was pretty clear to most that something unusual was happening, most epidemiologists, doctors, and scientists also thought initially that these cases were an aberration, probably related to some local, specific or limited exposure in some gay men.[11] Such wishful thinking waned as cases began to rapidly accumulate across the country. Also, in retrospect, as limited as these initial case reports were, it is amazing how prescient they were. The first report in 1981 of five cases[12] discussed the possibility of "disease acquired through sexual contact... in this [homosexual] population." By 1982 an *MMWR* report concluded that the distribution pattern of cases "strongly suggested" that AIDS was the result of an agent transmitted though sexual contact.[13]

This observation segues to another form of preliminary or initial analysis, the "ecologic study." In this type of analysis, two similar curves or two similar geographic distributions are compared and one deduces that there is a relationship or association between them. Some examples in the AIDS epidemic—that have had variable confirmation in subsequent studies of individual people—include: the graphic association of (lack of) circumcision and HIV/AIDS cases in Africa[14]; or distribution of AIDS cases and certain monkeys (e.g., Hooper, *The River*, 1999)[15]; or mosquitoes and the agent of AIDS (in studies as described by Leishman, 1987).[16] These "ecological fallacies" can be quite sophisticated and involve molecular analyses of unusual viruses[17] or complex statistical techniques.[18] Such articles can be dazzling and distract the reader from understanding that the units of analysis are not, for example, actual persons with a condition compared with persons without the condition. Rather, ecologic analyses are comparisons of lines on a graph or of maps or other distributions of conditions. Thus, it is wise to remember that two curves/lines may run in parallel yet have no relationship to one another —such as, say, refrigerator ownership in Poland and gun violence in Dubuque.

Accordingly, next in the hierarchy of credibility are case-control studies, especially those that report a strong association between a variable (x) and an outcome (y) in individual patients. These are often retrospective, and suffer from problems of memory or avoidance of questions by interviewees (per the example of the uniformed personnel asked about their sexual and drug-using behaviors within a military context); problems of confounding, bias, and error, of course, also plague these analyses. In such studies, though, big differences between cases and controls will always emerge and usually turn out to be true—that is, results duplicated by other researchers. Thus, the first national case-control studies of AIDS patients, as reported in a special August 1983 issue of *Annals of Internal Medicine,* found the many risk factors for getting AIDS that we now accept implicitly: gay men who had AIDS had had lymphopenia (low white blood cell counts) and many more lifetime and yearly sex partners and a history of more sexually transmitted diseases (STDs) than gay men without AIDS (which group must also have included some men with HIV infection who had not yet developed AIDS).[19, 20] Clearly, the indices of sexual activity and the increased numbers of STDs in the case-patients were related. Also, these reports included associations now thought to be "confounded" and incorrect, such as the association of AIDS and the use of illicit substances especially inhaled nitrites, so-called "poppers," to increase sexual stimulation (see Chapter 2).

Case-control studies may be adjusted in advance by "matching" the control persons with (usually a small number of) case patients: "controls" may be selected to be the same as "cases" on a number of potentially confounding factors such as age, sex, race/ethnicity, or geographical residence. However, such case–control "matching" has infrequently been done in HIV/AIDS studies over the past 25 years, except in small short-term clinical drug trials. More likely, the data are analyzed retrospectively by logistic or linear regression analysis (or stratification) such that if one is looking at a few potential risk factors, each stratum or cell of comparison is matched for the other variables before calculating the odds ratio (or relative risk) for the single variable of interest.

The currently preferred design of studies–the "gold standard" for assessing drug efficacy–is the randomized clinical trial (RCT); ideally, this is prospective (patients are followed forward in time), randomized (patients are randomly selected and assigned to receive or not receive the treatment of interest), and double-blind (neither treated patients or clinicians providing the treatment know which patients are receiving which treatment). In some cases, these RCTs can also be "placebo-controlled" as some patients receive pills or injections that look like the therapy but are, in fact, ineffective. However, provision of a placebo would be clearly unethical in AIDS, so all studies recently compare a new therapy to a currently available standard-of-care therapy or the addition of a drug to an "optimized" baseline therapy. Most HIV/AIDS clinical scientists believe that such well-controlled studies, with fixed, frequent, and intense examination and analysis of each patient over time, is the only valid way to *initially* assess drug efficacy.

It might help here to define the recognized "phases" to clinical trials. Phase I studies are primarily concerned with the drug's safety, and are the first time the drug is tested in humans. These studies are typically done in a small number of healthy volunteers (20–100), usually in a hospital setting where the volunteers can be closely monitored and treated should there be any side effects. Once an experimental drug has been proven to be safe and well tolerated in healthy volunteers, it must be tested in the patients who have the disease or condition to which the experimental drug is targeted to ameliorate or cure. In addition to ensuring that the experimental drug is safe and effective, Phase II studies are mainly of interest in evaluating the effectiveness of the drug. This second stage of study takes from several months to a few years—usually 24, 48, or 96 weeks in HIV/AIDS Phase II studies— and assesses several hundred patients within a controlled, randomized trial design. In a Phase III study, an experimental drug is tested in several hundred to several thousand patients with the disease/condition of interest. Because of their size, many Phase III studies are not blinded. The large-scale testing provides the pharmaceutical company, the FDA, and the medical community with a better understanding of the drug's effectiveness, benefits/risks, and range/severity of possible adverse side effects.

As the HIV/AIDS epidemic has progressed and issues of drug treatment become more important, phase I and II RCTs are increasingly used to es- timate the advantages and problems with new treatments. Yet there are limitations and problems with this study design. As in any case-control study, quality and accuracy of raw data, biases in comparison, and hidden method- ologic problems may beset these studies.[21] For example, in HIV therapeutic research of HIV (antiretroviral) drugs in the first decade or so, these therapies were usually tested in RCTs of people who were "treatment-naïve" and likely to respond well to any drug to which they first were exposed.

Additional theoretical problems with RCTs include that: repeated mea- surements over time increase the likelihood of finding a spuriously (ran- domly) significant p-value, and scientific data for the study may be confused with clinical data obtained on the patient.[22] RCTs are also expensive and time-intensive[23]: imagine the economic and time costs of having doctors and nurses examining and collecting laboratory data, often with the most recent technology, every week or two for a long period. Accordingly, these studies are often limited both in the number of patients examined and in time of observation, usually 24-, 48-, 72- or, at most and unusually, 96-weeks duration. Although NIH funds two important consortia—the AIDS Clinical Trials Group (ACTG) and the Community Programs for Clinical Research on AIDS (CPCRA)—many HIV-related RCTs have been "nested" as smaller and shorter studies within these clinical trial networks.

These considerations lead to the two biggest problems with RCTs from a larger population health point of view: they often end before true (individ- ual) efficacy, (population) effectiveness, occurrence, or impact of a drug or intervention over a prolonged period can be determined; and they frequently end well before the adverse effects of chronic and long-term treatment can be determined. This was, for example, the case with zidovudine (AZT), the first antiretroviral (anti-HIV) drug, as this drug trial was ended (truncated) based on interim statistical analysis at 24 weeks; most patients had only received 16 weeks' therapy[24] when the study was ended. The effectiveness of zidovudine in improving several laboratory and physical parameters was evident, and the drug needed to be approved for use in AIDS patients promptly. However, the big downside was that its effectiveness in treating HIV infection was limited and that some of its adverse effects—for example, final rates of anemia and neutropenia (low red and white blood cell counts) in treated patients, or the development of viral resistance to the drug—increased with time and became more evident after those first 24 (or, for most of the study-participants, 16) weeks of treatment in the original RCT (see Chapter 7).

Phase III studies unfold over a period of years and continue to randomize and blind both investigators and many patients as to who is receiving the drug of interest and who is receiving placebo or current-standard-of-care therapy; however, such long-term blinded, placebo-controlled are virtually never done in HIV/AIDS. The expense and difficulty are a major consideration; and placebo-control is unacceptable for a fatal infection, so comparison is usually to "standard-of-care" or "optimized" therapy. In a field as dynamic as HIV drug development, new and better drugs are continually being developed, rapidly displacing some drugs of interest of even the recent past.

Accordingly, longer term—say, three of more years' follow-up—observational cohort studies are also needed, especially to assess the eventual benefits and problems with treatments. There are currently over 20 FDA-approved antiretroviral drugs (see Appendix) and, while modern treatment for HIV is good in terms of substantially improving the quantity and quality of HIV patients' lives, the long-term therapeutic efficacy, toxicity, resistance, and other adverse effects are not known for all of these medicines. Most were approved for use after short-term intensive RCTs (see Chapter 8).

Most AIDS scientists believe that RCTs with their frequent, fixed-time analyses of patients are the only way to evaluate the worth of treatments specifically and perhaps other HIV-related conditions, too. Thus, leaders in the HIV/AIDS scientific community will often disparage the results from any of several government-sponsored long-term cohort studies of HIV patients that are not rigorously structured. However, most of what we understand about the epidemiology of HIV and even much of what we know about the clinical spectrum of HIV-related diseases and conditions and general benefits and adverse effects of long-term treatment come from such observational studies. These include, if one may be forgiven for not specifying important design differences in them (methodologies that can be found in the references) and for only indicating some of the larger and most productive cohorts to date: CDC's original study of 6,700 gay men in three cities (1982–1998) who were originally enrolled in studies of hepatitis B (HBV) and HBV vaccine in 1978–1981[25, 26]; NIAID's Multicenter AIDS Cohort Study (MACS) of almost 4,000 gay men in five cities from 1984 to the present[27]; the studies of HIV-infected women done in parallel–the CDC's HIV Epidemiology Study (HERS)[28] from 1993 to 2001, and the larger NIAID-funded Women's Interagency HIV Study (WIHS)[29] from 1994 to the present; and CDC's general HIV cohort studies that include the Adult and Adolescent Spectrum of Disease (ASD) Project from 1990 to 2004[30] and the HIV Outpatient Study (HOPS) of about 3,000 HIV-infected persons per year from 1993 to present.[31] As mentioned earlier, NIH also funds the AIDS Clinical Trials Group (ACTG) and the Community Programs for Clinical Research on AIDS (CPCRA), which have provided insights into the beneficial and adverse effects of antiretroviral drugs. There are many, many smaller cohort studies in the United States and Europe with various acronyms. Presently, most of these are of specific treatment questions, usually whether one drug or drug combination is better than another in treating HIV infection.

While long-term cohort studies are essential in the modern therapeutic era, they suffer from their own problems. One of the biggest practical problems is that they tend to be "convenience" samples of: the people most likely to persevere in any long-term study; persons diagnosed with HIV (only about 70% of Americans with the infection know they have HIV) and in care (only 50–60% of those diagnosed with HIV are in care); people who can afford to repeatedly visit a clinic; people most likely to remain in one geographic place; etc. If the factor being analyzed–say, a drug's biologic benefits–does not depend on the age, gender, race/ethnicity, body size, or stage of HIV infection of a person faithfully taking or exposed to it, and those effects or benefits are large and unlikely due to chance, we can have some modest confidence in the results. However, these are big assumptions and frequently made because most cohorts have had difficulty recruiting and maintaining indigent, substance-abusing, or homeless patients. Eligibility criteria for nested studies–for example, a case-control study–within persons in cohort studies may be too stringent and exclude important groups of interest, such as women.[32] Finally, as the epidemic has progressed, most HIV-infected patients enrolled in long-term studies have had extensive and complicated treatment histories that make finding comparable groups for comparison ever more difficult.

Still, all these sources of error, or "mis-science"–and there are more than can be reviewed in this book–can only delay the ultimate discovery, reporting, and acceptance of reality or scientific "truth."

The HIV/AIDS Epidemic Today

Background to this book would be incomplete without reference to the current state of the HIV/AIDS epidemic. There have indeed been many advances including good understanding of HIV and its epidemiology, pathogenesis, prevention, and treatment. For citizens of the developed world, current therapies may usually result in a near-normal life span and style in the HIV-infected patient. However, these scientific advances sometimes lead to complacency about an infection that, unless treated, will result in premature death for the currently estimated 40 million HIV-infected people worldwide; indeed, 3 million people are dying from AIDS every year, mainly in Africa and Asia.[33] Some areas of Africa, Asia, and eastern Europe are experiencing 50 percent or more increases in infection rates, despite our understanding of how HIV can be prevented. These grim figures underscore the importance of HIV prevention and treatment at all future stages of the epidemic.

Shifting our focus back to the United States, AIDS incidence (yearly rate) "peaked" in 1992–1993 and has subsequently plateaued at about 40,000–50,000 newly reported AIDS cases per year. Separate surveillance for newly diagnosed HIV infections from 29 states that collect and submit to CDC such (name-based and thus verifiable) reports tends to indicate current HIV infection rates at about 40,000 per year for the last 10 years. As seen in Figure 1.1 below, the shape of the AIDS epidemic curve is consistent with an explosive "common source" outbreak in gay men in the early 1980s leading to a peak in AIDS cases 10 years later, with a level "continuing source"

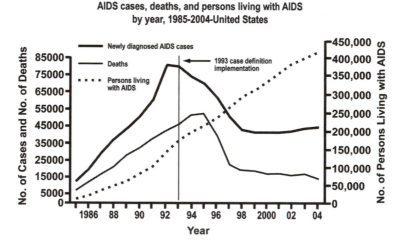

Figure 1.1 AIDS cases, deaths, and persons living with AIDS by year, 1985–2004–United States. Data available at www.cdc.gov/AIDS.

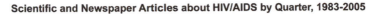

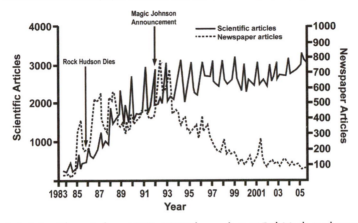

Figure 1.2 Scientific articles, 1983–2006 (——), per PubMed, and newspaper articles in 53 major English language newspapers, 1983–2006 (- - - -), per Lexis Nexis.

epidemic from steady infection rate from the mid-1980s on (see Chapter 3). Put another way, all our understanding of how HIV infection and AIDS can be prevented has not had a measurable impact on U.S. HIV incidence rates over the last decade or more. This depressing result has not been for lack of effort (see Chapter 6).

Public interest in HIV/AIDS has followed a trajectory in line with the number of newspaper and other media stories about it. In an admittedly ecologic analysis, the reader may consider Figure 1.2, that shows both scientific (solid) and newspaper (dashed) articles about HIV/AIDS over the past two decades.

Ignorance both in the scientific and lay community of the true scope of the epidemic was followed by frightened concern as the numbers of cases in San Francisco, New York, and elsewhere started to rapidly accumulate in the early 1980s. The death of movie star Rock Hudson in 1985 and the announcement by Magic Johnson, the talented basketball player, of his HIV infection in November 1991 generated pronounced spikes in media articles and stories. Hysteria in the late 1980s and early 1990s has been followed by "AIDS fatigue" on the public's part, followed by some complacency, "AIDS apathy," as HIV/AIDS disease may now be treated (but not cured). Currently, fewer than 100 newspaper stories are filed each quarter in the major English language newspapers of the world.

Still, the output of the scientific endeavor (solid line, Figure 1.2) increases each year: over 10,000 scientific articles about or mentioning HIV/AIDS are now published yearly in the medical and scientific English-language literature. A disease that initially was mainly of concern to those at the periphery of society[34] has become the center of a major scientific "industry."

With this background in mind, the objectives of this book are to examine, or "autopsy," some of the most egregious scientific errors and contentious controversies in HIV/AIDS science and prevention that (1) were important, visible, and took substantial research time to resolve; and (2) that have been resolved or almost resolved at the time of this writing.

References

1. Duesberg, P. 1988. HIV is not the cause of AIDS. *Science* 241:514, 517.

2. Rothenberg, R., M. Woelfel, R. Stoneburner, J. Milberg, R. Parker, and B. Truman. 1987. Survival with the acquired immunodeficiency syndrome. Experience with 5833 cases in New York City. *New England Journal of Medicine* 317:1297–1302.

3. Redfield, R.R., P.D. Markham, S.Z. Salahuddin, D.C. Wright, M.G. Sarngadharan, and R.C. Gallo. 1985. Heterosexually acquired HTLV-III/LAV disease (AIDS-related complex and AIDS). Epidemiologic evidence for female-to-male transmission. *Journal of the American Medical Association* 254:2094–2096.

4. Schultz, S., J.A. Milberg, A.R. Kristal, and R.L. Stoneburner. 1986. Female-to-male transmission of HTLV-III [letter]. *Journal of the American Medical Association* 255:1703–1704.

5. Redfield, R.R., D.C. Wright, P.D. Markham, S.Z. Salahuddin, M.G. Sarngadharan, and R.C. Gallo. 1986. Female-to-male transmission of HTLV-III [reply]. *Journal of the American Medical Association* 255:1705–1706.

6. Renzullo, P.O., J.G. McNeil, L.I. Levin, J.R. Bunin, and J.F. Brundage. 1990. Risk factors for prevalent human immunodeficiency virus (HIV) infection in active duty Army men who initially report no identified risk: A case-control study. *Journal of Acquired Immune Deficiency Syndromes* 3:266–271.

7. The Editors. The value of *P* 2001. *Epidemiology* 12:286.

8. Linden, J.V. 1994 Error contributes to the risk of transmissible disease. *Transfusion* 34:1016.

9. Busch, M.P., K.K. Watanabe, J.W. Smith, S.W. Hermansen, and R.A.Thomson. 2000. False-negative testing errors in routine viral marker screening of blood donors. The Retrovirus Epidemiology Donor Study. *Transfusion* 40:585–589.

10. Lackritz, E.M., G.A. Satten, J. Aberle-Grasse, et al. 1995. Estimated risk of transmission of the human immunodeficiency virus by screened blood in the United States. *New England Journal of Medicine* 333:1721–1725.

11. Altman, L.K. July 3, 2001 The doctor's world: The cause of the outbreak is unknown. *New York Times.*

12. CDC. 1981. Pneumocystis pneumonia- Los Angeles. *MMWR Morbidity and Mortality Weekly Report* 30:250–252.

13. CDC. 1982. A cluster of Kaposi's sarcoma and *Pneumocystis carinii* pneumonia among homosexual male residents of Los Angeles and Orange counties. *MMWR Morbidity and Mortality Weekly Report* 31:305–308.

14. Moses, S., J.E. Bradley, N.J. Nagelkerke, A.R. Ronald, J.O. Ndinya-Achola, and F.A. Plummer. 1990. Geographical patterns of male circumcision practice in Africa:

association with HIV seroprevalence. *International Journal of Epidemiology* 19:693–697.

15. Hooper, E. 1999. *The River: A Journey to the Source of HIV and AIDS*. Boston: Little, Brown and Company.

16. Leishman, K. September 1987. AIDS and insects. *The Atlantic Monthly* 260: 56–72.

17. Peeters, M., V. Courgnaud, B. Abela, et al. 2002. Risk to human health from a plethora of simian immunodeficiency viruses in primate bushmeat. *Emerging Infectious Diseases* 8:451–457.

18. Bozzette, S.A., C.F Ake, H.K. Tam, S.W. Chang, and T.A. Louis. 2003. Cardiovascular and cerebrovascular events in patients treated for human immunodeficiency virus infection. *New England Journal of Medicine* 348:702–710.

19. Jaffe, H.W., K. Choi, P.A. Thomas, et al. 1983. National case-control study of Kaposi's sarcoma and *Pneumocystis carinii* pneumonia in homosexual men, Part 1. Epidemiologic results. *Annals of Internal Medicine* 99:145–151.

20. Rogers, M.F., D.M Morens, J.A. Stewart, et al. 1983. National case-control study of Kaposi's sarcoma and *Pneumocystis carinii* pneumonia in homosexual men, Part 2. Laboratory results. *Annals of Internal Medicine* 99:151–158.

21. Feinstein, A.R., and R.I. Horowitz. 1982. Double standards, scientific methods, and epidemiologic research. *New England Journal of Medicine* 307:1611–1617.

22. Pocock, S.J., M.D. Hughes, and R.J. Lee. Statistical problems in the reporting of clinical trials. A survey of three medical journals. 1987. *New England Journal of Medicine* 317:426–432.

23. Ghani, A.C. 2003. Use of observational data in evaluating treatments: antiretroviral therapy and HIV. *Expert Review of Anti-infective Therapy* 1:551–562.

24. Fischl, M.A., D.D. Richman, M.H.Grieco, et al. 1987. The efficacy of azidothymidine (AZT) in the treatment of patients with AIDS and AIDS-related complex. A double-blind, placebo-controlled trial. *New England Journal of Medicine* 317:185–191.

25. Jaffe, H.W., W.W. Darrow, D.F. Echenberg, et al. 1985. The acquired immunodeficiency syndrome in a cohort of homosexual men. A six-year follow-up study. *Annals of Internal Medicine* 103:210–214.

26. Holmberg, S.D., S.P. Buchbinder, L.J. Conley, et al. 1995. The spectrum of medical conditions and symptoms before acquired immunodeficiency syndrome in homosexual and bisexual men infected with the human immunodeficiency virus. *American Journal of Epidemiology* 141:395–404.

27. Kaslow, R.A., D.G. Ostrow, R. Detels, J.P. Phair, B.F. Polk, and C.R. Rinaldo Jr. 1987. The Multicenter AIDS Cohort Study: rationale, organization, and selected characteristics of the participants. *American Journal of Epidemiology* 126:310–318.

28. Smith, D.K., D.L. Warren, D. Vlahov, et al. 1997. Design and baseline participant characteristics of the Human Immunodeficiency Virus Epidemiology Research (HER) Study: A prospective cohort study of human immunodeficiency virus infection in US women. *American Journal of Epidemiology* 146:459–469.

29. Barkan, S.E., S.L. Melnick, S. Preston-Martin, et al. 1998. The Women's Interagency HIV Study. WIHS Collaborative Study Group. *Epidemiology* 9:117–125.

30. Jones, J.L., D.L. Hanson, S.Y. Chu, P.L. Fleming, D.J. Hu, and J.W. Ward. 1994. Surveillance of AIDS-defining conditions in the United States. Adult/Adolescent Spectrum of HIV Disease Project Group. *AIDS* 8:1489–1493.

31. Moorman, A.C., S.D. Holmberg, S.I. Marlowe, et al. 1999. Changing conditions and treatments in a dynamic cohort of ambulatory HIV patients: The HIV Outpatient Study (HOPS). *Annals of Epidemiology* 9:349–357.

32. Gandhi, M., N. Ameli, P. Bacchetti, et al. 2005. Eligibility criteria for HIV clinical trials and generalizability of results: The gap between published reports and study protocols. *AIDS* 19:1885–1896.

33. UNAIDS/WHO. AIDS Epidemic Update: December 2006. Available at www.unaids.org/en/HIV_data/epi2006/.

34. Shilts, R. 1987. *And the Band Played On: Politics, People, and the AIDS Epidemic.* New York: St. Martin's Press.

CHAPTER TWO

Causes and Sources of AIDS

It is easy to forget that in the first few years of the HIV/AIDS epidemic no one knew the cause or source of the mysterious and lethal ailment. There were hopes that it would be a virus or other pathogen that was already known to medical science and that it would be easily treated with drugs or prevented through vaccination. As time went on, all these hopes faded, despite the relatively quick identification of HIV in 1983 and, 12 years later, effective drug treatment–highly active antiretroviral therapy (HAART)–that markedly improved both survival and quality of life if taken early and consistently enough. However, there was much confusion about the causes and sources of the "AIDS agent" throughout the 1980s.

Cytomegalovirus

All five patients described in this report had laboratory confirmed CMV [cytomegalovirus] disease or virus shedding within 5 months of the diagnosis of *Pneumocystis* pneumonia. CMV infection has been shown to induce transient abnormalities of *in vitro* cellular-immune function in otherwise healthy hosts.[1]

So reads part of the Discussion in CDC's original *Morbidity and Mortality Weekly Report* (*MMWR*) that described the first five AIDS cases in Los Angeles in June 1981.[1] At the time, two facts were known about cytomegalovirus (CMV) infection that made it attractive as the cause of the new syndrome: (1) it was ubiquitous in gay men, about 95 percent of whom had serologic evidence of infection[2]; and (2) it could lead to "transient abnormalities" in immunologic function.[3] Further, there may have been a perverse comfort in thinking that this new syndrome, immediately, briefly, and with prejudice known as "gay-related infectious disease" (GRID), was caused by an agent we knew.

Yet few scientists really thought that the new syndrome was really the result of just CMV infection. Immunologic evidence of CMV—that is, serum antibodies indicating prior infection—is seen in about 60 percent of the American population after age six.[4] How could it be that CMV was causing this odd disease in homosexual men, but a similar syndrome had not been seen much earlier and much more widely in the general population? Further, the experimental data indicated that CMV was only temporary in its adverse immunologic effects (measured in days), and these first five men with AIDS had been ill for weeks or months.

As cases started to rapidly accumulate from several cities and from people who were not gay men, as cases included the cancer Kaposi's sarcoma (KS) as well as *Pneumocystis carinii* pneumonia (PCP), and as the high prevalence of CMV became more evident in the general population, the tenuous thought that CMV was the proximal cause of AIDS quickly faded. However, some research laboratories were heavily invested in studies of CMV and other herpes group viruses, such as Epstein-Barr virus (EBV). Within the first year or two of the epidemic, some opined that KS was caused by CMV, that EBV was responsible for B-cell lymphoma, and that "[M]ultiple factors, rather than a novel virus, probably induce AIDS in male homosexuals."[5] This report and others like it was rapidly followed by the isolation of lympadenopathy-associated virus (LAV, later termed HIV) in 1983 by Luc Montagnier and his colleagues at Institut Pasteur in Paris.[6]

Accordingly, the CMV/EBV-hypothesis defenders shifted attention to looking at CMV and EBV as "cofactors" in HIV-related AIDS. So, for example, at a 1987 meeting of the American Society of Microbiology (ASM), Dr. Larry Drew from Mount Zion Medical Center in San Francisco summarized arguments that (1) CMV was a cofactor in immune suppression, PCP and KS[7]; and (2) that EBV was a cofactor in AIDS based on HIV and EBV interactions at the cellular level. Indeed, this latter thesis was entertained up until human herpesvirus 8 gene sequences (HHV-8, originally called the Kaposi's sarcoma herpes virus [KSHV]) were isolated from KS tissue, as reported first in 1994.[8]

Most researchers focused on the molecular aspects and did not advocate CMV or EBV as a cause of KS and other AIDS-associated cancers. For example, respected researchers at Massachusetts General Hospital in Boston and from other major medical centers reported on interactions between CMV and HIV, specifically that those interactions that enhanced HIVreplication occurred in certain cells coinfected with CMV.[9–11] However, concurrent and later work showed that a variety of viruses,[12] natural factors,[13, 14] and chemicals[15] might stimulate the "long terminal repeat" (LTR) segment of the HIV genome, indicating that CMV and EBV were not unique in this respect.

Finally, while the general attitude or impression has evolved that herpes group viruses may have a deleterious effect in HIV infection, the largest cohort studies of this issue concluded that actually "[c]oncurrent infection with more than one herpesvirus does not appear to have a significant effect on the course of HIV disease...." [16] Nonetheless, the role of herpesviruses in HIV disease was not just an academic or "in vitro" issue that simply distracted some research laboratories: some considerable effort in the 1990s was expended seeing if adding acyclovir, an anti-herpes drug, to zidovudine (AZT) would be efficacious AIDS treatment (see Chapter 7).

Human T-Cell Lymphotropic Virus Type III (HTLV-III)

The whole topic of human T-cell lymphotropic virus III (HTLV-III) is inextricably connected to the well known and described controversy between Robert Gallo of NIH's Tumor Retrovirology Lab and Luc Montagnier of Institut Pasteur as to who was the true discoverer of HIV. This is a somewhat complicated history and the purpose of this book is to examine how errors might divert or frustrate scientific advance; but, to do this topic justice, a brief overview will first be necessary. Those who wish to read much more about this are referred to the initial Pulitzer Prize winning *Chicago Tribune* exposé by John Crewdson in November 1989, "The Great AIDS Quest," that substantially undercut Gallo's claim as a codiscoverer of HIV.[17] A follow-up investigative report by Seth Roberts in the July 1990 issue of *Spy* (magazine), "Lab Rat," was, as the title suggests, a highly critical collection of comments by those who knew, worked with, and usually disliked Gallo and his aggressive, self-aggrandizing, sharp-elbowed style of lab politics.[18] Thus, this was a case where the scientific community ended up following the lead of journalists, who were able to obtain laboratory documents under federal Freedom of Information Act requests and interviews from people at the laboratories involved that were directly responsible for revealing the obfuscations and specimen contamination on which Gallo's claims rested. Long articles in *Science*[19, 20] treated in cautious terms the ongoing controversies that culminated in the American's May 1991 ceding of his claim of "discovery" of HIV. There have been later revisionist attempts to vindicate Gallo as a smart and productive senior researcher.[21] Still, a fog hangs over this episode that, even 15 years later, stands as an example of how errors, whether fraudulent or accidental, retarded American AIDS scientific efforts during the 7-year trans-Atlantic quarrel.

The briefest outline of the facts of this case, beyond the judgments derived, starts with Robert Gallo's early reputation. In the late 1970s and early 1980s, he had established his preeminence as the discoverer of human lymphotropic virus type 1 (HTLV-1), the first known human retrovirus: "lymphotropic" refers to the virus' attraction to human T-lymphocytes (white blood cells) which they infect and "immortalize" (cells so infected reproduce in the laboratory without end). Great excitement followed the discovery of HTLV-I because it linked an infectious agent to a rare human cancer, adult T-cell leukemia/lymphoma, mainly seen in southern Japan and a rare myelopathy, tropical spastic paraparesis. Even better, Gallo's lab developed a test for two products of HTLV-I-infected cells, p19 and p24, proteins found in "reverse transcriptase," an enzyme necessary to convert viral RNA to DNA, which latter can then insert itself into and "command" the human genome to make more of itself. Not long after, in 1982, "HTLV-II" was also described in two patients with another rare cancer, hairy cell leukemia.

Discovery of the HTLVs established Robert Gallo and his laboratory as pre-eminent in retrovirology, and, as HTLV-I proteins p19 and p24 were initially detected in one of the first AIDS patient's blood, this suggested to Gallo and others that AIDS might be the result of that or, more likely, another human T-cell lymphotropic virus[22]: thus came the naming of the AIDS virus on this side of the Atlantic HTLV-III. (In retrospect, it appears that the patient dubbed "CC" in the original report was in fact doubly infected with both HTLV-I and HIV.)

Meanwhile, in early 1983 Luc Montagnier and his group detected reverse transcriptase in cells from swollen lymph nodes (lymphadenopathy) of another AIDS patient and asked Gallo's lab to provide reagents to further distinguish their virus. Using those reagents, Montagnier showed that LAV was distinct from HTLV-I and HTLV-II. Shortly thereafter, in April 1983, Montagnier and his team published the first description of what we now know as HIV as LAV in *Science*.[6] Further, at about the same time, he also presented his findings to scientists at NIH, CDC, and elsewhere that substantially convinced almost everyone that the French group had indeed found the cause of AIDS. The virus that Montagnier described infected the specific T-cells, CD4-receptor bearing white cells, (CD4+ cells) and, unlike HTLV-I or HTLV-II that immortalized cells, LAV led to cell death. This would explain the targeting and depletion of CD4+ cells, a hallmark of AIDS.

In July 1983, Montagnier sent Gallo a sample of LAV/BRU as the former was having difficulty culturing the cell, that is, keeping cells containing the

AIDS virus alive and propagating in vitro (continuous mass cell culture). The track of this LAV virus thereafter is unclear, but Gallo and his associates, after trying various cells, found a cell line they called "H9" that allowed the continuous culture of virus taken from AIDS patients. This was critical in developing assays to detect protein products of the virally infected cells—proteins such as p24, p41, gp 120, and others—that would allow diagnosis of HTLV-III-infected persons. In May 1984, four publications in *Science* by Robert Gallo and his laboratory members, especially Mikulas Popovic, who had developed continuous H9 cell culture of the virus,[23] were pre-announced in a press conference by Margaret Heckler, then Secretary of the U.S. Department of Health and Human Services, as "a new miracle to the long honor roll of American medicine and science." Gallo was widely hailed as "codiscoverer" with Montagnier of the AIDS virus.

The fact that there had been a substantial American research investment in finding the cause of the rapidly accumulating AIDS cases being reported from all over the country; that Robert Gallo was first lauded as an American hero; and that he had discovered the retrovirus family (HTLVs) and a way of mass producing the "AIDS virus" that could then allow the detection of it with a profitable blood test (an enzyme immunoassay): all led to the convoluted reference by all of us in the American governmental agencies and in the institutions funded by the federal government to the AIDS virus as HTLV-III, or HTLV-III/LAV for the next few years. In 1986, an international body of nomenclature settled on the much more accurate and simple human immunodeficiency virus (HIV), and this nomenclature was formally adopted by U.S. researchers in 1988.[24]

However, the first major, general error in the 1984 announcement was that, even by then, lab notes obtained by John Crewdson at the *Chicago Tribune* make it clear that the virus that Gallo described in his publications and the LAV that had been sent him by Montagnier were the same virus. Subsequent genetic analysis showed these viruses to be only 1 percent different,[25, 26] which small difference would be an expected genetic "drift" over the year it was being analyzed. Clearly, the French virus had somehow contaminated or got confused with other samples in the American lab. Was this intentional fraud? One cannot second-guess or divine the motives of Gallo and all his laboratory colleagues, but clearly this major American "achievement" was, in fact, an error.

Even as the embarrassing error became more evident Gallo and Popovic still could claim that they had indeed developed a continuous cell culture necessary for producing enough virus to allow a way to test for products of that virus. This was an important achievement, and Gallo collected royalties at the rate of about $100,000 per year over the first years of an American licensed AIDS blood test. However, there were problems with this triumph as well. The French team had come up with a superior test—which they were using—4 months before the triumphant Gallo *Science* article and Secretary Heckler's announcement. The similarities between the French and American tests led to a lengthy and very expensive legal battle that initially delayed the test's availability in the United States. The dispute was ultimately settled out of court in 1987 with both American and French governments' sharing royalties of the blood test but without a statement as to whether the Gallo HTLV-III and the Montagnier LAV were the same. However, finally ending the 7-year dispute, Robert Gallo dropped his claim of prime discovery of the AIDS virus, HIV, in late May 1991.

Unfortunately, the American errors didn't stop there. The other major unpleasant discovery was that the "H9" cells needed for continuous cultivation/production of HIV were actually cells that had been developed in a separate laboratory, John Minna's Clinical Oncology Branch, then of the Veteran's Administration, by researchers Adi Gazdar and Paul Bunn. These calls, called "HUT78" were used in the original report on HTLV-1 and Minna, Gazdar, and Bunn were listed as coauthors. The HUT78 cells apparently had been shared with the Gallo laboratory predating Mikulas Popovic's arrival (January 1980); in any case, they were the cell line that Popovic found would not die when infected with 'HTLV-III.' Was this fraud on Popovic's part? It appears that he delayed doing tests to determine the identity of H9 and HUT78, but it will probably never be clear whether he made an unintentional error or purposely obfuscated his debt to the Minna lab. Cases have been made for both points of view.[20]

While it is difficult to write about this important episode without ascribing motivations, the purpose here is not to slip into the easy defamation of Gallo, who was aggressively and overtly chasing the Nobel Prize. In this case, the errors may not have been as grievous to scientific advance as the noncolleagial and uncooperative way that Gallo operated.

Probably the most disastrous import of the dispute between Gallo and the U.S. government vs. Montagnier and the French government was the delay of the introduction of an effective and available blood test for HIV for an estimated 6–12 months. During that time, some unknown number of recipients of blood and blood products—those getting transfusions, hemophilic men, and others with bleeding disorders—became infected when an available test may have screened out tainted blood and blood products. As well, many sexually active men and women who found they are infected have changed their behavior once aware of their infection, so there were probably some homosexual and heterosexual persons who, as it was widely understood even by late 1982 that AIDS was spread sexually, may have curtailed or changed their behaviors to protect partners—if there had been an available test.

Gallo's behavior also hindered research and public health in other ways. As became clear, based on examination of thousands of pages of documents obtained under the Freedom of Information Act (FOIA) and interviews with almost 200 scientists, Gallo published many misleading data and conclusions in late 1983 and early 1984 before suddenly "discovering" the virus lent him by the French.[17] This caused inevitable delays as scientists, especially in the United States, focused on HTLV-III. CDC and other researchers requested and did not receive necessary reagents and viral samples with which to expand research on this purported cause of AIDS. This delay in productive bench research seems to have been about a year long, the time Gallo and colleagues were focusing on HTLV. The "cost" of this delay would be hard to calculate, but, as discussed in the next Chapter, this came at a critical time of very high transmission and dissemination of HIV in this country and worldwide.

HIV-2, HTLV-IV (and . . . SIV and STLV . . .)

It would be hard to find a better example of how aberrant research results can lead to even more aberrant results than the discovery of another human T-cell lymphotropic virus, HTLV-IV. First, a review of confusing nomenclature.

HIV-1—the accepted term now for LAV, HTLV-III, and AIDS-related virus (ARV)—is the cause of the immunodeficiency that marks AIDS. The recovery of HIV-2, a virus distinct but related to HIV-1, was reported in 1986 by Francois Clavel, also of Luc Montagnier's laboratory at Institut Pasteur[27]; infection with this second HIV was reported from 30 West Africans, of whom 17 had AIDS or symptoms known to be precursors to AIDS (AIDS-related complex).[28] HIV-1 is found in all countries and accounts, we think, for more than 90 percent of all AIDS cases worldwide. It became evident that HIV-2 was mainly restricted to West Africa, and to a lesser extent South American and other countries to the degree of their contact with West African nations near the Bight of Benin; also, it appears that HIV-2 infection has a more indolent or less aggressive course than HIV-1.[29, 30]

If the story only involved HIV-1 and HIV-2, it would be easier to follow; but a confusing welter of acronyms sprang up in relation to simian viruses that appeared to be related to human immunodeficiency viruses. These former viruses, now known as simian immunodeficiency viruses (SIVs), are non-pathogenic (disease-causing) in their natural host, African green monkeys. These viruses can productively infect and induce in macaques and other simian species disease that is very similar to acquired immunodeficiency seen in humans. Thus, the SIV/macaque provides a useful animal model for HIV/humans and is the model in which experimental HIV vaccines are tested first.

In the spring of 1986, Phyllis Kanki and Max Essex of Harvard's School of Public Health reported that a new human retrovirus that they termed HTLV-IV had been recovered from apparently healthy Senegalese prostitutes and that HTLV-IV shared a number of major antigens with an SIV strain.[31] Following the continued American predilection to show the link between HTLV-III and AIDS, they termed that simian virus "simian T-lymphotropic virus III" (STLV-III or STLV-IIIAGM). This group plus Franchini and others in Robert Gallo's laboratory showed that STLV-III and HTLV-II were by serologic (antibody) tests remarkably similar to LAV-2 (Montagnier's group's original term for HIV-2)[32−34]: that is, it was known early on from this and other work that somehow SIV and HIV-2 and HTLV-IV were similar by all available contemporaneous, mainly serologic typing, tests. In fact, this new HIV was sometimes called HTLV-4/HIV-2 by the discoverers of HTLV-IV.[34] So, in summary, it looked like there was another AIDS virus in Africa, HTLV-IV, which apparently did not cause disease in people: could this novel virus act as a vaccination against HIV, a la vaccinia (cowpox) immunization for smallpox? As had Robert Gallo for his early work with HTLV-1 and -2, Max Essex received the Lasker award, perhaps the most prestigious American award for biomedical research, for his work with HTLV-IV.

However, by early 1988, work by other Harvard Medical School researchers found that the STLV-III$_{AGM}$ from African green monkeys and the HTLV-IV isolated from humans were more than 99 percent genetically identical: "These results and other observations provide strong evidence that isolates previously referred to as STLV-III$_{AGM}$ and HTLV-IV by others are not authentic, but were derived from cell cultures infected with SIV$_{MAC−251}$."[35] The report did not wholly invalidate the serologic studies of Kanki and Essex that showed prevalence of a virus related to HIV-1 among West African prostitutes. However, it was now clear that the virus that those researchers referred to as HTLV-4 was SIV, and HTLV-4/HIV-2 was, in fact, simply HIV-2. In response to the research results of Kestler et al., Kanki and Essex agreed that HTLV-IV was the result of inadvertent contamination of their cell cultures.[36] Indeed, in retrospect, several studies by them[31, 34, 36, 37] indicate that SIV (their STLV-III) and HTLV-IV were essentially the same in several genetic and serologic characterizations. Studies to find HTLV-IV in persons who had symptoms of AIDS had been generally unfruitful.[38]

The end of all this work seems to be that researchers and those in the wider AIDS community are relieved that there are only two HIV types, HIV-1 and HIV-2, and that our therapies and prevention efforts can be directed to them alone (Figure 2.1).[39]

Does HIV-2 Protect against HIV-1?

Phyllis Kanki and colleagues were intrigued by the fact that HTLV-IV had been recovered from persons without signs or symptoms of AIDS: could HTLV-IV infection protect against HIV infection? Or, could HTLV-IV "super-infection" retard the progression of HIV-1 disease? Even after HTLV-IV was found to be SIV (or by their terminology, STLV-III), because HTLV-IV, STLV-III, SIV, and HIV-2 appeared to be so similar, the question remained if HIV-2 might exhibit some of the properties of SIV (STLV-III)–that is, could HIV-2, an "SIV-like virus" protect against HIV-1?

Karin Travers, Kanki, and other researchers at Harvard's School of Public Health then published data that purported to show "natural protection" against HIV-1 by prior infection with HIV-2.[40, 41] Essentially, the Travers study presented data that HIV-2-infected African women had about one-third the risk of acquiring HIV-1 than women without HIV-2 infection.[40] If true, this would be big news for developing an HIV-1 vaccine as it indicated that infection with the milder retrovirus–or perhaps, better, its noninfectious components–could somehow be used as a vaccine to protect against HIV-1 infection.

However, this analysis appeared to have a large "selection bias." By comparing data between the Kanki and Travers papers,[40, 41] Alan Greenberg and his colleagues at CDC showed that about half of the HIV-1- and HIV-2-uninfected women in the original 1994 (Kanki) analysis were somehow assigned to the HIV-2-infected group in the second 1995 (Travers) analysis.[42] Thus, the numbers of women who were both reportedly HIV-1- and HIV-2-uninfected were about halved, making the incidence (occurrence) of HIV-1 in them seem to be double the real rate; conversely, the HIV-1-uninfected but HIV-2-infected women had doubled in size, halving the incidence rate of HIV-1 in them. Put another way, if the two groups described in the initial 1994 article (HIV-2-infected vs. HIV-2-uninfected women) had not been reassigned by suspicious allocation procedures, the rates of HIV-1 occurrence (incidence rate) in the two groups would be essentially the same.

Accordingly, a reanalysis by the Travers/Kanki researchers of the larger group of HIV-1 uninfected women was performed, and this, again, indicated a protective effect of about 64 percent in HIV-2-infected women against

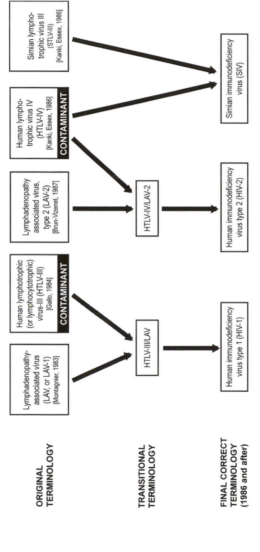

Figure 2.1 Evolution of terminology for human (HIV-1, HIV-2) and simian (SIV) immunodeficiency viruses.

acquiring HIV-1 infection.[43] In turn, this follow-up report stimulated research teams working in West Africa, where HIV-2 is endemic, to examine their data on Africans they had followed over time (longitudinally). They looked at the possible protective effect of HIV-2 in six additional populations including female sex workers, urban and rural adults, postpartum women, and police officers from 1987 through 1998. In each of these populations, the HIV-1 infection rate/incidence was actually *higher* in the previously HIV-2-infected vs. HIV-2-uninfected persons.[44] Further, work in the laboratory showed that, if anything, HIV-2 coinfection stimulated HIV-1 replication, leading to higher "viral loads" of HIV-1.[45]

At present, the many West Africans with dual HIV-1 and HIV-2 infections now stand testament to the fact that infection with one HIV does not substantially protect against infection with the other.

"Poppers" and Kaposi's Sarcoma

One of the most common AIDS-defining illnesses was Kaposi's Sarcoma (KS), which before 1981 was a rare tumor seen mainly on the skin of elderly men from the Mediterranean. "Poppers" is a street name for small bottles of amyl nitrite, or less frequently butyl nitrite, used for sexual stimulation and popular with gay men in the early 1980s. These were frequently used in gay bathhouses. When the original case-control studies of men with HIV infection were performed, poppers were associated with having AIDS,[46] but there were concerns that this was the result of confounding with indices of sexual activity.[47] That is, those who were using poppers were more sexually active, more likely to be having sex with anonymous partners in bathhouses, and, so, more likely to have AIDS. Still, there quickly arose advocates for a special relationship between amyl or butyl nitrites and KS.

Michael Marmor and colleagues performed an early case-control study that showed that those in the highest strata of amyl nitrite use had a crude odds ratio of 8.6 for having KS; when this association was adjusted for sexual activity, the association between poppers and KS actually rose (adjusted odds ratio of 12.3).[48] This finding was unexpected if popper use was indeed associated with number of sex partners or other parameters of sexual activity as the odds ratio should have decreased when the analysis adjusted for sex partners or activity. Also, the association between amyl nitrite use and KS was adjusted for sexual activity (numbers of sex partners per month), not, as might have been more appropriate, between this measure of sexual activity and KS, adjusted for popper use. This was somewhat strange since a concurrent publication by the same authors[49] studied risk factors for 19 homosexual men with KS and found the strongest associations were with indices of sexual activity, such as sexually transmitted diseases. Also, in terms of recreational drug use, all 19 men had used amyl or butyl nitrites, but all had also used alcohol and marijuana, and 18 admitted cocaine use. Singling out popper use was never explained, but was one of the two items unique to these gay men as opposed to others in the general population. However, the other unique risk factor was the very high number of lifetime sex partners these men had, often numbering in the hundreds.

It was also unclear how amyl or butyl nitrites, used for their vasodilatory properties, would lead to the rare cancer. Work by Jim Goedert and colleagues at the National Cancer Institute found a modest immunosuppressive effect–measured at the time as helper/suppressor T- lymphocyte ratios in amyl nitrite inhaler users–when compared to nonpopper users.[50] As this would not explain the levels of immunosuppression seen in the early AIDS patients, these investigators proposed that inhalants were suppressive "in the setting of repeated antigenic stimulation" by CMV and other viruses.[50] This "biologically plausible" mechanism was not confirmed by later work, and was essentially forgotten once the viral cause of KS (mentioned below) was described.

Several years later, the senior author of the report, a well respected researcher, Bill Blattner, conceded that they had "overstated" the association between amyl nitrite and immune suppression:

> We went wrong in our analysis in that paper because we were looking at the various behaviors, and one of the behaviors associated with immune deficiency was the use of amyl nitrite inhalants. In retrospect, we can think about this differently. It was a mark of a high risk behavior for HIV infection. You have to understand that when you are going through this kind of process and living it, as opposed to looking back on it, things were not that clear. There were very few of us who were living it, because there were not very many people working in the area. It is very clear to people in retrospect how 'stupid' we were, but ultimately the problem got solved through the process of scientific research.[51]

Indeed, within a few months, this process of scientific research convincingly showed that HIV was the cause of the immunosuppression seen in AIDS, followed in 1994 by the demonstration of herpes virus group-like DNA sequences in KS tissue.[8] This KSHV, now known as human herpes virus type 8 (HHV8), acts as an opportunistic infection in the immunocompromised person (also in persons therapeutically immunosuppressed for purposes of kidney transplantation in whom KS is sometimes seen as well). HHV8 can be recovered frequently from the HIV risk groups in which it appears as a manifestation of AIDS, namely homosexual men in the United

States and other developed countries and heterosexual men in sub-Saharan Africa.

If HHV8 had not been discovered, this controversy may have continued without resolution, because, even at this date, there are a few scientists who find multifactorial causation of AIDS an attractive hypothesis and think inhaled nitrites might be somehow involved as "cofactors" in KS or other AIDS diseases.[52] For most scientists and certainly clinicians, though, treatment of HIV with modern antiretroviral therapy has eliminated KS in those treated early enough and successfully, so that, even if there are cofactors for KS, these would be considered of less than direct practical significance.

African Swine Fever Virus

From 1982 though 1986, an odd battle of letters to the British journal *The Lancet* disputed the role of African swine fever virus (ASFV), a DNA virus that causes a indolent and chronic infection in feral African pigs (such as warthogs) spread by direct contact or ticks, and human AIDS. In the late 1950s the virus was transmitted to Portugal and Spain where it became endemic in some domestic swine populations, and then to pigs in Haiti in the late 1970s. In 1983, Jane Teas, a microbiologist at Harvard's School of Public Health posited that AIDS could be caused by a variant of ASFV. She noted: the coincident appearance of the first cases of AIDS in Haiti in 1978 and the first confirmed appearance of ASFV in Haiti[53]; and some similar signs and symptoms of ASFV in pigs and AIDS in humans—fever, loss of weight, and swollen lymph nodes. She also proposed a possible mode of introduction of ASFV to human populations, "Perhaps an infected pig was killed and eaten either as uncooked or cooked meat. One of the people eating the meat who was both immunocompromised and homosexual would be the pivotal point, allowing for the disease to spread to the vacationing 'gay' tourists in Haiti."[53]

African swine fever or its causative agent ASFV had never been detected in the United States despite surveillance by the U.S. Department of Agriculture (USDA). No humans anywhere had ever been found to be infected with the virus, but this was a double-edged piece of information. While it was reassuring, this meant there could be no standardized approaches to serologic testing of humans: that is, only the serologic tests used on swine could be used.

Still, the Teas letter was followed also in 1983 by two others in *Lancet* reporting the inability to detect or isolate ASFV from human AIDS patients in Haiti itself[54] and Belgium.[55] Skeptics of these reports could always counter that it was an ASFV *variant* in humans that would not be detected by cross-reactivity with the porcine ASFV serologic tests. Not only would this be unlikely, but also the "variant" would have to be so substantially different from ASFV that it would perhaps be another virus altogether. Further, no large icosahedral DNA virus-like particles (ASFV) had been seen in electron microscopy of serum and blood from the original laboratory investigation of AIDS patients in 1983.[56] Between 1983 and 1985, CDC testing of serum from 160 persons, 50 of whom had AIDS, showed a few weak, nonspecific reactions on ASFV serologic testing that was actually more frequent in the non-AIDS controls than in the AIDS patients. Thus, the interest in this agent would have normally waned, except for a few events in 1986.

In March 1986, John Beldekas of Boston University Medical School published with Jane Teas another *Lancet* letter[57] reporting they had found antibodies to ASFV in plasma from 9 of 21 people with AIDS and 2 of 12 persons with lymphadenopathy syndrome (considered part of AIDS-related complex in 1986), but in only 1 of 16 control persons. This came shortly after two Miami physicians, Caroline MacLeod and Mark Whiteside, presented data showing high AIDS rates and impoverished living conditions in Belle Glade, Florida, at the First International Conference on AIDS in 1985 in Atlanta. MacLeod and Whiteside—originally thinking and eventually discarding that a variant of dengue, a mosquito-borne virus, was the cause of AIDS in Belle Glade—eventually focused their and press attention in 1986 to ASFV after discussions with Jane Teas.[58]

In March of 1986, following the Beldekas letter, *The New York Native* published an article with the headline "Is the Reign of Error over? Swine fever found in AIDS patients,"[59] and questioned whether CDC was merely incompetent or engaged in a cover-up. And in June Jeremy Rifkin, long-time activist and head of the Foundation on Economic Trends in Washington, sent a letter to Richard Lyng, Secretary of the USDA, and James Mason, Director of CDC, asking why no further testing had been done after a September 1985 report from the New York State Department of Laboratories showed that ASFV antibody was discovered in 4.5 percent of serum tested. Even *The New York Times* editorial page somewhat praised the work of MacLeod and Whiteside in Belle Glade "to seek a cause [for AIDS] in overcrowded, unsanitary conditions, or blood-biting insects."[60] The *Times* was careful to note that Belle Glade "may prove a false lead for AIDS as for African swine fever. But dead ends are unavoidable in traversing the maze of this deadly disease."

John Bennett, then Acting Director of CDC's Center for Infectious Diseases, outlined responses to each of these concerns in reply to Jeremy Rifkin (John V. Bennett, Letter to Jeremy Rifkin, July 16, 1986), including that: ASFV had never been recovered or isolated from humans with or without AIDS symptoms; while macrophages are target cells for ASFV in swine, cultures of specimens from 33 AIDS patients in the pig macrophage-monocyte system, a highly sensitive assay for the presence of ASFV, did not result in detection of the virus[61]; and the indirect immunofluoresence serologic assay used by the NY Department of Health laboratories were noted for frequently producing nonspecific "spurious" positive reactions. He also cited several technical shortcomings in the Beldekas article, as pointed out in another *Lancet* letter following it.[62] Researchers from CDC, USDA, NIH, and other agencies met in Cold Spring Harbor, Long Island, NY, in 1986 and released a statement noting, in addition to the above, that serologic reactions to ASFV had not been found with consistency in AIDS patients and, when reactivity was sometimes seen, it was weak and nonspecific: "In our opinion, USDA and other agencies have considered the hypothesis seriously, and should not expend further resources exploring it."[63] Subsequent to these statements and open letters, and after a flurry of intense and unproductive research, this issue has been dormant for the last two decades.

HIV Does Not Cause AIDS

In a series of articles over many years and starting in 1987, Peter Duesberg of the University of California at Berkeley has repeatedly argued that HIV, "a passenger virus," could not be the cause of AIDS, and that the adverse effects of (recreational) drugs were being attributed to harmless retroviruses."[64] The main lines of argument were initially the violation of one or more of Koch's postulates–namely, that at the time of his writing, HIV could not be reliably isolated from all AIDS cases.[64, 65] Other claims, such as that "HIV does not reproduce AIDS when inoculated into chimpanzees or accidentally into humans"[65]–elided over the species-specificity of HIV for humans and SIV for chimpanzees and the chronic nature of HIV infection with its decade-long incubation between HIV infection and AIDS. In 1988, a Policy Forum in *Science* carried Duesberg's concise argument[64] but also a similarly concise response from William Blattner and Robert Gallo of NCI and Howard Temin from the University of Wisconsin.[66] The champions of the "germ theory" (HIV) of AIDS pointed out, among other things, the "absolute requirement for HIV infection for the development of AIDS." This article and other dissections and refutations of Duesberg's theories[67] seemed to have settled the issue finally for the HIV/AIDS scientific community by 1990.

As it became clearer over the subsequent years that HIV would eventually cause AIDS in HIV-test-positive persons followed for long enough and as new tests and techniques made identification and recovery of HIV possible from all AIDS patients, the argument against HIV-as-the-sole-cause-of-AIDS shifted. By knocking down several theoretical "straw men"–for example, that proponents of HIV as the cause of AIDS had predicted explosive growth of HIV/AIDS into the general population—and ignoring that other predictions—for example, that prostitutes would get HIV from their clients and hemophilic men from blood transfusions—had turned out to be true, Duesberg concluded that "American and European AIDS is caused by the long-term consumption of recreational drugs and the anti-HIV drug AZT"[68] (even though zidovudine had not been available to cause AIDS before 1987). As late as 1998, by pointing inaccurately to chaotic facts of unclear import to his argument—for example, that AIDS is nonrandom in its victims, or that the epidemic proceeded nonexponentially—Duesberg continued to make the case for recreational drugs such as amyl nitrite, cocaine, etc. as the underlying etiology of AIDS.[68, 69]

These arguments were appealing for many HIV-infected persons who did not want to believe that HIV infection was necessarily fatal and strongly supported, for example, "the effort to re-examine the hypothesis that HIV causes AIDS, a hypothesis that has yet to save a single human life."[70] It is unknown how many thought based on such criticisms of HIV and HIV therapy that zidovudine (AZT) and later antiretroviral drugs were toxic or poisonous, and so avoided them. It is known that in surveys of gay men[71] and of heterosexual women,[72] many described concerns with toxicity of zidovudine as the reason they did not take that drug.

The Source of HIV and AIDS

Where did HIV come from? Despite the initial confusion of identifying HIV as a human T-lymphocytotrophic/leukemia virus (HTLV-III), it was clear that this "American" virus, the "French" virus, LAV, SIV (or STLV), and HIV-2 were all genetically similar. As these viruses were all traceable to West Africa, this early suggested a common origin of HIV-1 and HIV-2 from that area. By the late 1980s, computer programs, mainly those run at the Los Alamos labs in New Mexico, calculated envelope protein differences between HIV-1 and HIV-2, based on observed rates of "genetic drift,"[73, 74] indicated that HIV-1 and HIV-2 may have diverged about 70 years ago or even earlier.[75–78] The "molecular clock" data usually place the emergence of HIV-1 (and HIV-2) around 1930.

This genetic evidence was somewhat confusing: where was HIV all those years until it became epidemic in the early 1980s? Intriguing reports appeared in the medical literature, sometimes corroborated by (rarely) saved clinical specimens that showed the presence of HIV before the 1980s. Thus, HIV clinical manifestations present as early as 1966 in one Norwegian family were confirmed by HIV antibody tests available in the late 1980s.[79] In New York City, several female intravenous drug-using women clearly had symptoms fulfilling the CDC case definition of "AIDS" between 1977 and 1980.[80] Testing of serum collected in 1976 from 659 Zaireans[81] and of gay men in San Francisco who were part of studies of hepatitis B and its vaccination[82] (CDC, unpublished data) showed the presence of HIV in both these quite disparate populations in the 1970s. (Some, however, could not find such serologic evidence of HIV in a limited number of specimens from 1970 to 1974 in South Africa.[83])

With time, even earlier cases of HIV infection were reported. Frozen specimens from a teenage boy in St. Louis who apparently died of KS and CMV infection in 1968 showed the presence of HIV when specimens from him were tested years later.[84, 85] However, the initial excitement about positive findings from samples from a British sailor who reputedly acquired HIV infection during visits to West African prostitutes in the 1950s[86] were later followed by the retraction of results from the original researchers: " . . . We must conclude that we can find no evidence, in the light of our failure to repeat our original HIV-PCR findings on tissue recently supplied by [the Manchester hospital], to suggest that the 1959 Manchester patient carried the HIV genome."[87]

However, the accumulating cases convinced most in the HIV scientific community that, if one looked hard enough, one could find cases that fulfilled the CDC's AIDS diagnostic criteria for many years before the original AIDS report in 1981. One review that accorded with this growing conviction was an analysis by three Israeli doctors who examined the medical literature, mainly from the *Index Medicus,* starting in 1950.[88, 89] They found 19 "probable" AIDS cases before 1981, the beginning of the "AIDS era." The earliest case of CMV pulmonary infection in a young American man dated from 1953.[90] None of these "AIDS cases" were, obviously, suspected to be the beginnings of a new infectious disease epidemic, but were individual and scattered case reports from puzzled clinicians and pathologists. Indeed, 28 cases of disseminated KS in immunocompromised patients in Europe and North America between 1902 and 1966 were discovered in one review[91]; these authors, perhaps because of sensitivity to the "blaming" of AIDS on Africa and African Americans, hypothesized a possibly European or North American origin of the disease.

Still, by the 1990s, most investigators considered the presence of HIV-2 in West and Central Africa and not elsewhere and the apparent derivation of both HIV-1 and HIV-2 from a progenitor virus as strong indication of the likely origin of HIV from related SIV in that part of sub-Saharan Africa.[92]

This attitude was substantially confirmed by work 10 years later by Beatrice Hahn and colleagues at the University of Alabama at Birmingham.[93] HIV-1 probably originated from introductions to humans of a common ancestor of those viruses and SIVcpz, a SIV that, as its name suggests, is recovered from chimpanzees. The primate reservoir of HIV-2 had already been clearly identified as the sooty mangabey (*Cercocebus atys*). These findings were hailed at scientific meetings in the late 1990s and early 2000s, partly because they confirmed the view that these viruses had evolved over a long period of time before their epidemicity. For example, some European researchers have suggested that the simian ancestor of HIV-1 and its SIVcpz relative must have diverged in the seventeenth century.[94] While some have questioned this "molecular clock," in any case, these viruses are "old," which leads to two important questions.

First, how did these (precursor) viruses originally get introduced from chimpanzees to men? While we will never know for certain the route of chimpanzee-to-man, given our understanding of HIV transmission it is unlikely to have been from eating simian meat, as cooking, factors in the mouth and high gastric acidity all inactivate HIV. Some had proposed that it might have occurred through injection of monkey blood for sexual stimulation,[95] but this is very rarely practiced. Thus, most HIV/AIDS scientists subscribe to the view that transmission of the HIV-1 (ancestor) to humans was most likely "by contamination of a person's open wound with the infected blood of a chimpanzee."[96] This may have occurred in the preparation of "bushmeat" or of hides from infected apes.[97]

Second, why did the AIDS epidemic occur now? Most subscribe to the view that large social dislocations of Africans in the twentieth century and increasing international traffic fostered the AIDS epidemic in Africa and its spread elsewhere. Increased sexual activity in homosexual communities in the United States and Europe and of greater markets for injection drugs–with attendant sharing of contaminated needles–in many U.S. and European cities triggered an explosive and unsuspected growth of HIV before its identification and an understanding of its routes of spread.

Any alternate theory–for example, that HIV arose recently or was actually spread from humans to chimpanzees–had difficulty fitting the data. ("Modern" SIVcpz does not infect humans although SIV$_{MAC}$ has transiently infected two lab workers.[98]). Nonetheless, a major alternative theory of monkey-to-man transfer was proposed in 1999.

The River

Edward Hooper, a radio journalist for BBC covering AIDS in Africa, read a 1992 *Rolling Stone* magazine article by Tom Curtis that postulated that HIV was inadvertently related to testing of an oral polio vaccine (OPV) in the Belgian Congo in the 1950s. According to his 1999 book *The River: A Journey to the Source of HIV and AIDS,*[99] African green monkey kidney cells, the source of cells used for cultivating the vaccine, may have harbored SIVcpz, which then underwent rapid molecular evolution after introduction to human populations. This view significantly faulted Hillary Koprowski of Philadelphia's Wistar Institute who developed the early OPV trials, particularly for alleged mysteries about the donor species and ultimate fate of that vaccine. That Hooper's book was 852-pages-long bespoke his deep research into the circumstances surrounding the original OPV trials in Africa. Conjectures in the book are frequently presented in a seemingly open-minded way, although those scientists who were interviewed by Hooper describe a brow-beating zealot.[100]

According to Hooper's argument, a type 1 strain "CHAT" poliovirus was produced in cells from chimpanzees that were contaminated with the SIVcpz, the simian precursor of HIV-1 Group M, the major agent of AIDS. The first assertion is that CHAT vaccine was prepared in kidney cells from SIV-infected chimpanzees from a colony established in the Belgian Congo. The second claim is essentially an "ecologic" argument that there was a coincidence in the sites where OPV was administered and where early AIDS cases were identified. There are other assertions, but these two seem to provide the basis of the argument.

These allegations culminated in a meeting in London in September 2000, in which many protagonists were present.[101] The concern in the scientific community was stated to be the amount of distraction created in disputing the conspiracy theory presented in *The River.* In the public health community, there was the fear that public concern about all vaccines—considered, with antibiotics, the greatest medical infectious disease advances of the twentieth century—were already causing low levels of vaccination in suspicious populations.

Stanley Plotkin of the University of Pennsylvania presented an extensive analysis and review[102] of both the claims at the center of *The River.* Scientists interviewed by Plotkin complained that statements they made to Hooper were edited and misinterpreted in a manner opposite the interviewee's intention—especially about the fact that chimpanzee tissue and cells were used to make the "CHAT" OPV. Plotkin reviewed testimony of eye witnesses, documents from the 1950s, epidemiologic, and molecular biologic data and found that "the kidneys from chimpanzees were not used in the production of polio vaccine" and that, even if they had been, trypsinization of the cell lines would have acted as a potent destroyer of HIV-SIV.[102] Cross-infection between primate species can occur and presumably has over a prolonged time and, as indicated above, several lines of evidence suggest cases would have occurred before OPV vaccination trials.

Plotkin also concluded that the second main argument about "the supposed geographical correlation between vaccination and AIDS is an illusion." Perhaps a more accurate observation was that events up to 175 miles away could be interpreted by Hooper as occurring in the same locality. Again, ecologic arguments are generally suspect by most epidemiologists, especially those who know how many different tribal boundaries and geographic obstacles may accrue in even a few miles in Africa.

Other Theories

A still persistent belief that HIV/AIDS was created by government scientists to victimize African Americans, gay men, and others is still current. This disinformation started with an article in the Soviet newspaper, *Literary Gazette*, in 1985, which claimed that AIDS was a product of germ warfare developed at Fort Dietrick, Maryland. In turn, the *Gazette*'s source was *The Patriot*, an Indian newspaper that the U.S. government has charged was a frequent conduit for Soviet KGB disinformation. This rumor never gained credence within the AIDS scientific community, which dismissed it as a conspiracy theory without any plausible basis. (It does not fit with either the origins of AIDS now believed to be 80 or more years' old, or the inability of scientists to identify, let alone create, a retrovirus in the 1970s.) However, a substantial portion—usually more than 25 percent of those surveyed—of the African American community still believes that the U.S. government created HIV.[103, 104] As well, 20 percent or more of Asians and whites and about 10 percent of Asians surveyed also subscribe to the conspiracy theory of AIDS.[103]

A different and clearly incorrect impression is that the U.S. AIDS epidemic started with a Canadian airline steward, Gaëtan Dugas, who for purposes of a network analysis was termed "Patient 0"[105] and later as "Patient Zero" in Randy Shilts' 1987 book, *And The Band Played On*,[106] as well as in the 1993 HBO movie version of that book. One effect of this popularization of the story of the start of the American AIDS outbreak was the misimpression that Dugas, who infected at least 40 of his 248 sex partners, was the original source of AIDS in the United States. In fact, many gay men in San Francisco, Los Angeles, New York, and other U.S. cities were HIV-infected by the late 1970s[107] and, as described above, sporadic AIDS cases had apparently been occurring in the decades before the 1980s.

Despite these several theories that have distracted both the public and HIV researchers, AIDS scientists accept HIV as the sufficient primary cause of AIDS and are dedicated to finding treatments, cures, and vaccinations for this virus. As time has progressed, as more and more HIV-infected persons have succumbed to AIDS, the alternate theorists of AIDS' cause and origin have become less vocal, or perhaps simply less reported.

References

1. CDC. *Pneumocystis* Pneumonia–Los Angeles. 1981. *Morbidity and Mortality Weekly Report* 30:250–252.

2. Drew, W.L., L. Mintz, R.C. Miner, M. Sands, and B. Ketterer. 1981. Prevalence of cytomegalovirus infection in homosexual men. *Journal of Infectious Diseases* 143:188–192.

3. Rinaldo Jr., C.R., W.P. Carney, B.S. Richter, P.H. Black, and M.S. Hirsh. 1980. Mechanisms of immunosuppression in cytomegaloviral mononucleosis. *Journal of Infectious Diseases* 141:488–495.

4. Staras, S.A., S.C. Dollard, K.W. Radford, W.D. Flanders, R.F. Pass, and M.J. Cannon. 2006. Seroprevalence of cytomegalovirus infection in the United States, 1988–1994. *Clinical Infectious Diseases* 43:1152–1153.

5. Sonnabend, J., S.S. Witkin, and D.T. Purtilo. 1983. Acquired immunodeficiency syndrome, opportunistic infections, and malignancies in male homosexuals. A hypothesis of etiologic factors in pathogenesis. *Journal of the American Medical Association* 249:2370–2374.

6. Barré-Sinoussi, F., J.-C. Chermann, F. Rey, et al. 1983. Isolation of a T-lymphotropic retrovirus from a patient at risk for acquired immune deficiency syndrome (AIDS). *Science* 220:868–871.

7. Drew, W.L., J. Mills, J. Levy, et al. 1985. Cytomegalovirus infection and abnormal T-lymphocyte subset ratios in homosexual men. *Annals of Internal Medicine* 103:61–63.

8. Chang, Y., E. Cesarman, M.S. Pessin, F. Lee, J. Culpepper, D.M. Knowles, and P.S. Moore. 1994. Identification of herpesvirus-like DNA sequences in AIDS-associated Kaposi's sarcoma. *Science* 266:1865–1869.

9. Skolnik, P.R., B.R. Kosloff, and M.S. Hirsch. 1988. Bidirectional interactions between human immunodeficiency virus type 1 and cytomegalovirus. *Journal of Infectious Diseases* 157:508–514.

10. Duclos, H., E. Elfassi, S. Michelson, F. Arenzana-Seisdedos, U. Hazen, A. Munier, and J.-L. Virelizier. 1989. Cytomegalovirus infection and transactivation of HIV-1 and HIV-2 LTRs in human astrocytoma cells. *AIDS Research and Human Retroviruses* 5:217–224.

11. Fiala, M., J.D. Mosca, P. Barry, P.A. Luciw, and H.V. Vinters. 1991. Multi-step pathogenesis of AIDS–Role of cytomegalovirus. *Research in Immunology* 142:87–95.

12. Ostrove, J.M., J. Leonard, K.E. Weck, A.B. Rabson, and H.E. Gendelman. 1987. Activation of the human immunodeficiency virus by herpes simplex virus type 1. *Journal of Virology* 61:3726–3732.

13. Furth, P.A., H. Westphal, and L. Hennighausen. 1990. Expression from the HIV-LTR is stimulated by glucocorticoids and pregnancy. *AIDS Research and Human Retroviruses* 6:553–560.

14. Kobayashi, N., Y. Hamamoto, Y. Koyanagi, I.S. Chen, and N. Yamamoto. 1989 Effect of interleukin-1 on the augmentation of human immunodeficiency virus gene expression. *Biochemical and Biophysical Research Communications* 165:715–721.

15. Li, Y.C., J. Ross, J.A. Scheppler, and B.R. Franza Jr. 1991. An in vitro transcription analysis of early responses of the human immunodeficiency virus type 1 long terminal repeat to different transcriptional activators. *Molecular and Cell Biology* 11:1883–1893.

16. Suligoi, B., M. Dorrucci, J. Uccella, M. Andreoni, G. Rezza, and the Italian Seroconversion Study. 2003. Effect of multiple herpesvirus infections on the progression of HIV disease in a cohort of HIV seroconverters. *Journal of Medical Virology* 69:182–187.

17. Crewdson, J. November 19, 1989. The great AIDS quest (part 1: science under the microscope). *Chicago Tribune.*

18. Roberts, S. November 1990. Lab rat: What AIDS researcher Dr. Robert Gallo did in pursuit of the Nobel Prize, and what he didn't do in pursuit of a cure for AIDS. *Spy.*

19. Culliton, B.J. 1990. News report: Inside the Gallo probe. *Science* 248:1494–1498.

20. Rubinstein, E. 1990. Inside the Gallo probe. II. The untold story of HUT78. *Science* 248:1499–1507.

21. Coppola, V. June 1996. Robert Gallo wants to fight. *Worth.* Available at http://www.virusmyth.net/aids/data/vcgallo.htm.

22. Gallo, R.C., P.S. Sarin, E.P. Gelmann, et al. 1983. Isolation of human T-cell leukemia virus in acquired immune deficiency syndrome (AIDS). *Science* 220:865–867.

23. Popovic, M., M.G. Sarngadharan, E. Read, and R.C. Gallo. 1984. Detection, isolation, and continuous production of cytopathic retroviruses (HTLV-III) from patients with AIDS and pre-AIDS. *Science* 224:497–500.

24. CDC. 1988. Agent summary statement for human immunodeficiency viruses (HIVs) including HTLV-III, LAV, HIV-1, and HIV-2. *Morbidity and Mortality Weekly Report* 37(suppl 4):1–17.

25. Wain-Hobson, S., J.P. Vartanian, M. Henry, et al. 1991. LAV revisited: Origins of the early HIV-1 isolates from Institut Pasteur. *Science* 252:961–965.

26. Chang, S.Y., B.H. Bowman, J.B. Weiss, R.E Garcia, and T.J. White. 1993. The origin of HIV-1 isolate HTLV-IIIB. *Nature* 363:466–469.

27. Clavel, F., M. Guyader, D. Guetard, M. Salle, L. Montagnier, and M. Alizon. 1986. Molecular cloning and polymorphism of the human immune deficiency virus type 2. *Nature* 324:691–695.

28. Clavel, F., K. Mansinho, S. Chamaret, et al. 1987. Human immunodeficiency virus type 2 infection associated with AIDS in West Africa. *New England Journal of Medicine* 316:1180–1185.

29. Pepin, J., G. Morgan, D. Dunn, et al. 1991. HIV-2-induced immunosuppression among asymptomatic West African prostitutes: Evidence that HIV-2 is pathogenic, but less so than HIV-1. *AIDS* 5:1165–1672.

30. Wilkins, A., D. Ricard, J. Todd, H. Whittle, F. Dias, and A. Paolo Da Silva. 1993. The epidemiology of HIV infection in a rural area of Guinea-Bissau. *AIDS* 7:1119–1122.

31. Kanki, P.J., F. Barin, S. M'Boup, et al. 1986. New human T-lymphotropic retrovirus related to simian T-lymphotropic virus III (STLV-IIIAGM). *Science* 232:238–242.

32. Brun-Vezinet, F., M.A. Rey, C. Katlama, et al. 1987. Lymphadenopathy-associated virus type 2 in AIDS and AIDS-related complex. Clinical and virological features in four patients. *Lancet* 1:128–132.

33. Francini, G., E. Collalti, S.K. Arya, et al. 1987. Genetic analysis of a new subgroup of human and simian T-lymphotropic retroviruses: HTLV-IV, LAV-2, SBL-6669, and STLV-IIIAGM. *AIDS Research and Human Retroviruses* 3:11–17.

34. Kanki, P.J., J.R. Hopper, and M. Essex. 1987. The origins of HIV-1 and HTLV-4/HIV-2. *Annals of the New York Academy of Science* 511:370–375.

35. Kestler 3rd, H.W., Y. Li, Y.M. Naidu, et al. 1988. Comparison of simian immunodeficiency virus isolates. *Nature* 331:619–622.

36. Barin, F., F. Denis, A. Baillou, et al. 1987. A STLV-III related human retrovirus, HTLV-IV: Analysis of cross-reactivity with the human immunodeficiency virus (HIV). *Journal of Virologic Methods* 17:55–61.

37. Hoxie, J.A., B.S. Haggarty, S.E. Bonser, J.L. Rackowski, H. Shan, and P.J. Kanki. 1988. Biological characterization of a simian immunodeficiency virus-like retrovirus (HTLV-IV): Evidence for CD4-associated molecules required for infection. *Journal of Virology* 62:2557–2568.

38. Kanki, P.J., J. Allan, F. Barin, et al. 1987. Absence of antibodies to HIV-2/HTLV-4 in six central African nations. *AIDS Research and Human Retroviruses* 3:317–322.

39. Lucey, D.R. 1991. The first decade of human retroviruses: A nomenclature for the clinician. *Military Medicine* 156:555–557.

40. Travers, K., S. M'Boup, R. Marlink, et al. 1995. Natural protection against HIV-1 infection provided by HIV-2. *Science* 268:1612–1615.

41. Kanki, P.J., K.U. Travers, S. M'Boup, et al. 1994. Slower heterosexual spread of HIV-2 than HIV-1. *Lancet* 343:943–946.

42. Greenberg, A.E., S.F. Wiktor, K.M. DeCock, P. Smith, H.W. Jaffe, and T.J. Dondero Jr. 1996. HIV-2 and natural protection against HIV-1 infection [technical comments]. *Science* 272:1959.

43. Kanki, P.J., G. Eisen, K.U. Travers, et al. 1996. HIV-2 and natural protection against HIV-1 infection [letter]. *Science* 272:1960.

44. Greenberg, A.E. 2001. Possible protective effect of HIV-2 against incident HIV-1 infection: Review of available epidemiological and *in vitro* data [editorial comments]. *AIDS* 15:2319–2321.

45. Nkengasong, J.N., L. Kestens, P.D. Ghys, et al. 2000. Dual infections with human immunodeficiency virus type 1 and type 2: Impact on HIV type 1 viral load and immune activation markers in HIV-seropositive female sex workers in Abidjan, Ivory Coast. *AIDS Research and Human Retroviruses* 16:1371–1378.

46. Jaffe, H.W., K. Choi, P.A. Thomas, et al. 1983. National case-control study of Kaposi's sarcoma and *Pneumocystis carinii* pneumonia in homosexual men, Part 1. Epidemiologic results. *Annals of Internal Medicine* 99:145–151.

47. CDC Task Force on Kaposi's Sarcoma and Opportunistic Infections. 1982. Epidemiologic aspects of the current outbreak of Kaposi's sarcoma and opportunistic infections. *New England Journal of Medicine* 306:248–252.

48. Marmor, M., A.E. Friedman-Kien, L. Laubenstein, et al. 1982. Risk factors for Kaposi's sarcoma in homosexual men. *Lancet* 1:1083–1086.

49. Friedman-Kien, A.E., L.J. Laubenstein, P. Rubinstein, et al. 1982. Disseminated Kaposi's sarcoma in homosexual men. *Annals of Internal Medicine* 96(part 1):693–700.

50. Goedert, J.J., C.Y. Neuland, W.C. Wallen, et al. 1982. Amyl nitrite may alter T lymphocytes in homosexual men. *Lancet* 1:411–416.

51. Harden, V.A., and D. Rodrigues. March 2, 1990. Interview with Dr. William A. Blattner, NIH Historical Office, Available at http://history.nih.gov/NIHInOwnWords/docs/page_08.html.

52. Haverkos, H.W. 2004. Viruses, chemicals and co-carcinogenesis. *Oncogene* 23:6492–6499.

53. Teas, J. 1983. Could AIDS agent be a new variant of African swine fever virus [letter]? *Lancet* 1:923.

54. Arnoux, E., J.M. Guerin, R. Malebranche R, et al. 1983. AIDS and African swine fever [letter]. *Lancet* 1:110.

55. Colaert, J., J. Desmyter, J. Goudsmit, N. Clumeck, and C. Terpstra. 1983. African swine fever antibody not found in AIDS patients. *Lancet* 1:1098.

56. Rogers, M.F., D.M. Morens, J.A. Stewart, et al. 1983. National case-control study of Kaposi's sarcoma and *Pneumocystis carinii* pneumonia in homosexual men, Part 2. Laboratory results. *Annals of Internal Medicine* 99:151–158.

57. Beldekas, J., J. Teas, and J.R. Herbert. 1986. African swine fever virus and AIDS [letter]. *Lancet* 1:564.

58. Leishman, K. September 1987. AIDS and insects. *Atlantic Monthly* 55–72.

59. Ortleb, C.L. March 17, 1986. AIDS linked to African Swine Fever Virus. *New York Native*, 8–9.

60. Pigs, AIDS and Belle Glade [editorial]. June 3, 1986. *The New York Times* A26.

61. Feorino, P., G. Schable, G. Schochetman, et al. 1986. AIDS and African swine fever virus [letter]. *Lancet* 2:815.

62. Martins, C.V., and M.J.P. Lawman. 1986. African swine fever and AIDS [letter]. *Lancet* 1:1504.

63. Consensus Statement. ASF/AIDS Workshop. Cold Spring Harbor, NY, September 11, 1986.

64. Duesberg, P.H. 1987. Retroviruses as carcinogens and pathogens: Expectations and reality. *Cancer Research* 47:1199–1220.

65. Duesberg, P. 1988. HIV is not the cause of AIDS [policy forum]. *Science* 241:514, 517.

66. Blattner, W., R.C. Gallo, and H.M. Temin. 1988. HIV causes AIDS [policy forum]. *Science* 241:515.

67. Weiss, R.A., and H.W. Jaffe. 1990. Duesberg, HIV and AIDS. *Nature* 345:659–660.

68. Duesberg, P., and D. Rasnick. 1998. The AIDS dilemma: Drug diseases blamed on a passenger virus. *Genetica* 104:85–132

69. Duesberg, P. 1994. Infectious AIDS–Stretching the germ theory beyond its limits. *International Archives of Allergy and Immunology* 103:118–127.

70. Schoch, R. August 17, 1992. Dad, I'm HIV positive. *Newsweek* 9.

71. Holmberg, S.D., L.J. Conley, S.P. Buchbinder, et al. 1993. Use of therapeutic and prophylactic drugs for AIDS by homosexual and bisexual men in three U.S. cities. *AIDS* 7:699–704.

72. Siegel, K., and E. Gorey. 1997. HIV-infected women: barriers to AZT use. *Social Science and Medicine* 45:15–22.

73. Balfe, P., P. Simmonds, C.A. Ludlam, J.O. Bishop, and A.J. Brown. 1990. Concurrent evolution of human immunodeficiency virus type 1 in patients infected from the same source: Rate of sequence change and low frequency of inactivating mutations. *Journal of Virology* 64:6221–6233.

74. Li, W.-H., M. Tanimura, and P.M. Sharp. 1988. Rates and dates of divergence between AIDS virus nucleotide sequences. *Molecular Biology and Evolution* 5:313–330.

75. Myers, G., A.B. Rabson, S.F. Josephs, et al. (eds.). 1989. *Human Retroviruses and AIDS 1989. A Compilation and Analysis of Nucleic and Amino Acid Sequences.* Los Alamos, NM: Los Alamos National Laboratory.

76. Srinivasan, A., D. York, D. Butler, et al. 1989. Molecular characterization of HIV-1 isolated from a serum collected in 1976: Nucleotide sequence comparison to recent isolates and generation of hybrid HIV. *AIDS Research and Human Retroviruses* 5:121–129.

77. Doolittle, R.F., D.F. Feng, M.S. Johnson, and M.A. McClure. 1989. Origins and evolutionary relationships of retroviruses. [Review] *Quarterly Review of Biology* 64:1–30

78. Krause, R.M. 1992. The origin of plagues: Old and new. *Science* 257:1073–1078.

79. Frøland, S.S., P. Jenum, C.F. Lindboe, K.W. Wefring, P.J. Linnestad, and T. Böhmer. 1988. HIV-1 infection in Norwegian family before 1970 [letter]. *Lancet* 1:1344–1345.

80. Thomas, P., R. O'Donnell, and R. Williams. 1988. HIV infection in heterosexual female intravenous drug users in New York City, 1977–80 [letter]. *New England Journal of Medicine* 319:374.

81. Nzilambi, N., K.M. De Cock, D.N. Forthal, et al. 1988. The prevalence of infection with human immunodeficiency virus over a 10-year period in rural Zaire. *New England Journal of Medicine* 318:276–279.

82. Jaffe, H.W., P.M. Feorino, W.W. Darrow, et al. 1985. Persistent infection with human T-lymphotropic virus type III/lymphadenopathy-associated virus in apparently healthy homosexual men. *Annals of Internal Medicine* 102:627–628.

83. Sher, R., S. Antunes, B. Reid, and H. Falcke. 1987. Seroepidemiology of human immunodeficiency virus in Africa from 1970 to 1974 [letter]. *New England Journal of Medicine* 317:450–451.

84. Witte, M.H., C.L. Witte, P.R. Finley, and W.L. Drake. 1984. AIDS in 1968 [letter]. *Journal of the American Medical Association* 251:2657.

85. Garry, R.F., M.H. Witte, A. Gottlieb, et al. 1988. Documentation of an AIDS virus infection in the United States in 1968. *Journal of the American Medical Association* 260:2085–2087.

86. Corbitt, G., A.S. Bailey, and G. Williams. 1990. HIV infection in Manchester, 1959 [letter]. *Lancet* 336:51.

87. Bailey, A.S., and G. Corbitt. 1996. Was HIV present in 1959 [letter]? *Lancet* 347:189.

88. Huminer, D., J.B. Rosenfeld, and S.D. Pitlik. 1987. AIDS in the pre-AIDS era. *Reviews of Infectious Diseases* 9:1102–1106.

89. Huminer, D., and S.D. Pitlik. 1988. Further evidence for the existence of AIDS in the pre-AIDS era [correspondence]. *Reviews of Infectious Diseases* 10:1061.

90. Wyatt, J.P., T. Simon, M.L. Turnbull, and M. Evans. 1953. Cytomegalic inclusion pneumonitis in the adult. *American Journal of Clinical Pathology* 23:353–362.

91. Katner, H.P., and G.A. Pankey. 1987. Evidence for a Euro-American origin of human immunodeficiency virus (HIV). *Journal of the National Medical Association* 79:1068–1072.

92. McClure, M.O., and T.F. Schulz. 1989. Origin of HIV [editorial]. *British Medical Journal* 298:1267–1268.

93. Gao, F., E. Bailes, D.L. Robertson, et al. 1999. Origin of HIV-1 in the chimpanzee *Pan troglodytes troglodytes. Nature* 397:436–441.

94. Salemi, M., K. Strimmer, W.W. Hall, et al. 2001. Dating the common ancestor of SIVcpz and HIV-1 Group M and the origin of HIV-1 subtypes by using a new method to uncover clock-like molecular evolution. *Federation of American Societies for Experimental Biology Journal* 15:276–278. Available at http://www.fasebj.org/cgi/doi/10.1096/fj.00-0449fge.

95. Noireau, F. 1987. HIV transmission from monkey to man [letter]. *Lancet* 1:1498–1499.

96. Fauci, A.S. 1999. The AIDS epidemic–Considerations for the 21st century. *New England Journal of Medicine* 341:1046–1050.

97. Peeters, M., V. Courgnaud, B. Abela, et al. 2002. Risk to human health from a plethora of simian immunodeficiency viruses in primate bushmeat. *Emerging Infectious Diseases* 8:451–457.

98. Khabbaz, R.F., H. Walid, J.R. George, et al. 1994. Brief report: Infection of a laboratory worker with simian immunodeficiency virus. *New England Journal of Medicine* 330:172–177.

99. Hooper, E. *The River: A Journey to the Source of HIV and AIDS.* Boston: Little, Brown and Company, 1999.

100. Cohen, J. October 2000. The hunt for the origin of AIDS. *Atlantic Monthly* 88–104.

101. Weiss, R., and S. Wain-Hobson (eds.). 2000. The origins of AIDS. In *Philosophical Transactions of the Royal Society (London).* London: Royal Society.

102. Plotkin, S.A. 2001. CHAT oral polio vaccine was not the source for human immunodeficiency virus type 1 Group M for humans. *Clinical Infectious Diseases* 32:1068–1084.

103. Ross, M.W., E.J. Essien, and I. Torres. 2006. Conspiracy beliefs about the origin of HIV/AIDS in four racial/ethnic groups. *Journal of the Acquired Immune Deficiency Syndromes* 41:342–344.

104. Bogart, L.M., and S. Thorburn. 2006. Relationship of African Americans' sociodemographic characteristics to belief in conspiracies about HIV/AIDS and birth control. *Journal of the National Medical Association* 98:1144–1150.

105. Auerbach, D.M., W.W. Darrow, H.W. Jaffe, and J.W. Curran. 1984. Cluster of cases of the acquired immune deficiency syndrome. Patients linked by sexual contact. *American Journal of Medicine* 76:487–492.

106. Shilts, R. 1987. *And The Band Played On: Politics, People, and the AIDS Epidemic.* New York: St. Martin's Press.

107. Jaffe, H.W., W.W. Darrow, D.F. Echenberg, et al. 1985. The acquired immunodeficiency syndrome in a cohort of homosexual men. A six-year follow-up study. *Annals of Internal Medicine* 103:210–214.

CHAPTER THREE

Counting Cases

Surveillance of public health problems, especially infectious diseases, is a major function of CDC in cooperation with state and local health departments. Counting cases may be used to act as "early alert" of an emerging outbreak or to monitor progress in controlling ongoing health problems, such as conditions as diverse as *Salmonella* infection, injuries, childhood obesity, or smoking. At the beginning of the AIDS epidemic, it was thought that surveillance would function as the former, that is detecting and understanding a hoped-for limited outbreak. Twenty-five years later, surveillance for AIDS and HIV infection acts as an index of how well prevention and treatment are (or are not) working. As Epidemic Intelligence Service (EIS) Officers in CDC's program, which trains about 60 practical epidemiologists every year from various disciplines, learn early, defining what constitutes a "case" is a critical early step in evaluating and controlling an epidemic.

The definition of "case," the AIDS case definition, has big implications for the "sensitivity" and "specificity" of the AIDS surveillance system—that is, the ability to detect all true cases (sensitivity), and the exclusion of "cases" not truly AIDS (specificity). There have been problems with the sensitivity of AIDS surveillance from the beginning. Many cases were not detected early in the epidemic as gay men and intravenous drug users would avoid identification, especially the added stigma and emotional stress of a fatal disease acquired through socially proscribed activity; early on, physicians sometimes colluded in hiding the identity of people with this fatal and stigmatizing disease. This situation of diminished sensitivity still pertains as, for example, many "do not want to know" if they are HIV-infected. (Oddly, the opposite sometimes occurs—psychiatric patients with the delusion they have AIDS when they don't.[1]) Presently this problem of undercounting HIV infections is acute in the South where African American heterosexual spread continues,[2] as best anyone can tell, unabated and increasing. The most recent estimates are that about 30 percent of all HIV-infected Americans do not know they are infected. At the turn of the century, of the estimated 900,000 HIV-infected U.S. residents, with or without clinical AIDS, 280,000 were thought to be undiagnosed and unaware of their HIV status–and potentially spreading HIV. [3, 4] Thus, the "sensitivity" of AIDS surveillance persists as a problem.

"Specificity" of AIDS surveillance was even more of a problem early, as there were so many manifestations of AIDS, many of which required special or invasive testing such as biopsy. However, as diagnosis of HIV itself has become ever easier, faster, and cheaper, and testing of immunologic function, especially CD4+ cell counts, now gives an indication of how advanced HIV disease is, the specificity of the HIV/AIDS surveillance system has steadily improved. That is, very few would be incorrectly diagnosed as having HIV infection, "false positive" serological (enzyme immunoassay) testing, and these would be eliminated on confirmatory (Western blot) testing.

There were many controversies about what constituted the "AIDS case definition" in the first 15 years. Counting AIDS cases turns out to be more complicated than it might seem. The basic problems relate to several issues. One of these is that the signs and symptoms of AIDS–such as fever or lymphadenopathy (swollen lymph glands)–are nonspecific and may occur with many other diseases or conditions. Another is that the various opportunistic infections (OI) and cancers associated with AIDS may occur without underlying HIV. For example, tuberculosis, still the most common AIDS-associated "OI" in the world, usually occurs independent of HIV infection in most patients. Other AIDS-associated conditions engendered by low CD4+ cell counts, such as internal Kaposi's sarcoma (KS) or esophageal candidiasis, may require special and comparatively expensive diagnostic tests or procedures. Finally, the long incubation period between infection and overt disease also somewhat frustrated early case counting and was a big problem for initially anticipating the future shape of the epidemic. The time between HIV infection and AIDS-defining disease is usually estimated to be 8–11 years, [5, 6] and this might occasionally confuse case-counting–for example, someone had not had sex or shared needles in injection drug abuse for many years and so there was patient or physician uncertainty and reluctance to diagnose AIDS.

The first major concern in the AIDS epidemic was finding the extent and scope of the problem. By September 1982, CDC had already received 593 reports of AIDS from all over the country, and 243 (41%) of the patients had died.[7] This was clearly a major public health emergency. Almost daily AIDS "cases" were being expanded to include more and more associated diseases, potential transmission risk groups and reporting states and localities.

By September 1982, 88 percent of cases had either *Pneumocystis carinii* pneumonia (PCP), Kaposi's sarcoma (KS), or both.[7] However, even worse, it was now being recognized that an ever-expanding list of other OIs could signal serious, acquired immune deficiency. These might include a veritable textbook of infectious disease.

> These infections include pneumonia, meningitis, or encephalitis due to one or more of the following: aspergillosis, candidiasis, cryptococcosis, cytomegalovirus, nocardiosis, strongyloidosis, toxoplasmosis, zygomycosis, or atypical mycobacteriosis (species other than tuberculosis or lepra); esophagitis due to candidiasis, cytomegalovirus, or herpes simplex virus; progressive multifocal leukoencephalopathy; chronic enterocolitis (more than 4 weeks) due to cryptosporidiosis; or unusually, extensive mucocutaneous herpes simplex of more than 5 weeks duration. CDC encourages reports of any cancer among persons with AIDS and of selected rare lymphomas (Burkitt's or diffuse, undifferentiated non-Hodgkins lymphoma) among persons with a risk factor for AIDS.[7, 8]

This expanding list of AIDS-associated conditions included diseases that were ubiquitous—such as pneumonia that was initially or ultimately of an unknown cause—and others that would not be seen by a lifetime of medical practice in the United States (e.g., progressive multifocal leukencephalopathy, or strongyloidosis).

Ominously, CDC was now also requesting "reports of AIDS cases regardless of the absence of risk factors."[7] This implied that while AIDS cases in the United States were still predominantly reported from gay or bisexual men it was undeniable that cases were also occurring in intravenous drug users, persons of Haitian origin (presumably from heterosexual transmission) and, now, two men with hemophilia A, who had received blood transfusions. A cold analysis of the data coming in was sobering: the unknown agent of AIDS could be spread sexually—both by homosexual and heterosexual contact—and by blood. (Pediatric AIDS from perinatal—that is, mother-to-infant—spread had not yet been established.) By the end of 1982 cases had been reported from 27 states and the District of Columbia, and reports were now coming in at the rate of about two per day. Even if some were ultimately not AIDS, it was clear that a major and fatal epidemic had begun.

From a scientific and epidemiologic viewpoint, the rapidly expanding AIDS case definition was necessary. However, it resulted in confusion and controversy about what should be included in the definition. In retrospect, the definition even by 1982 was pretty good, especially absent the knowledge of the cause of AIDS or a way to specifically test for it.

The first problem for the AIDS case definition was that it was not broad enough to include many AIDS cases in the developing world. Thus, a special workshop on expanding the case definition of "AIDS" was convened in Bangui, Central Africa, in 1985. This meeting decided that major but nonspecific clinical signs of AIDS included weight loss, asthenia (weakness), chronic diarrhea, and prolonged or recurring fever.[9] The Bangui conference did not list tuberculosis as an AIDS-defining illness, but was important in providing an easy, referable case definition for situations in most of the world where laboratory testing was not available—for example, the presence of unexplained wasting, diarrhea, and fever.

Tensions between the CDC and the WHO definitions were unavoidable as the manifestations of AIDS were different in developed countries where lab indices of immunodeficiency and verified diagnosis of AIDS conditions could be determined and developing countries where, at best, one would need a "sensitive" definition of "AIDS" in which Africans with, say, wasting of another cause would be lumped in with the ever burgeoning AIDS cases clinically (presumptively) diagnosed.

In the early 1990s, it was clear that the CDC definition needed to broaden under two distinct forces. The first force was scientific, in the sense that better testing for HIV and for CD4+ cell counts had become easier and cheaper. For example, in CDC studies in the late 1980s, CD4+ cell counts, usually by Coulter counter, typically cost $170 for each CD4+ cell count. This testing was a major cost burden to any cohort study but did serve to (1) provide good laboratory parameters in which to assess HIV disease in study-participants; and (2) paying for this (at the time) expensive test and providing results to study-participants was an inducement for them to join and remain in studies. The decision to include all persons with a CD4+ cell count less than 200 cells/mm^3 as having AIDS[10] reflected that almost no one would naturally have such a low CD4+ cell count—or a CD4+ T-lymphocyte percentage of less that 14 percent of total lymphocytes—unless he or she was HIV-infected (see idiopathic CD4 lymphocytopenia [ICL] below). So, in addition to dropping a few diagnoses—such as the fungal infection nocardiosis—the definition was expanded to include tuberculosis and low CD4+cell counts.

The other force was almost entirely political and social. In AIDS, the definition of a "case" also has import in terms of who qualifies for federal (e.g. Ryan White) or local funding for their medical care. In the mid-1980s, women accounted for only 8 percent of all AIDS cases reported in the United States, but by the 2000s the percentage had jumped to nearly 25 percent.

Activists were concerned and angry that women were not being included sufficiently in getting diagnosed and treated for AIDS. That is, in the 1980s, focus on gay men, (male) drug users, and hemophilic men, who made up the overwhelming majority of the first AIDS cases in the United States, provided the diseases that constituted an AIDS diagnosis. Some of these, such as KS, occurred virtually exclusively in gay men.

Thus, there was real concern that women with immunodeficiency were being excluded from the AIDS diagnosis. Some women with immunodeficiency might not qualify for compensated medical care because they did not have conditions seen in men. Highly visible demonstrations, with several arrests, were conducted in Washington.[11] Concern about expanding the AIDS case definition continued to increase,[12] but adjusting the case definition in the context of increasing and realigning federal funding for AIDS care was problematic.[13]

On one hand, this growing worry about women with AIDS concern led, for example, to the First National Women and HIV Conference in 1989, where differences in female and male AIDS were compared in the venue of a scientific meeting. It also led in the same year to protests at CDC by the advocacy and protest group ACT UP (AIDS Coalition To Unleash Power) to open the AIDS case definition to woman-specific and common pelvic conditions, including vaginal candidiasis and pelvic inflammatory disease (usually from gonorrhea or chlamydial infection). For example, at a meeting held at the American Public Health Association (APHA) in 1992, public officials, academic doctors and others who were meeting to discuss changing the AIDS case definition were disrupted and literally held hostage for a over two hours—a few were handcuffed—by a splinter group of ACT UP (which disavowed the actions of the disrupters).

One result of this activism was that in the late 1980s the idea was disseminated that vulvovaginal candidiasis (VVC)—that is, "yeast" infection of the female vaginal tract—could be a manifestation of immunodeficiency from HIV infection and that women with recurrent VVC should be tested for HIV. While no public health official would discount the importance of HIV testing, there was a concern that opening the AIDS diagnosis to this common condition would inappropriately suggest that millions of women with common yeast infection could be considered as having or possibly having HIV/AIDS. The earliest studies of this issue suggested that women with HIV might be more likely than those without infection to have recurrent VVC; but these studies were small, used inconsistent criteria for diagnosing VVC, and reflected biased selection of women.[14] In fact, later, more stringent, and larger cohort studies of HIV-infected women failed to show elevated attack rates of symptomatic *Candida vaginitis* in HIV-infected vs. uninfected women.[15, 16]

Another condition advocated by the activists, cervical cancer, caused by strains of human papillomavirus (HPV), was not common and might indicate immunodeficiency. HPV causes stages of progressive cell changes that are "precancerous" on Papanicolaou (Pap) smear. The earliest studies of the relatively few HIV-infected women showed that, indeed, they were more likely to show these changes on Pap smear than women without HIV infection.[17–19] Studies of cancer incidence in the 1980s were mainly of men and demonstrated the increased likelihood of KS and non-Hodgkins lymphoma. Squamous cell carcinomas of the anus and rectum, also caused by HPV, had been observed in much increased frequency in HIV-infected gay men, [20, 21] and it was reasonable to conclude that an increased predilection for cervical cancer would be seen in HIV-infected women.

It is interesting to note that at the time of the greatest debate no one had or–given the comparatively few women identified as HIV-infected at the time–could actually document that cervical cancer itself was more likely to occur in HIV-infected than HIV-uninfected women. The debate in the late 1980s and early 1990s centered around rates of cervical cell (Pap smear) change in HIV-infected women compared with similar HIV-uninfected women. Here, the epidemiology was tricky. Since many women had acquired both HIV and HPV from increased sexual activity, finding comparable women with increased sexual activity, who did not have HIV infection and who would agree to act as comparison study-subjects was not easy. The women being recruited for studies were often injection drug users, women who traded sex for money or drugs, and others unlikely or unwilling to be recruited to any study.

As epidemiology is a science of comparisons, making sure that the populations being compared–HIV-infected vs. uninfected women–were as similar to one another as possible was problematic. If the comparison (control) women were equally sexually active but did not have HIV infection, would they nonetheless have comparable rates of HPV infection? Nonetheless, by 1990, it was pretty clear that intraepithelial neoplasia, carcinoma in situ (CIS), and other precancerous conditions were more likely, more advanced, and more difficult to treat in HIV-infected than uninfected women.[17, 22, 23]

After the 1992 decision to include cervical cancer in the AIDS case definition (starting in 1993), several federally sponsored cohort studies of HIV-infected women demonstrated the greater likelihood of precancerous conditions and cervical cell changes both in the CDC's HIV Epidemiology Research Study (HERS)[15, 24, 25] and the NIAID's Women's Interagency HIV Study (WIHS).[19, 26, 27] It was several years later that any study of women actually demonstrated increased occurrence of cervical cancer itself in HIV-infected than uninfected women.[28] This was not possible until enough cervical cancer cases had accrued.

However, it is fair to state that the "[N]atural history, progression, survival, and HIV-associated illnesses—except for those of the reproductive tract—thus far appear to be similar in HIV-infected women and men."[29]

What Is the Future of AIDS? Modeling the Past to Estimate the Future

Probably no question in the HIV/AIDS epidemic has been more pressing from a public health and policy viewpoint than its future course. From the beginning, there have been many different attempts and approaches to trying to estimate the "epidemic curve" of AIDS. In looking back at the many different conclusions modelers and estimators arrived at, it is good to remember that estimating into the future has major constraints. The first is the accuracy and completeness of AIDS reporting, especially early in the epidemic. While reported cases were accumulating rapidly in the early 1980s, how many more were going undetected? Estimates of undetected and unreported cases would markedly change one's estimate of the true numbers of HIV/AIDS cases.

A second major factor in estimating the future of AIDS in the 1980s and 1990s was the length of the "incubation period," classically defined as time from HIV infection to the onset of AIDS. (Before 1993, "AIDS" would be any AIDS-defining condition, irrespective of CD4+ cell count). If one thinks about the first 100 or 1,000 AIDS cases observed, did these represent infection acquired weeks, months, or years ago? If the incubation was short—say, days, weeks, or even months—the first cases may signal a limited outbreak. If, however, as we now know, cases were the result of an infection acquired a decade previously, the rapidity and number of AIDS cases being observed signaled a much larger, more ominous epidemic. (Note that it was not necessary to know the exact agent of AIDS, HIV, in the first such estimates as any "AIDS agent" could act for purposes of modeling the future course of the epidemic.) In fact, assuming a normal distribution of incubation period, one would need to see a peak, then decline, in reported AIDS cases to start making more accurate estimates of incubation time, because many cases with long or longest incubation periods had not yet been diagnosed.

Further, both the beginning of the incubation period, HIV infection, and the end, AIDS-defining illness, were quite fluid and hard to pin down. That is, the date of infection was almost impossible to specify in gay men or injection drug users who had many sex or needle-sharing partners and contacts. (Again, the average number of lifetime sex partners in the first AIDS cases in San Francisco gay men often numbered in the hundreds.[30]) So, many of the initial exercises to estimate incubation time focused on the relatively few people whose infection dated from a blood transfusion:

was their incubation period, from infection to AIDS, similar to that as seen in persons acquiring HIV through sexual contact? Nor was the end-point, AIDS, a single point in time. Men with KS, for instance, might have much higher CD4+ cell counts (say, 250 cells/mm^3) and be considerably earlier in their disease than men or women with atypical mycobacterial infections, usually seen at very low CD4+ cell counts (almost always, fewer than 50 cells/mm^3) and quite late in disease.

All estimates before 1993 or 1994, when AIDS cases "peaked" in the United States (see Figure1.1), would have to model the various incubation periods in persons with known or suspected dates of HIV infection and dates of AIDS, and calculate probable distribution of incubation period. Given the relatively few cases with known or putative dates of HIV infection, this kind of calculation required clever mathematics and a trust in the representativeness of the limited data (known incubation periods) available. Those with transfusion-acquired AIDS may have received a huge "slug" of virus directly to the bloodstream, compared with sexually acquired AIDS, and so might have a relatively short incubation to developing AIDS.

Thus, CDC investigators concluded that the simple mean of incubations they had observed (2.6 years) in transfusion-infected persons underestimated the true mean, as the epidemic had not progressed long enough to see how long the longest incubation periods might be. So, they used maximum likelihood techniques to assess that the AIDS incubation period would be 4.5 years (90% CI, 2.6–14.2 years) in transfusion-infected persons.[31] Their similar calculations using a truncated Weibull distribution of incubation periods observed in children who had transfusion-acquired AIDS found a median incubation period of only 2.4 years (90% CI, 1.5–7.2 years).[31] In retrospect, as indicated above, the true average incubation period between HIV infection and AIDS is closer to 9 or 10 years,[32] the upper confidence interval bounds in transfusion-acquired AIDS in adults. This was a classic instance where the data analyzed early in the epidemic were simply insufficient.

Even by the mid-1980s, it was clear that the incubation period of AIDS was much longer and more variable than for almost any other known viral infection of humans other than for "slow viruses" such as those of kuru or Jacob-Creutzfeldt disease. By 1990, enough cases had accumulated to allow accurate calculation of the incubation period, for adults, of about 8–11 years.[33] So, it was also evident by the mid- and late-1980s that the first thousands of AIDS cases represented only the proverbial tip of an iceberg.

Estimating the Impact of AIDS

There have been wildly different, correct and incorrect, assessments of the future shape of the "epidemic curve" such as: AIDS would follow the trajectory of other epidemics and wane of its own accord; AIDS was controlled with zidovudine (AZT) therapy, that was markedly reducing the epidemic; or, AIDS cases would continue to increase, unabated, even at an exponential rate. As AIDS case reports reflect HIV infections acquired many years before, attempting to understand the current true HIV prevalence (the percentage of population with HIV), and, harder, trying to extrapolate into the future from infections acquired long ago have been fraught with problems.

A watershed meeting of major health and infectious disease leaders was held in June 1986 in Berkeley Springs, West Virginia. Named after the conference center where it was held, the Coolfont Conference represented a so-called Delphi method of estimating AIDS in the United States. The assembled epidemiologists, clinicians, policymakers, basic research scientists and other experts were asked to estimate the dimensions of the AIDS epidemic in the mid-1980s. The resulting estimate "by extrapolating all available data" was that there were at that time 1.0–1.5 million Americans "with HTLV-III/LAV infection."[34] The Coolfont estimates would inform basic policy and prevention debates in the United States for the next decade and more. The lower bound of this estimate–about 1 million HIV-infected U.S. residents– was actually reasonably accurate, especially considering that the absence of good data or parameters to estimate numbers of active gay men or injection drug users in the country.

A seminal article by Jim Curran and others at CDC[35] built on the Coolfont Conference report and extrapolated the near future of the AIDS epidemic. The basic epidemiology–spread by sexual contact, or, less frequently, blood-to-blood contact through sharing needles, transfusion, or birth to an HIV-infected mother–was well understood by 1988. "Black and Hispanic adults and children have reported rates 3 to 12 times as high as whites."[35]

Of course, there were skeptics. Based on respondents who said they knew someone with AIDS in their General Social Survey, Ed Laumann and colleagues at the University of Chicago argued in a 1989 *Science* article that "data provided by the Centers for Disease Control may underestimate by a substantial margin the prevalence of AIDS in the white population of higher socioeconomic status" and in those in the Midwest.[36] This conclusion was based on very few respondents ($N=133$), and did not consider factors such that gay men in substantial numbers moved from the Midwest to the Coasts. The deductions based on such scant data were clearly wrong, even by the late 1980s, and especially so as the HIV/AIDS epidemic has increasingly been centered in indigent, minority populations over the last 20 years.[37] Even at the time, CDC officials acknowledged that while AIDS cases were undeniably being undercounted in the 1980s, based on the then-available data, such underestimates were, if anything, probably greater for women and minorities than for white men.[38, 39]

For CDC personnel, the most painful dissent from the Coolfont and CDC estimates was the public argument by Dennis Bregman and Alex Langmuir that AIDS cases would peak in late 1988 and would only include 200,000 cases.[40] Their application of Farr's Law of Epidemics–that AIDS cases would wane as susceptibles were infected and removed from the population at risk and would eventually decline to a continuing, low level of incidence (rate of infection)–was irritating for two reasons. First, it was clear by 1990 that "susceptibles" at risk of HIV infection such as sexually active and needle-sharing populations were large and unlikely to substantially decline in the subsequent few years. It was also clear to all other analysts of the epidemic that many, many more than 200,000 AIDS patients would eventually accrue in the United States.

The second problem was especially painful. Alex Langmuir was prominent in the pantheon of CDC "greats." The originator of the Epidemic Intelligence Service (EIS), mentor to successive waves of EIS Officers, intimately involved in CDC's practical approach to epidemic investigation and control, this intellectual giant was very difficult to gainsay. Imperious, condescending, sometimes truculent, "Alex" was greatly respected, admired, and feared. New EIS Officers presenting at the annual April EIS Conference at CDC in the 1970s and 1980s would quake as he rose: they knew that his insight would home in on whatever soft underbelly their study had. At least two visits by him to the then nascent "AIDS Activity"–by the late 1980s, still only a handful of active investigators–resulted in deadlock and polite disagreement.

In the end, publication of this clearly wrong analysis in the prominent journal *JAMA*[40] (compare the curves of Figure 1.1 and Figure 3.1) was demoralizing, even embarrassing, for CDC personnel. However, editorials accompanying the Bregman and Langmuir article questioned many aspects of their hypothesis, such as: the rationale for applying a bell-shaped curve to the AIDS epidemic; the reasons why AIDS cases had, if anything, been underestimated by Bregman and Langmuir; and the fact the AIDS epidemic in 1990 had not declined after 1988 but was still demonstrably increasing in many population groups.[41, 42]

Because of the vagaries of counting AIDS cases and extrapolating from them into the future, CDC convened a workshop in October 1989, dubbed "Projectfest '89."[43] This was mainly a convocation of statisticians, who were asked to model future AIDS from past AIDS incidence. Given the long incubation period, it was understood by all at the meeting that AIDS cases currently enumerated were a window into HIV infections acquired a decade before. Thus, any model projecting from past incidence would have to credibly include current AIDS cases and try to estimate, based on the long and variable incubation period, what was happening with

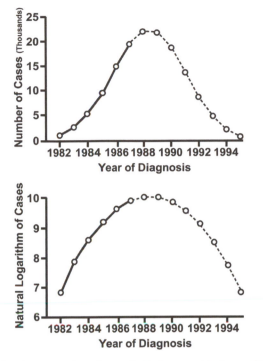

Figure 3.1 "Epidemic curves" as shown in Reference 40. Annual incidence (solid line) from 1982 to 1987 with projections to 1995 based on Farr's Law (dashed line). The upper panel was charted on an arithmetic scale, and the lower panel on a logarithmic scale (first approximations for both). "Epidemic curves," as postulated by Bregman and Langmuir, 1990, is reproduced by permission of *The Journal of the American Medical Association.*

HIV infections acquired presently. This was a very tall order, and all models would necessarily have very wide "confidence limits" when projecting into the future.

The dominant model or paradigm at the meeting was the so-called back-calculation procedure used by Ron Brookmeyer and colleagues at Johns Hopkins University.[44] As the name suggests, back-calculation requires taking current AIDS cases and, based on incubation periods, estimating when they would have occurred in the past and, from those past points, extrapolating incidence into the present and near future.[45] Critical to the back-calculation technique are good estimates of the incubation period distribution.[44, 46]

Brookmeyer and other statistical modelers–notably, John Karon of CDC and Mitch Gail of the National Cancer Institute–correctly predicted that HIV incidence was declining in the late 1980s and early 1990s, but that AIDS cases

acquired years ago—that can be used for the rational distribution of pre-vention, health and medical resources locally. By the early 1990s, scattered studies had looked at risk groups in certain cities and provided some help for health officials, but, by and large, everyone thought that there might be about one million HIV-infected persons, and considering ever-declining trends in AIDS yearly incidence, there was a general impression that HIV yearly incidence in the United States might have plateaued at about 40,000 new infections per year.

There are at least two approaches to estimating HIV (not AIDS) preva-lence and incidence. The mathematical modeling approach has dominated the intellectual landscape. In this approach, the most reliable datasets—say, reported AIDS cases—are back-calculated to estimate times of HIV infection, then projected into the future based on best-fitted curves. Given uncertain-ties, going back in time, then forward in time, creates ever larger confidence intervals—less surety—about the present situation.[53] Similarly, taking another database, such as known HIV infections in women testing for HIV before they give birth (CDC's Survey of Childbearing Women [SCBW]) provides a sparse dataset—that is, few infected women—from which to try to impute the larger picture of HIV infection in the community. Yet another database, the National Health and Nutrition Examination Survey (NHANES), randomly selects, interviews, and tests respondent households for health and disease. However, participation by contacted households is voluntary, and persons who fit the demographic profile of people most likely to be HIV-infected are also unlikely to give consent to interview and blood testing. Thus, it has been understood that this database unavoidably underestimates true HIV prevalence.[54]

To all these warts and inconsistencies in the databases must be added the problem of trying to estimate how these data relate to final estimates. For example, what can we reasonably deduce about all HIV infections in a given locality from, say, a few infections in African American women and one in a white woman from one of these databases?

> Perhaps most common among abuses, and not always easy to recog-nize, are situations where mathematical models are constructed with an excruciating abundance of detail in some aspects, whilst other impor-tant facets of the problem are misty or a vital parameter is uncertain to within, at best, an order of magnitude.[55]

Colleagues at CDC estimated the national prevalence of HIV from 1984 to 1992 by using exactly the three databases listed above—reported AIDS cases, infected women in the SCBW, and infected persons detected from NHANES.[56] While they did not make any assumptions that would be "an order of magnitude" off, they did not mention in their article that they were making national imputations from a database of about 7,000 HIV-infected women nationally in the SCBW and from many fewer HIV infections in the NHANES.[56] Thus, for the reader of the article, the logic and assumptions described were reasonable, but the actual imputations were "misty." In any case, these CDC colleagues estimated that there were between 650,000 and 900,000 HIV-infected persons in the United States in 1992.

This broad estimate of U.S. HIV prevalence has been generally accepted as a good refinement of the original Coolfont estimate of 1 million infected Americans, and it has been helpful for federal and national agencies trying to estimate the national or "big picture" impact of HIV. But what was the incidence and prevalence of HIV in particular risk groups and in individual American cities? What was the health department in, for instance, Akron, Ohio, or Tampa, Florida, supposed to do?

From 1993 to 1995 I collected data to construct a more granular picture of HIV prevalence and its incidence (rate of new cases) in the three major risk groups—gay men, injection drug users, and heterosexuals at high risk (i.e., those with many partners in localities where HIV infection was frequent)—in the 96 biggest metropolitan statistical areas (MSAs) per the U.S. Census.[57]

My approach started with the attitude that more data is always better than less data. Almost all information points to an estimate that "fits" the various datasets. I thought that decent estimates might be derived from integrating the data from several sources of information and that this would yield more useful information for city, local, and state planning than more sophisticated statistical manipulations of a single or even a few datasets to arrive at a general national picture.

Accordingly, I talked with over 200 local health officials and sifted through hundreds of documents and articles and several large datasets. I used not only the results of specific epidemiologic studies in each city but also data from: AIDS case reports from each MSA; U.S. Census data (e.g., numbers of never-married men as an index of gay male population in the MSA); rates of HIV prevalence in the risk groups as they presented to sexually transmitted disease clinics,[58] substance abuse treatment centers, and HIV counseling and testing sites in the MSAs; etc. Prevalence and incidence rates were adjusted based on insights and impressions from local health officials and documented rates of associated behaviors such as "crack" cocaine smoking, rates of reported syphilis, drug-related visits to emergency rooms, or, even, where appropriate, the numbers of gay bars in a city. The estimated numbers of gay men, injection drug users, and heterosexuals at risk, and the HIV prevalence and incidence in them, were estimated for each of the 96 MSAs.

Adding them up in this "components model" indicated that there were about 700,000 HIV infections and about 41,000 new HIV infections each year in the United States as of 1996.[57] Studies and AIDS reports in the succeeding years have confirmed these estimates about national prevalence (about 700,000, increasing in the last 10 years as more survive on better therapy) and incidence (about 40,000 per year, unchanged in a decade [Figure 3.2]), and, as there were specific estimates for the 96 largest MSAs and the risk populations in them, there were hundreds of requests for these estimates from state, county, and city health departments for purposes of their health planning and prevention.

Objective analysis of actual AIDS cases 10 years later—again, as they reflect HIV incidence 8–11 years before, when I was making my estimates—indicates that most estimates were reliable and confirmed by later trends in HIV and AIDS cases. However, the notable exception was that I think I overestimated the number of injection drug users in Northeastern cities and Puerto Rico and HIV infection rates in them. I inflated the numbers of injection drug users based on only a few indices of their known prevalence (per AIDS cases, emergency room reports of overdoses, etc.) and received high estimates of the numbers of injection drug users in their localities from health departments and substance abuse treatment agencies. I also underestimated that many were now sniffing heroin rather than injecting it, or obtaining clean, nonshared needles for injection in many instances from needle or syringe exchange programs.[59] While my estimates accorded with those of Bob Hahn and CDC colleagues who also thought there were somewhat over 1.2 million injection drug users in the United States in the late 1980s,[60] in retrospect those estimates, too, must have been inflated. In both cases, overestimates of numbers of injection drug users in the United States, and of HIV prevalence and incidence in them, resulted from the very high rates indicated by the sparse data from a few studies available in the mid- and late-1980s A common source of error in HIV epidemiologic research, there was simply not enough accurate data at the time.

Idiopathic CD4-Lymphocytopenia (ICL), or the "AIDS, Not!" Syndrome

At the Eighth International Conference on AIDS in Amsterdam in July 1992, Jim Curran, CDC's HIV/AIDS Director, Tony Fauci, and other public health and medical notables were aggressively questioned why CDC was not investigating cases of lymphocytopenia (low white blood cell counts) or immunodeficiency absent HIV infection. Curran had taken the brunt of activist criticism for 10 years—much of this was ad hominem attacks in *The Village Voice*—especially in relation to problems about changing the AIDS definition (see above). At the Conference, Jeff Laurence of Cornell's Medical School reported five cases of immunodeficiency for which there was no HIV infection or other explanation, and he advocated aggressive investigation.[61, 62] It was also known that Sudhir Gupta of the University of California at Irvine had reported he had found intracisternal retrovirus-like particles in both a mother and daughter with immunodeficiency but without HIV infection.[63] (However, such particles were suspected of being nonviral or otherwise artifactual; in any case, they were not subsequently seen or corroborated by any other researcher.) Jim Curran followed, adding that the CDC knew of six other cases of unexplained low CD4+ cell counts in persons without HIV infection. At this point, members of the audience started to describe other examples of such HIV-test-negative immunodeficient persons, and some began to shout questions about CDC's failure to investigate the phenomenon. This time even the normally cautious *New York Times* trumpeted that "C.D.C. Is Embarrassed By Its Tardy Response to AIDS-like Illness."[64]

If CDC had inappropriately delayed investigating such cases, this error or failing was potentially very detrimental to public health. Was another HIV-like pathogen spreading through the population, causing immunodeficiency and death? How many patients had been evaluated for immunodeficiency, been found HIV-antibody-test "negative," and perhaps omitted from public health and medical concern? The cases reported were few, from all areas of the country, and not specific to any risk or particular demographic group. However, everyone agreed that concern was warranted.

Accordingly, the Epidemiology Branch of CDC's Division of HIV/AIDS was asked to evaluate this immediately upon our return from the International Conference in Amsterdam. Within a few weeks, several EIS Officers were dispatched to investigate all possible such cases across the country; updates were provided on a near-daily basis as data came in on the first such patients identified, interviewed, and investigated. Within a few months, a clearer picture of this odd syndrome was found to include a hodgepodge of different diagnoses, conditions, and nonconditions in persons of all ages and sexes, some of whom appeared to be completely normal.[65]

A series of reports in the February 11, 1993, issue of *The New England Journal of Medicine* essentially reassured those worried about a new epidemic. We (CDC) reported the results of epidemiologic and laboratory investigations of the 31 persons we identified with this condition, now called "idiopathic CD4+ lymphocytopenia (ICL, low white blood cell counts in the absence of any known cause)." The case definition adopted was persistent CD4+ cell counts less than 300 cells/mm^3 in the absence of HIV infection or other known cause (such as immunosuppressive drugs), and the cases who met this definition were rare and represented various clinical and immunologic states. As no household, blood, or sexual contacts of the ICL cases had themselves developed ICL, there was "no evidence of a new transmissible agent that causes lymphocytopenia."[65]

Other investigators, such as David Ho and his colleagues from the Aaron Diamond Research Center and Robert Duncan and his colleagues from Boston University and elsewhere, reported that their laboratory investigations were likewise "negative" for any virus or for a viral product (such as reverse transcriptase) indicative of a novel virus.[66, 67] Sten Vermund and his colleagues from NIH's Multicenter AIDS cohort (MACS) looked at 22,643 measurements of CD4+ cells performed in 2,713 HIV-seronegative (uninfected) men who have sex with men and could find no man who had counts persistently less than 300 CD4+ cells/mm^3 not explained by HIV infection or cancer chemotherapy.[68] Louis Aledort and others examined low CD4+ cell counts in 4,018 persons enrolled in the Transfusion Safety Study and saw no instances of AIDS-defining illness in 20 persons with known causes for immunosuppression (such as chemotherapy) or in 12 who did not have a known cause for low CD4+ cell counts and fulfilled the ICL case definition, but who were clinically and otherwise normal.[69]

These many investigations were summarized in an editorial in the same issue of *The New England Journal of Medicine* by Tony Fauci. ICL was extremely rare, heterogenous in its clinical manifestations, unlikely to be a new condition, and very unlikely to be caused by a transmissible agent:

> Public officials were accused of being "asleep at the wheel" as a new mystery virus was spreading throughout the world. Serious concern was expressed about the safety of the blood supply. Fortunately, the scientific investigations proceeded in an orderly fashion, and solid data were collected. This experience should underscore the fact that the best answers to important questions come from the scientific process . . . and not from a media frenzy.[70]

Almost 15 years later, only a few more instances of this "lump" designation have been reported.[71–74] It is intriguing that in the original[65] and later investigations many patients with low CD4+ cell counts had cryptococcal meningitis, and it has not been possible to determine whether low CD4+ cell counts precede this infection, or vice versa. In any case, the most recent reviews of ICL continue to describe very few cases and no evidence of a new infectious disease outbreak.[75, 76]

HIV Reporting

As AIDS cases represent the later manifestations of HIV infection, counting AIDS cases is really enumerating a subset of HIV infection. Name-based reporting of HIV cases would be preferable for a few reasons. HIV diagnoses precede AIDS diagnoses, so the former should give us a better idea of recent HIV incidence. As more HIV patients are treated well before they develop AIDS manifestations of HIV, HIV reporting would give policymakers and health providers better insight into health and other resources needed to treat the epidemic. Improved knowledge of HIV status and access to care and prevention services is important to decrease the number of new HIV infections among populations most affected.[77]

HIV reporting has been left to the discretion of the individual States.[78] Some, such as Arizona and Colorado, instituted name-based HIV reporting before 1990. This gave them a better knowledge of the true populations of HIV-infected persons in their state but even their "name-based" reporting was flawed. For example, many who presented for "confidential" testing in the 1980s gave their names as "Mickey Mouse" or "Ronald Reagan" (both popularly and frequently used), and it was difficult to mesh these "named" reports with the names of those who had AIDS. Many HIV and AIDS cases move or are otherwise lost to a state's record keeping. Thus, adjustments have to be made, as simply trying to add HIV plus AIDS case reports could give an inaccurate picture. Also, while 31 states had instituted name-based reporting by the mid 1990s, these did not include some states with a substantial number of HIV infections, such as California.

The two sides of the policy debate have been forced to cite relatively sparse data to support their arguments.[79] Accordingly, this particular controversy has been mainly political or policy-associated, and less a debate about a scientific issue. States who prefer "anonymous" (non-named-based) vs. "confidential" (name-based) HIV test result reporting argue that for many knowing that their name will now enter a state or federal database makes them more reluctant to get tested.[80, 81] This fear of being included in name-based registry may be greater in some localities and populations than others. However, there are some limited data to support the view that the 25–30 percent of HIV-infected Americans who avoid getting HIV tested and diagnosed are not mainly doing so because of fears about the reporting system.[82, 83] The effects of a tested person's fears about confidentiality, in this view, will have little effect on his or her getting tested.

Again, this has mainly been a policy rather than purely scientific dispute, and it appears that it will be resolved by de facto federal fiat rather than by scientific debate and resolution. As of this writing, the federal Health Resources and Services Administration (HRSA), that administers the Ryan White Care Act funding, plans to start allocating such monies based on total HIV cases rather than on reported AIDS cases alone. Among the reasons for the shift in targeted funding base is that some states (California and

New York) have had many AIDS patients who have now died, whereas other states, such as in the South, are experiencing increases in HIV infections that have not yet been enumerated in an AIDS reporting system but who need care and prevention services. In any case, the practical impact is that states and cities that need Ryan White Care funding will be required to collect the names or otherwise distinguish the identities of HIV as well as AIDS patients.

HIV reporting may help undergird rational and fair resource allocation, but it will still be only an indirect way of divining current HIV incidence. Most HIV tested and diagnosed persons will be discovered at some time well after actual HIV infection. Theoretically, factoring the rates at which a large group of HIV patients progress to AIDS—now complicated by retarded disease progression from highly active antiretroviral therapy (HAART)—one could try to model recent HIV incidence (say in the past 5 years). Still, such calculation would be very difficult and fraught with such wide estimates that it would probably lend only limited insight.

Obviously, the best way to determine current incidence is to actually measure it as it is occurring. From a public health viewpoint, finding recently infected patients—especially as they may be more likely to transmit to others at this time[84] (see also Chapter 4)—and notifying and testing recent partners may be an important, focused intervention. Thus, for the past few years, some projects and studies have evaluated the originally called "detuned assay" to detect how many HIV-antibody-tests reflect recent HIV infections.[85] The detuned assay relies on the fact that antibodies to HIV are increasingly produced in the first several weeks of infection. As per Figure 3.3, one uses a highly sensitive antibody test—that is, one that detects very low levels of such antibody—and couples it with a relatively insensitive test—one that only detects much higher levels of antibody later in HIV infection. Anyone whose serum "lights up" on the more sensitive but not the less sensitive assay is presumably recently infected—that is, within the "window period" of infection. This sensitive/less sensitive testing strategy could facilitate studies and treatment of early HIV infection; [85] and knowing the actual incidence (occurrence) of new HIV infections can help assess the impact of HIV prevention efforts.

Evaluations of the originally described detuned test indicated that it might be overly sensitive (reduced positive predictive value—many who were positive on the assay were, in fact, not undergoing acute HIV infection). Some patients who were not recently infected also had low levels of HIV antibody, such as, ironically, persons who were moribund or very late in HIV infection. Accordingly, there has been interest and effort to evaluate more specific sensitive/less sensitive tests in a variety of settings.[86-88]

Window Period by Various Methods

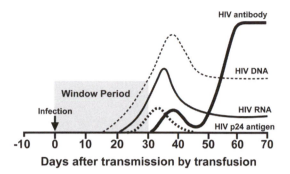

Figure 3.3 The HIV "window period" showing development and times to detection of HIV genetic material (DNA, RNA), p24 antigen, and HIV antibody following known infection date (for transfusion recipients). Note that early in infection HIV RNA and p24 antigen can be detected before antibody-test-positive status.

Both p24 antigen and HIV nucleic acids will be detectable in an infected person in the "window period" before development of detectable HIV antibody (see Figure 3.3). Based on these principles, p24 antigen testing in March 1996, then HIV nucleic-acid-amplification testing (NAT) in 1999, were introduced for screening of all donated blood in the United States. Another recent approach has been to measure actual HIV RNA—which is also low in untreated early infection but can be detected earlier than HIV antibodies—as a means of detecting how many tested-positive persons are recently infected.[89, 90] Pioneering work in this arena has been done by the North Carolina Department of Health, which demonstrated that plasma or serum could be pooled and tested for HIV RNA, speeding up detection of it when it relatively infrequently occurs in serologic specimens that are HIV-antibody negative.[91] Still, this test, too, would have the same problem as the sensitive/less sensitive assay—namely that people very late in infection may have low antibodies (because of immune suppression) and be antibody-test negative, yet have much detectable HIV RNA.

In summary, the area of HIV reporting and efforts to detect early HIV infection or incidence are still areas of rapid evolution and flux. Earlier HIV detection may inform our thinking about current HIV incidence, but will not likely give definitive answers. In the end, for the near future we will probably continue to have difficulty understanding the impact of education and prevention efforts on HIV incidence except in retrospect.

References

1. Mahorney, S.L., and J.O. Cavenar Jr. 1988. A new and timely delusion: The complaint of having AIDS. *American Journal of Psychiatry* 145:1130–1132.

2. Wortley, P.M., and P.L. Fleming. 1997. AIDS in women in the United States. Recent trends. *Journal of the American Medical Association* 278:911–916.

3. Fleming, P., R.H. Byers, P.A. Sweeney, et al. HIV prevalence in the United States, 2000. In *Program and Abstracts of the 9th Conference on Retroviruses and Opportunistic Infections* [abstract 11]. Seattle, WA: Foundation for Retrovirology and Human Health, 2002, p. 56.

4. Fleming, P.L., P.M. Wortley, J.M. Karon, K.M. DeCock, and R.S. Janssen. 2000. Tracking the HIV epidemic: Current issues, future challenges. *American Journal of Public Health* 90:1037–1041.

5. Porter, K., A.M. Johnson, A.N. Phillips, and J.H. Darbyshire. 1999. The practical significance of potential biases in estimates of the AIDS incubation period distribution in the UK register of HIV seroconverters. *AIDS* 13:1943–1951.

6. Muñoz, A., C.A. Sabin, and A.N. Phillips. 1997. The incubation period of AIDS. *AIDS* 11(suppl A):S69–S76.

7. CDC. 1982. Current trends update on Acquired Immune Deficiency Syndrome (AIDS)–United States. *Morbidity and Mortality Weekly Report* 31:507–508, 513–514.

8. CDC. 1982. Diffuse, undifferentiated non-Hodgkins lymphoma among homosexual males–United States. *Morbidity and Mortality Weekly Report* 31:277–279.

9. World Health Organization. Workshop on AIDS in Central Africa, Bangui, Central African Republic, October 22–25, 1985. Available at http://www.who.int/hiv/strategic/en/bangui1985report.pdf.

10. CDC. 1993. Revised classification system for HIV infection and expanded surveillance case definition for AIDS among adolescents and adults. *Morbidity and Mortality Weekly Report* 41(RR-17):1–17.

11. Mesce, D. October 2, 1990. Eighteen arrested for protesting lack of benefits for women AIDS victims. Associated Press.

12. Knox, R.A. December 11, 1991. Proposed definition of AIDS drawing fire. *The Boston Globe.*

13. Navarro, M. February 10, 1992. Agencies slowed in effort to widen definitions of AIDS. *The New York Times.*

14. White, M.H. 1996. Is vulvovaginal candidiasis an AIDS-related illness? *Clinical Infectious Diseases* 22(suppl 2):S124–S127.

15. Schuman, P., J.D. Sobel, S.E. Ohmit, et al. 1998. Mucosal candidal colonization and candidiasis in women with or at risk for human immunodeficiency virus infection. HIV Epidemiology Research Study (HERS) Group. *Clinical Infectious Diseases* 27:1161–1167.

16. Sobel, J.D. 2002. Vulvovaginal candidiasis: A comparison of HIV-positive and -negative women. *International Journal of STDs and AIDS* 13:358–362.

17. Palefsky, J.M. 1991. Human papillomavirus-associated anogenital neoplasia and other solid tumors in human immunodeficiency virus-infected individuals. *Current Opinions in Oncology* 3:881–885.

18. Schäfer, A., W. Friedman, M. Mielke, B. Schwartländer, and M.A. Koch. 1991. The increased frequency of cervical dysplasia-neoplasia in women infected with

the human immunodeficiency virus is related to the degrees of immunosuppression. *American Journal of Obstetrics and Gynecology* 164:593–599.

19. Palefsky, J.M., H. Minkoff, L.A. Kalish, et al. 1999. Cervicovaginal human papillomavirus infection in human immunodeficiency virus-1 (HIV)-positive and high-risk HIV-negative women. *Journal of the National Cancer Institute* 91:226–236.

20. Rabkin, C.S., and F. Yellin. 1994. Cancer incidence in a population with a high prevalence of infection with human immunodeficiency virus type 1. *Journal of the National Cancer Institute* 86:1711–1716.

21. Tirelli, U., E. Vaccher, V. Zagonel, et al. 1988. Malignant tumors other than lymphoma and Kaposi's sarcoma in association with HIV infection. *Cancer Detection and Prevention* 12:267–272.

22. Vermund, S.H., K.F. Kelley, K.S. Klein, et al. 1991. High risk of human papillomavirus infection and cervical squamous intraepithelial lesions among women with symptomatic human immunodeficiency virus infection. *American Journal of Obstetrics and Gynecology* 165:392–400.

23. Maiman, M., R.G. Fruchter, E. Serur, J.C. Remy, G. Feuer, and J. Boyce. 1990. Human immunodeficiency virus and cervical neoplasia. *Gynecologic Oncology* 38:377–382.

24. Cu-Uvin, S., J.W. Hogan, D. Warren, et al. 1999. Prevalence of lower genital tract infections among human immunodeficiency virus (HIV)-seropositive and high-risk HIV-seronegative women. HIV Epidemiology Research Study Group (HERS). *Clinical Infectious Diseases* 29:1145–1150.

25. Jamieson, D.J., A. Duerr, R. Burk, et al. 2002. Characterization of genital human papillomavirus infection in women who have or who are at risk of having HIV infection. *American Journal of Obstetrics and Gynecology* 186:21–27.

26. Massad, L.S., K.A. Riester, K.M. Anastos, et al. 1999. Prevalence and predictors of squamous cell abnormalities in Papanicolaou smears from women infected with HIV-1. Women's Interagency HIV Study Group. *Journal of Acquired Immune Deficiency Syndromes* 21:33–41.

27. Massad, L.S., L. Ahdieh, L. Benning, et al. 2001. Evolution of cervical abnormalities among women with HIV-1: evidence from surveillance cytology in the Women's Interagency HIV study. *Journal of Acquired Immune Deficiency Syndromes* 27:432–442.

28. Phelps, R.M., D.K. Smith, C.M. Heilig, et al. 2001. Cancer incidence in women with or at risk for HIV. *International Journal of Cancer* 94:753–757.

29. Hader, S.L., D.K. Smith, J.S. Moore, and S.D. Holmberg. 2001. HIV infection in women in the United States: Status at the Millenium. *Journal of the American Medical Association* 285:1186–1192.

30. Jaffe, H.W., W.W. Darrow, D.F. Echenberg, et al. 1985. The acquired immunodeficiency syndrome in a cohort of homosexual men. A six-year follow-up study. *Annals of Internal Medicine* 103:210–214.

31. Lui, K.J., D.N. Lawrence, W.M. Morgan, T.A. Peterman, H.W. Haverkos, and D.J. Bregman. 1986. A model-based approach for estimating the mean incubation period of transfusion-associated acquired immunodeficiency syndrome. *Proceedings of the National Academy of Sciences USA* 83:3051–3055.

32. Lui, K.J., T.A. Peterman, D.N. Lawrence, and J.R. Allen. 1988. A model-based approach to characterize the incubation period of paediatric transfusion-associated acquired immunodeficiency syndrome. *Statistics in Medicine* 7:395–401.

33. Alcabes, P., A. Muñoz, D. Vlahov, and G.H. Friedland. 1993. Incubation period of human immunodeficiency virus. *Epidemiologic Reviews* 15:303–318.

34. U.S. Public Health Service. 1986. Coolfont Report: A PHS plan for prevention and control of AIDS and the AIDS virus. *Public Health Reports* 101:341–347.

35. Curran, J.W., H.W. Jaffe, A.M. Hardy, W.M. Morgan, R.M. Selik, and T.J. Dondero. 1988. Epidemiology of HIV infection and AIDS in the United States. *Science* 239:610–616.

36. Laumann, E.O., J.H. Gagnon, S. Michaels, R.T. Michael, and J.S. Coleman. 1989. Monitoring the AIDS epidemic in the United States: A network approach. *Science* 244:1186–1189.

37. Durant, T., K. McDavid, X. Hu, et al. 2007. Racial/ethnic disparities in diagnoses of HIV/AIDS–33 States, 2001–2005. *Morbidity and Mortality Weekly Report* 56:189–193.

38. Berkelman, R., J. Curran, W. Darrow, T. Dondero, and M. Morgan. 1989. Monitoring the U.S. AIDS epidemic [letter]. *Science* 245:908.

39. Stoneburner, R.L., D.C. Des Jarlais, D. Benezra, et al. 1988. A larger spectrum of severe HIV-1-related disease in intravenous drug users in New York City. *Science* 242:916–919.

40. Bregman, D.J., and A.D. Langmuir. 1990. Farr's Law applied to AIDS projections. *Journal of the American Medical Association* 263:1522–1525.

41. Gail, M.H., and R. Brookmeyer. 1990. Projecting the incidence of AIDS [editorial]. *Journal of the American Medical Association* 263:1538–1539.

42. Morgan, M., J.W. Curran, R.L. Berkelman. 1990. The future course of AIDS in the United States [editorial]. *Journal of the American Medical Association* 263:1539–40.

43. Karon, J.M., and T.J. Dondero Jr. 1990. HIV prevalence estimates and AIDS case projection for the United States: Report based upon a workshop. *Morbidity and Mortality Weekly Report* 39(RR-16):1–18.

44. Brookmeyer, R., and A. Damiano. 1989. Statistical methods for short-term projections of AIDS incidence. *Statistics in Medicine* 8:23–34.

45. Brookmeyer, R. 1991. Reconstruction and future trends of the AIDS epidemic in the United States. *Science* 253:37–42.

46. Brookmeyer, R. 1989. More on the relation between AIDS cases and HIV prevalence [letter]. *New England Journal of Medicine* 321:1547–1548.

47. Andrews, E.B., T. Creagh-Kirk, K. Pattishall, and H.H. Tilson. 1990. Number of patients treated with zidovudine in the limited distribution system, March–September, 1987 [letter]. *Journal of Acquired Immune Deficiency Syndromes* 3:460.

48. Holmberg, S.D., L.J. Conley, S.P. Buchbinder, et al. 1993. Use of therapeutic and prophylactic drugs for AIDS by cohorts of homosexual and bisexual men in three U.S. cities. *AIDS* 7:699–704.

49. Gail, M.H., P.S. Rosenberg, and J.J. Goedert. 1990b. Therapy may explain recent deficits in AIDS incidence. *Journal of Acquired Immune Deficiency Syndromes* 3:296–306.

50. Jaffe, H.W., P.M. Feorino, W.W. Darrow et al. 1985. Persistent infection with human T-lymphotropic virus type III/lymphadenopathy-associated virus in apparently healthy homosexual men. *Annals of Internal Medicine* 102:627–628.

51. Byers Jr., R.H., W.M. Morgan, W.W. Darrow, et al. 1988. Estimating AIDS infection rates in the San Francisco cohort. *AIDS* 2:207–210.

52. Schneider, E., M.K. Glynn, T. Kajese, and M.T. McKenna. 2006. Epidemiology of HIV/AIDS–United States, 1981–2005. *Morbidity and Mortality Weekly Report* 55:689–692.

53. Gigli, A., and A. Verdecchia. 2000. Uncertainty of AIDS incubation time and its effects on back-calculation estimates. *Statistics in Medicine* 19:175–189.

54. McQuillan, G.M., D. Kruszon-Moran, B.J. Kottiri, et al. 2006. Prevalence of HIV in the US household population: The National Health and Nutrition Examination Surveys, 1988–1992. *Journal of the Acquired Immune Deficiency Syndromes* 41:651–656.

55. May, R.M. 2004. Uses and abuses of mathematics in biology. *Science* 303:790–793.

56. Karon, J.M., P.S. Rosenberg, G. McQuillan, M. Khare, M. Gwinn, and L.R.. Petersen. 1996. Prevalence of HIV infection in the United States, 1984 to 1992. *Journal of the American Medical Association* 276:126–131.

57. Holmberg, S.D. 1996. The estimated prevalence and incidence of HIV in 96 large US metropolitan areas. *American Journal of Public Health* 86:642–654.

58. Weinstock, H.S., J. Sidhu, M. Gwinn, J. Karon, T.R. Petersen. 1995. Trends in HIV seroprevalence among persons attending sexually transmitted disease clinics in the United States, 1988–1992. *Journal of Acquired Immune Deficiency Syndromes* 9:514–522.

59. Friedman, S.R., S. Lieb, B. Tempalski, et al. 2005. HIV among injection drug users in large US metropolitan areas, 1998. *Journal of Urban Health* 2005; 82:434–435.

60. Hahn, R.A., I.M. Onorato, T.S. Jones, and J. Dougherty. 1989. Prevalence of HIV infection among intravenous drug users in the United States. *Journal of the American Medical Association* 261:2677–2684.

61. Laurence, J., F.P. Siegal, E. Schattner, I.H. Gelman, and S. Morse. 1992. Acquired immunodeficiency without evidence of infection with human immunodeficiency virus types 1 and 2. *Lancet* 340:273–274.

62. Laurence, J. 1993. T-cell subsets in health, infectious disease, and idiopathic CD4+ T lymphocytopenia. *Annals of Internal Medicine* 120:168–169.

63. Gupta, S., C.E. Ribak, S. Gollapudi, C.H. Kim, and S.Z. Salahuddin. 1992. Detection of a human intracisternal retroviral particle associated with CD4+ cell deficiency. *Proceedings of the National Academy of Science USA* 89:7831–7835.

64. Altman, L.K. July 28, 1992. C.D.C. is embarrassed by its tardy response to AIDS-like illness. *The New York Times* B6.

65. Smith, D.K., J.J. Neal, S.D. Holmberg, and the Centers for Disease Control Idiopathic CD4+ T-lymphocytopenia Task Force. 1993. Unexplained opportunistic infections and CD4+ T-lymphocytopenia without HIV infection. An investigation of cases in the United States. *New England Journal of Medicine* 328:373–379.

66. Ho, D.D., Y. Cao, T. Zhu, et al. 1993. Idiopathic CD4+ T-lymphocytopenia–Immunodeficiency without evidence of HIV infection. *New England Journal of Medicine* 328:380–385.

67. Duncan, R.W., C.F. von Reyn, G.M. Alliegro, Z. Toossi, A.M. Sugar, and S.M. Levitz. 1993. Idiopathic CD4+ T-lymphocytopenia–Four patients with opportunistic infections and no evidence of HIV infection. *New England Journal of Medicine* 328:393–398.

68. Vermund, S.H., D.R. Hoover, and K. Chen. 1993. CD4+ counts in seronegative homosexual men [correspondence]. *New England Journal of Medicine* 328:442.

69. Aledort, L.M., E.A. Operskalski, S.L. Dietrich, et al. 1993. Low CD4+ counts in a study of transfusion safety [correspondence]. *New England Journal of Medicine* 328:441–442.

70. Fauci, A.S. 1993. CD4+ T-lymphocytopenia without HIV infection–No lights, no camera, just facts [editorial]. *New England Journal of Medicine* 328:429–431.

71. Ramirez, J.A., L. Srinath, S. Ahkee, A.K. Huang, and M.J. Raff. 1994. HIV-negative "AIDS" in Kentucky: A case of idiopathic CD4+ lymphocytopenia and cryptococcal meningitis. *Southern Medical Journal* 87:751–752.

72. Matsuyama, W., T. Tsurukawa, F. Iwami, et al. 1998. Two cases of idiopathic CD4+ T-lymphocytopenia in elderly patients. *Internal Medicine* 37:891–895.

73. Lepur, D., Z. Vranjican, B. Barsic, J. Himbele, and I. Klinar. 2005. Idiopathic CD4+ T-lymphocytopenia–Two unusual patients with cryptococcal meningitis. *Journal of Infection* 51:E15–E18.

74. López-Medrano, F., J.M. Aguado, J. Ruiz-Contreras, et al. 2007. Idiopathic CD4+ T lymphocytopenia disclosed after the diagnosis of visceral leishmaniasis [letter]. *Clinical Infectious Diseases* 44:1522–1523.

75. Wortley, P.M., and S.D. Holmberg. 1994. No evidence of blood-borne transmission of idiopathic CD4+ T-lymphocytopenia. *Transfusion* 34:556.

76. Walker, U.A., and K. Warnatz. Idiopathic CD4 lymphocytopenia [review]. 2006. *Current Opinion in Rheumatology* 18:389–395.

77. CDC. 2005. Trends in HIV/AIDS diagnoses–33 states, 2001–2004. *Morbidity and Mortality Weekly Report* 54:1149–1153.

78. Anonymous. 1998. CDC calls name reporting a local issue. *AIDS Alert* 13:15–16.

79. Colfax, G.N., and A.B. Bindman. 1998. Health benefits and risks of reporting HIV-infected individuals by name. *American Journal of Public Health* 88:876–879.

80. Dolbear, G.L., and L.T. Newell. 2002. Consent for prenatal testing: A preliminary examination of the effects of named HIV reporting and mandatory partner notification. *Journal of Public Health Management Practice* 8:69–72.

81. Charlebois, E.D., A. Maiorana, M. McLaughlin, et al. 2005. Potential deterrent effect of name-based HIV infection surveillance. *Journal of Acquired Immune Deficiency Syndromes* 39:219–227.

82. Osmond, D.H., A.B. Bindman, K. Vranizan, et al. 1999. Name-based surveillance and public health interventions for persons with HIV infection. *Annals of Internal Medicine* 131:775–779.

83. Schwarz, S., J. Stockman, V. Delgad, and S. Sheer. 2004. Does name-based HIV reporting deter high-risk persons from HIV testing? Results from San Francisco. *Journal of the Acquired Immune Deficiency Syndromes* 35:93–96.

84. Pilcher, C.D., H.C. Tien, J.J. Eron Jr., et al. 2004. Brief but efficient: Acute HIV infection and the sexual transmission of HIV. *Journal of Infectious Diseases* 189:1785–1792.

85. Janssen, R.S., G.A. Satten, S.L. Stramer, et al. 1998. New testing strategy to detect early HIV-1 infection for use in incidence estimates and for clinical and prevention purposes. *Journal of the American Medical Association* 280:42–48.

86. Parekh, B.S., D.J. Hu, S. Vanichseni, et al. 2001. Evaluation of a sensitive/less-sensitive testing algorithm using the 3A11-LS assay for detecting recent HIV seroconversion among individuals with HIV-1 subtype B or E infection in Thailand. *AIDS Research and Human Retroviruses* 20:453–458.

87. Kothe, D., R.H. Byers, S.P. Caudill, et al. 2003. Performance characteristics of a new less sensitive HIV-1 enzyme immunoassay for use in estimating HIV seroincidence. *Journal of the Acquired Immune Deficiency Syndromes* 33:625–634.

88. Taylor, M.M., K. Hawkins, A. Gonzalez, et al. 2005. Use of the serologic testing algorithm for recent HIV seroconversion (STARHS) to identify recently acquired HIV infections in men with early syphilis in Los Angeles County. *Journal of the Acquired Immune Deficiency Syndromes* 38:505–508.

89. Fiebig, E.W., D.J. Wright, B.D. Rawal, et al. 2003. Dynamics of HIV viremia and antibody seroconversion in plasma donors: Implications for diagnosis and staging of primary HIV infection. *AIDS* 17:1871–1879.

90. Patel, P., J.D. Klausner, O.M. Bacon, et al. 2006. Detection of acute HIV infections in high-risk patients in California. *Journal of Acquired Immune Deficiency Syndromes* 42:75–79.

91. Pilcher, C.D., S.A. Fiscus, T.Q. Nguyen, et al. 2005. Detection of acute infections during HIV testing in North Carolina. *New England Journal of Medicine* 352:1873–1883.

CHAPTER FOUR

Epidemiologic Controversies

The basic epidemiology of HIV infections has been understood almost since the beginning, in that transmission of the infectious agent of AIDS mainly occurs by: sexual contact (homosexual or heterosexual); or blood-to-blood contact, usually by needles shared between injection drug abusers. Today, in the United States, other modes of transmission are much less frequent, such as: by blood or blood-product transfusion, which mainly occurred before screening of the blood supply after March 1985 with progressively better HIV enzyme immunoassays (EIAs); from mother to infant during or near the time of birth, especially before screening and antimicrobial prophylaxis (pretreatment) of parturient women was widely practiced; or, very rarely, from needlestick accidents in the clinical care or laboratory setting.

Despite the overwhelming agreement on the basic epidemiologic "W's"—
who was getting infected, *what* was infecting them, and *why* they were getting infected—false reports, misconceptions, and slow comprehension have sometimes distracted both the scientific and public communities. Several topics and questions have led at times to great public and scientific anxiety and confusion, although almost all of the controversial initial reports or concerns have eventually been discredited, and initial skepticisms about the basic epidemiology of HIV have now long since been addressed.

For example, Michael Fumento's 1989 book provocatively titled *The Myth of Heterosexual AIDS* argued essentially that heterosexually transmitted AIDS cases were few and mainly limited to African Americans and sex partners of injecting drug users.[1] His thesis was that the potential threat to mainstream Americans had been oversold by the media and public policy officials and had distracted and panicked too many Americans. This argument, while true to some extent, was subtly demeaning as it was clear that HIV was spreading rapidly and by heterosexual contact through minority communities, but was not a concern for white citizens. In any case, the contention that concern about the heterosexual epidemic was overblown was never seriously entertained by public health and other scientists who were and remain truly worried about the continuing increase in heterosexually transmitted HIV.

Their fears have been unfortunately vindicated, as heterosexuals are the one transmission risk group in which HIV and AIDS have shown an inexorable increase over the past 20 years (see Figure 3.1); they are being recorded ever more frequently than cases in injection drug use and now rival cases in men who have sex with men as a transmission risk group. Many such AIDS and HIV cases are being reported in the rural and small-city South, which is the one area of the country that continues to show increases in AIDS and HIV cases. The rising incidence in the South and in heterosexual men and women reflect the current epidemiology of AIDS in America.[2] If persons not at real risk were unduly panicked about the heterosexual epidemic in 1989, they are conversely now unduly sanguine about the epidemic in the South. Despite efforts to highlight this problem,[3, 4] it has been difficult to get public or major scientific journal attention to and action against this distressing trend. "We maintain that for a region of the country with the highest absolute numbers of HIV-infected individuals and the largest proportionate increases, research and attention has been relatively scant."[5]

Another public but not exactly scientific controversy has been the recent attention to African American men who are on the "down low," meaning bisexual men, especially African American men who do not disclose their homosexual activities to their female partners. The *New York Times* article in 2003 by Benoit Denizet-Lewis raised the issue that such men,[6] closeted by their community's attitudes toward gay men, served as an important bridge for infecting their female partners. Not to diminish the importance of this observation, still, bisexual men of all races have generally not disclosed their homosexual behaviors to their heterosexual partners since the beginning of the AIDS epidemic.[7-10] The public perception that bisexual men are responsible for many or most HIV infections in black women may distract from the much greater likelihood that these women will acquire HIV infection from heterosexual male partners who have acquired their infections from heterosexual women or from intravenous drug use.[11, 12]

These and other controversies that have roiled the media or the general public have been quite different from those that have interested the HIV/AIDS scientific, epidemiologic and public health communities.

Issues in Sexual Transmission

Almost all HIV infections have been acquired through sexual contact, whether by homosexual contact in the United States and other developed nations or by heterosexual contact in the rest of the world. A few sometimes counterintuitive points have been clear since early in the epidemic. For example, the per-contact risk (without condom use) of heterosexual transmission from an HIV-infected man to a susceptible HIV-uninfected woman has been very low, despite the fact that the result of heterosexual transmission has been worldwide endemicity of HIV infection. We found early that only 15–20 percent of the wives of HIV-infected men were themselves HIV-infected despite that these were sexually active couples.[13] Assuming (a low estimate of) an average of 100 vaginal sex acts between them, we calculated that the (binomial) probability of HIV transmission during a single sex act between an HIV-infected man to a woman is less than 0.3 percent,[13] a population-based estimate that has generally been confirmed in several later studies,[14–17] though rates of male-to-female transmission may be substantially higher in sub-Saharan Africa than in the United States and Europe.[18]

But are all sexual contacts the same? Clearly not, as transmission is not solely a function of the number of sex contacts in a given couple: some transmissions occur with a single sex contact; others may not occur despite repeated, even hundreds of, contacts.[13, 19] Further, studies indicate that it is the number of different sex partners, not the number of actual sex acts between a given couple, that is a greater determinant of risk of infection.[20–22] So it seems that some people are better at spreading the virus than others. Or, is it the timing of the exposure relative to the time of the (index) infectious person's infection?

Incident infection of susceptible female partners may decline over time despite repeated exposure to their HIV-infected male partner.[23] Are some men, or women, "super-spreaders",[18] such as Gaëtan Dugas, the notorious "Patient Zero" in the first cluster of HIV infections investigated?[24] Or, does infectiousness of the HIV-infected partner fluctuate with time?[25]

Highest viremia occurs early in infection, and transmission between couples seems more likely to occur early after the index partner is infected, when measured virus is high and CD4+ cell counts are low.[19, 20, 23, 25] These same conditions of high viremia and immunodeficiency occur very late in infection, but, putatively, at times the patient is quite ill and much less likely to be sexually active. Thus, many consider that it is the period right after HIV infection when infectiousness is highest, when the patient is asymptomatic and sexually active, that accounts for much or even most HIV transmission.[26, 27]

These deductions may be true, but the few cohort studies of sexually active "discordant" (one HIV-infected, the other not) couples show they changed their behavior markedly once enrolled in a cohort study, and counseled to only have sex protected by a condom.[22, 28] That is, long-term-cohort studies have seen few transmission events because people have much less unprotected sex once enrolled in such a study and, if they seroconvert, do so early, just before, at, or soon after study enrollment. (HIV-discordant partners must receive counseling to reduce the risk of HIV transmission between them.) Therefore, imputations from such studies with this bias of ascertainment might incorrectly suggest that transmissions occur early in the natural situation as well. In any case, from a public health viewpoint, an HIV patient is considered infectious at all periods of patient viremia, and HIV can be recovered from semen and genital secretions throughout infection.

What no longer seems to be controversial is that factors that thin or disrupt the mechanical barriers of the (recipient) sex organ predispose to passage or infection of HIV. For example, few now question that herpes simplex type 2 or syphilis—that leave shallow ulcers that would facilitate the passage of HIV—increase one's risk of acquiring HIV.[29–32] Early in the epidemic, this association was challenged by some Multicenter AIDS Cohort Study (MACS) investigators,[33] but their analysis had many problems[34] and swam against the great tide of data indicating that genital ulcerative disease indeed facilitates HIV sexual transmission.[35]

If one thinks about the three elements in transmission of HIV, per Table 4.1, it seems at present that the probability of transmission of any sex act between an infected and an uninfected person will be a function of many variables,[13] most of which arguably we still know little about.

Biologic factors that can lead to easier transmission and wider dissemination through a population have long been interests of many researchers, but identifying such factors, especially ones that are modifiable, has been very difficult and debated. The major obstacle in uncovering the biologic determinants of HIV sexual transmission has been that it has been easy to find HIV-infected persons, but it has been inordinately harder to identify (and get permission to test) the person who transmitted infection. Most sexually infected people in this country have had multiple partners, many or most of whom were of unknown HIV infection status. In countries where transmission is occurring between stable, identifiable partners (as in, for example, some traditional African couples), such transmissions are rarely uncovered close to the time that they actually occurred. Thus, critical biologic parameters, such as the levels or type of virus in the transmitter's blood or semen at the time of transmission, are not known. Likewise, as HIV continually evolves into a multitude of quasi-species during the course of infection, it is

Table 4.1 Putative and Possible Biologic Factors in the Sexual
Transmission of HIV

INFECTIOUS PERSON →	VIRUS INFECTIVITY →	SUSCEPTIBLE PERSON
Factors that may enhance transmission	**Factors that may enhance transmission**	**Factors that may enhance acquisition**
High HIV viremia (or low CD4+ cells)	Syncytia-forming virus	Thinning/abrasion of vagina, anus, prepuce Older age Lack of circumcision GUD, e.g., herpes, syphilis
Factors that may retard transmission	**Factors that may retard transmission**	**Factors that may retard acquisition**
Antiretroviral therapy	Antiretroviral drug resistance mutations in the virus	Postexposure antiretroviral drug prophylaxis HLA mismatching

Note: GUD, genital ulcerative disease; HLA, Human leukocyte antigen.

impossible to specify which viral quasi-species recovered from the man or woman was (were) actually transmitted.

If these questions seem academic, one need only think of the benefit for developing vaccines or even drugs for the most infective strains of HIV, or the value of public health steps that could identify and intervene close to the time a person is infected and presumably more infectious.

Thus, investigators have leapt at the very few times we have been allowed an insight into transmission at the time it is occurring. An investigation of a cluster of very young women infected by one man in upstate New York was hampered by our inability to collect blood for analysis from the perpetrator.[36] However, molecular epidemiology was able to indicate that these mainly adolescent girls were infected by the same virus and, so, presumably the same young man.[37]

A second investigation of a cluster of HIV infection in very young women aged 12–17 years–infected by two men in their 20s in rural Mississippi– yielded a unique insight into factors that may lead to HIV infection.[38] As replicating HIV "buds" from its host CD4+ cell, it picks up a many cell membrane proteins including human leukocyte antigens (HLAs). It is little appreciated that one fifth of HIV surface proteins are the alpha and beta chains of HLA DR.[39] In transplant medicine, these HLAs determine acceptance or rejection of surgically transplanted tissues or organs, that is, transplants must first be "HLA-matched" before successful transplantation. This suggested to us that virus membrane coated with HLA antigens may be "accepted" or "rejected," as it were, by a susceptible, uninfected person based on HLA-matching or mismatching. Indeed, in the clusters of HIV transmissions in which the HLA type of the infecting and infected/not infected partners were known, discordance at HLA DR B3, was associated with "protection" against getting infected.[40] Did those susceptible persons who did not get infected "reject" an HIV carrying a discordant HLA, as they would reject a similarly mismatched transplant?

To date, this intriguing epidemiologic "lead" has not been followed, probably because it is so difficult to find enough couples who have clearly transmitted HIV or not between them. However, Larry Arthur and his AIDS vaccine program at the National Cancer Institute have demonstrated that HIV-bearing HLA-DR is biologically active and important to pathogenicity and immunogenicity[41]; in fact, in the most widely used animal model for human HIV, macaques immunized with HLA-DR were protected from infection on challenge with simian immunodeficiency virus.[42, 43] Currently, this unit is exploring inactivation methods that might allow (whole inactivated) virus, with it full complement of surface protein antigens, to serve as an effective, immunogenic vaccine.[44]

It is difficult to describe the "next level" of risk of HIV transmission beyond biologic characteristics, as this really is an integration of the several biologic variables. For example, transmission by insertive oral sex, which may occur because semen has infected white blood cells and the recipient may have (as many do) "breaks" in the integrity of the oral or gingival mucosa.[45] Most AIDS scientists now think that such oral-sex transmission occasionally occurs. This was at one time somewhat "controversial" as the first reports of oral transmission[46–50]—meaning, insertive fellatio from an HIV-infected man to an uninfected man or woman, unprotected by condom use—were met with some open-minded skepticism. However, as so many anecdotes have accumulated of persons getting infected by receptive oral intercourse (again, unprotected by condom use), it has gradually been generally accepted that such transmission can occur. There are factors in the mouth that tend to inactivate HIV, and the normal (unbroken) oral mucosa is much less likely to be infected than the vagina or anus.[51] However, in unvoiced acceptance that such infection may nonetheless occur, this transmission is listed as the "reference" risk activity in CDC publications on reducing risk behaviors from 1993, per Table 4.2.[52]

Table 4.2 Estimated Per-Act Relative Risk
(RR) for a Person without HIV Infection
Acquiring Such Infection, Based on Type of
Sex Act and Condom Use

Risk factor	Relative risk
	Sex act
Insertive fellatio	1
Receptive fellatio	2
Insertive vaginal sex	10
Receptive vaginal sex	20
Insertive anal sex	13
Receptive anal sex	100
	Condom use
Yes	1
No	20

Source: From Table 5, Reference 52.

On the other end of the spectrum is the risk of transmission by condom-unprotected receptive anal intercourse, that involves a friable membrane easily disrupted, allowing the passage of HIV more easily. After much internal debate and discussion over several years, CDC finally weighed in as to its crude estimation of the risk of HIV infection with the several sex acts.

One way of viewing these relative risks is to consider certain types of sex acts as "overwhelming" any natural biologic defenses.

Blood and Blood Products

It is fair to say that the American blood banking community initially "didn't get it." In a well known case, [24] at an all day meeting on January 4, 1983, at CDC, prominent blood bankers from organizations responsible for almost all blood collection in the United States–Gerry Sandler and Paul Cumming from the American Red Cross, Joe Bove from the American Association of Blood Banks, and Jay Menitove of the Council of Community Blood Centers–were reluctant to credit the concerns of public health officials and infectious disease epidemiologists from CDC, FDA, and NIH. These latter, mainly government doctors, were concerned about five cases of AIDS in hemophilic men who had no risk factor other than receipt of blood products in the previous 2 years.[53] The meeting was held only a few months before the April 1983 description of HIV (termed lymphadenopathy-associated virus [LAV]) by Luc Montagnier and collaborators at Institute Pasteur.[54] However, by the end of 1982 most researchers were already convinced, based on network and other analyses, that the cause of AIDS must be an infectious agent spread sexually. Like other sexually transmitted diseases, such as syphilis or hepatitis B, there was also a distinct possibility that this then unknown agent could be spread by blood-to-blood contact, such as by transfusion.

At the meeting, the blood bankers had doubts regarding: the likelihood that AIDS was spread by a transmissible agent; the risk of AIDS from blood transfusion; and the best approach for adapting guidelines of blood donation and donor screening.[53]

It was suggested that blood donations could be screened for hepatitis B core (HBc) antibody, found in about 90 percent of serum specimens from the first definitive AIDS cases in CDC's Serum Bank. As it now known, actually fewer than 10 percent of all HIV/AIDS patients in the United States currently are HBV- as well as HIV-co-infected. In any case, this method of eliminating persons infectious for the unknown "AIDS agent" (as well as for hepatitis B) was rebuffed. Concerns from the blood bankers centered around the availability and the cost of such testing, which was not inconsiderable; the other was that some centers would need to discard up to 5 percent of blood donations that would test "positive" for anti-HBc antibody. Even a subsequent meeting at a closed session of FDA in February 1983–2 of the 12 panel members were blood bankers–likewise concluded that the then available evidence was not sufficient to support a conclusion that AIDS was blood transmitted. As Roger Dodd, current Vice President at the ARC Holland Laboratory–who was not actually part of the early CDC or FDA meetings– has indicated his estimation of the source of error:

> [T]he one thing that really led us all astray, however, was the extremely long incubation period for AIDS. This concealed the true size of the epidemic and generated a very unfamiliar situation. I remember being in the middle of it all, and I do think that most people were trying to do the right thing in terms of what they knew and believed. (Roger Dodd, personal communication, April 15, 2007).

It should be noted, that, as if in contradiction to their stated disbelief that there was a widespread national infection that could be spread by blood, as early as December 1982 plasma collection agencies were excluding potential donors from high risk groups for hepatitis or AIDS (such as gay men and injection drug users). Taking a precautionary stance, in January 1983, blood banking organizations also issued a joint statement recommending donor-screening questions to detect early symptoms of AIDS for all blood donors. A separate issue was the heat-treatment of coagulation factors used for treating hemophilic men (and a few women, almost all hemophilic persons are men). Heat had been shown to inactivate "serum hepatitis" (hepatitis B) in plasma derivatives by 1981, and by 1985 all coagulation products were heat inactivated.

This transition period between "AIDS denial" by the blood banking community and screening donors who had risk factors for AIDS was brief–that is immediately after the first descriptions of AIDS and suspicion that it might be blood-borne in 1982 and ending with documentation in 1983 of 64 AIDS cases whose only risk was receipt of blood or blood-product transfusion in the previous few years.[55] The end of the era of agonizing about which donors to exclude and which blood screening tests to use ended in March 1985. At that time a serum antibody test for HIV was first available and was immediately adopted to screen donated blood; this dramatically reduced risk from acquiring HIV from the blood supply (now estimated at about one infection in 2 million donated units[56]–see below).

However, the initial reluctance on the part of American blood banking organizations to adopt strategies or tests that would prevent transmission of HIV in blood and blood products had profound negative consequences. The first major political fall-out was the damage to the reputation of the American blood banking community. The reticence to screen potential donors for AIDS in the early 1980s particularly hit the American Association of Blood Banks (AABB), the largest blood banking organization in the United States, as this organization was successfully sued by a man who was infected with HIV by receipt of blood during open-heart surgery in 1984.[57, 58] Eventually, AABB was able to successfully appeal this decision, as most blood banks in 1984 did not screen for hepatitis B, and HIV antibody (ELISA or EIA) tests were not commercially available.[59] Still, the perception in the AIDS and general community was that the major blood banking organizations had been remiss in their grasping that the AIDS agent could be blood-borne and that practical steps should be taken immediately.

In the public mind, there was also perhaps some conflating of the American situation with the criminal behavior of government officials Drs. Michel Garretta and Jean-Pierre Allain in France's National Center for Blood Transfusions, who knowingly let HIV-test-positive blood units be distributed and who were ultimately convicted of a crime in the French legal system, "deception over the basic quality of a product."[60] (It was grimly ironic that this occurred in the same country where Luc Montagnier and others of Institut Pasteur had developed a prototype test to screen blood for antibodies to HIV as early as 1983.)

By the time antibody test screening added to donor deferral strategies had made the blood supply safe after 1985, tens of thousands of persons had become infected; specifically, about 80 percent of hemophilic men who had relied on clotting factors derived from thousands of donated blood units had become infected. Hemophilia activists strove, successfully, to challenge the blood bankers' assertions that what had happened had been an unavoidable and awful tragedy. According to a 1995 Institute of Medicine report,[61] the response to the possibility of HIV in the blood supply was unnecessarily tardy:

> Paternalistic assumptions about medical decision-making led to failures to adequately disclose the risk of continuing use of AHF [antihemophilic factor] concentrate and enable individuals to make informed decisions for themselves. [This led to] ancillary failures to warn possibly infected individuals of the risks they might pose to others through sexual contact.[61]

The second consequence to the blood banking communities' perceived tardiness in addressing AIDS can perhaps be considered a reaction to the reactive anger of the hemophilic[62] and the wider HIV/AIDS public community. While stressing that hindsight had been harsh in evaluating the blood banking organizations,[63, 64] following this controversy, all blood banking organizations nonetheless immediately adopted a "zero risk" strategy for any other potential pathogen.

At the present time, blood is not only screened for common endemic infections in the United States, such as HIV-1, hepatitis B and C viruses and syphilis, but also for extremely rare conditions in the United States such as: Chagas disease (*Trypanosoma cruzi*), a parasitic infection seen in Brazil;[65] human T-lymphotropic virus type 1 (HTLV-I), the causative agent of a rare leukemia (see Chapter 2); and HTLV-II, still not firmly associated with any specific human medical condition.[66] The recent investigation of West Nile virus in the blood supply[67-69] also serves as an illustration of the impact of criticism on the blood banking community to their initial delayed response to the AIDS epidemic. The brevity of the time between the recognition of transfusion-transmitted infection in 1999 and the development and full-scale implementation of a blood-screening test—by June 2003 all blood in the United States was being screened for WNV—bespeaks the seriousness with which all infectious disease outbreaks are now viewed by blood banking organizations.

In terms of HIV, EIAs that were initially used to screen blood for HIV-1 and HIV-2, although the latter is very rare in the United States,[70, 71] have been developed with increasing sensitivity. Still, there is a "window period" when a newly infected person may not yet screen "positive" by EIA and still donate blood (see Figure 3.3). Some HIV-infected individuals thus slip through normal screening. Accordingly, new tests for virus and viral products have been used to try to narrow this window period. Testing for HIV p24 antigen—detectable in the "window period" HIV antibody—adopted in March of 1996 was thereafter supplanted in 1999 by nucleic acid-amplification testing (NAT).

About 14 million units of blood are donated each year: these are processed into 20 million blood products that are given to about 3.6 million recipients. (Most blood—about 60 percent—is donated to patients who die of the underlying condition for which they received blood, such as trauma or surgery.) Because of NAT testing for HIV and for hepatitis C virus (HCV), current risks of these infections are thought to be one in 2 million transfused blood units.[72] As of 2004, only four transfusion-transmitted HIV infections had been identified since such screening was adopted in 1999.[68] It is not widely appreciated that inherent human error such as from transfusion of mismatched blood, with serious health results, currently poses a risk up to 100 times greater than from undetected HIV in donated blood.[73]

"Silent Sequences"

New laboratory techniques may be double-edged in their value: while many are ultimately very helpful, new techniques in the hands of inexperienced researchers may lead to spurious and alarming results. This seems to have been the case with the introduction of the polymerase chain reaction (PCR) tests for HIV. This test uses oligonucleotide primers (short lengths of DNA) to attach to HIV DNA (provirus), if viral DNA is there within the host's genome. The gene sequence flanked by the primers is then replicated in many, usually 30 "cycles"—that is, the flanked DNA is repeatedly "read"—by a specific polymerase such that the many copies of the HIV DNA sequence can then be detected by probes. Thus, this test for HIV, originally developed by Chin-Yi Ou and his colleagues,[74] is a very sensitive assay for the presence of HIV gene sequences and can be used to discover HIV infection before the production of HIV antibodies detectable by usual serum screening assays,[75] such as very early after HIV infection.

This was a big breakthrough as it made possible the detection of minute quantities of HIV DNA, and later RNA, in a person's blood. For example, infants born to HIV-infected mothers will passively acquire anti-HIV-antibodies and so will test "positive" on an immunoassay, even though they are not infected. Usually, it takes about 9 months, when the maternal antibodies have cleared, to determine if an infant is infected. However, with PCR for HIV DNA sequences, true HIV infection can be determined early in the roughly 20–30 percent of infants who will get HIV from their untreated mother or in the roughly 5 percent or less of infants of mothers receiving chemoprophylaxis (see Chapter 6, *Preventing Mother-to-Infant Spread* section).

PCR is certainly faster, easier, and perhaps even more reliable than laborious and time-consuming HIV viral culture techniques. However, PCR's exquisite sensitivity is such that minute quantities of DNA in the laboratory, even small amounts airborne, can contaminate a test specimen and lead to a "false positive" PCR result. This potential for contamination was not immediately appreciated when PCR testing was first introduced. In addition, handling of many field specimens leads inevitably to some errors of classification, labeling, and storage.

These sources of error were, in retrospect, important factors in major controversies about "immunosilent sequences" reported in the early 1990s—that is, persons who tested serologically (by antibody assay) "negative" but who purportedly had HIV gene sequences that could be "amplified" and detected by PCR. This was far from an academic debate, as many people who had tested "negative" on standard HIV antibody tests and their clinicians now had to worry that they nonetheless harbored HIV.

In 1988, Houmy Farzadegan and fellow MACS investigators reported that rare persons with HIV-1 "may not remain seropositive, but may remain latently infected with HIV-1."[76] This loss of antibodies—but not PCR-detectable HIV infection—was observed in four (0.4%) of 1,000 MACS cohort participants and was of grave concern to the safety of the blood supply.[77] Although it was known that seriously moribund patients late in HIV infection may lose antibodies,[78] this was the first report of HIV-infected persons with few or no symptoms who might be able to donate (infectious) blood. Following the Farzadegan article, we immediately looked at 660 persons who had 1,658 antibody tests done as participants in CDC cohort studies in San Francisco, Boston, and New York.[79] Indeed, we too initially found 16 possible "seroreverters" but our examination of records and retesting of serum specimens showed 19 errors—11 clerical and 8 due to early and insensitive immunoassay tests—that accounted for all 16 "seroreversions."

As PCR technology has become more standardized, mechanical, easier, and more widely done, no more cases of unexplained seroreversion have been reported. A later analysis of six potential "seroreverters" in the U.S. Army Data system revealed that five were the result of sample mix-up and one reflected a testing error.[80] To date, no further cases of seroreversion not attributable to specimen mix-up or nonspecific test reaction have been reported,[81] and this issue is now essentially quiescent.

A much greater scientific furor attended the 1989 report by David Imagawa and other researchers of the Los Angeles Multicenter AIDS Cohort Study (MACS) that by PCR they had detected HIV-1 from fully 31 men (23%) of 133 HIV-seronegative (antibody-test-negative) men, and that 27 of these men had remained HIV antibody-test seronegative up to 36 months.[82] This report was met with great consternation and many questions. An accompanying editorial in the same issue of *The New England Journal of Medicine* by the respected researcher William Haseltine of the Dana-Farber Cancer Institute in Boston seemed to accept the Imagawa report at face value; long-term "silent HIV infections," undetectable by usual screening tests, were considered a distinct pattern of HIV infection.[83] That is, he considered that some infected persons might go many, many months before generating enough HIV antibody to be detected by usual serologic tests. As the PCR technique was still new, not standardized, and still tricky to perform at the time, the call for "reliable, cost-effective methods for detecting silent infections" [83] was a distant dream. Certainly, it was not reassuring for the tens of thousands of Americans who had tested negative by HIV antibody tests, but up to one quarter of whom might nonetheless be infected if the report by Imagawa and his colleagues was true.

An immediate flurry of letters in a subsequent issue of *The New England Journal* focused not on developing new tests or expanding PCR use for all testing, but instead first verifying that "silent infections" were actually occurring. For example, Bob Horsburgh and his CDC coworkers performed similar PCR to detect HIV in 78 highly sexually active (more than 250 lifetime sex partners) gay men in San Francisco who had tested HIV-antibody-negative. Two PCR-positive seronegative men were "found" but clinical and other follow-up data indicated these were "false positive" results.[84] Similar attempts to detect HIV infection in 24 seronegative men by Li-Zhen Pan and others from the University of California similarly found no virus detected by PCR (or viral culture) in them: "We believe that either the antibody tests conducted by Imagawa et al. missed subjects who were already seropositive, or the subjects they studied came from a highly selected group generally not observed in other parts of the country."[85] Letters from blood bankers were similarly cautious,[86] and one was frankly skeptical of the Imagawa results "until further studies document the phenomenon."[87]

Indeed, no group of investigators was able to find persistently seronegative but HIV-infected men, whether: 59 sexually active homosexual men;[88] 27 homosexual and 12 hemophilic men;[75] 15 men and their 37 sexual contacts;[89] 36 men from the Pittsburgh arm of the MACS[90]; or from 945 injection drug users in a Johns Hopkins University study (ironically by some of the same researchers who reported "seroreversion").[91] Researchers in Geneva, Switzerland, were likewise unable to detect HIV provirus in 127 study-participants who tested HIV-antibody-assay negative except in two instances of persons in the process of seroconverting to antibody-test positivity. By 1992, it was clear that the results reported by Imagawa et al. were radically different from the findings of any other research team that looked for "silent sequences" in HIV-antibody-test-negative persons.

Accordingly, Imagawa's team re-investigated three men of the 27 with silent infection and found that HIV-1 DNA was detected by PCR in three of eight specimens from one man, in one of nine serial specimens from a second man, and from none of 14 specimens from a third man. No HIV-1 could be re-isolated from the frozen supernatants of the "positive" cultures from the original 31 men an average of 40 months later.[92] While Imagawa and Roger Detels of UCLA's School of Public Health concluded in their letter that these results were "more consistent with the hypothesis of incomplete infection than with latent, persistent infection," this was not the conclusion of most scientists. It seemed to almost all that the original results were more consistent with specimen mislabeling or contamination. Indeed, the national sigh of relief was almost audible, especially from the blood banking community who were worried about HIV transmission in blood products collected from "silently" infected HIV persons.

A Florida Dentist

One of the oddest controversies in the transmission of HIV revolved around an investigation of patients of a Florida dentist, David Acer, who died of AIDS in 1990 at age 40 years. Kimberly Bergalis, a 22-year-old college student who had no other risk for HIV infection, came forward a few months before Acer's death and insisted that she had been infected as his patient. The reaction in the public health, dental, and other communities was mixed. On one hand, if this young woman had been infected by an HIV-infected dentist who took usual precautions (mask, gloves) during routine tooth extraction yet nevertheless infected her, were our notions of the (low) transmissibility of HIV completely wrong? On the other hand, if she had been infected by unacknowledged, unknown, or unremembered exposure, yet had blamed the dentist, what would be the impact on dentists and, beyond them, any surgeon or physician? Either way, would many patients avoid an HIV-infected doctor or dentist as their clinician; conversely, would doctors and dentists shun HIV-infected patients?

The reaction of Jim Curran, then Director of the HIV/AIDS Division at CDC, was perspicacious: he saw this event as, at a minimum, a public health and public perception disaster. Hopes that this was a lone, aberrant case faded as investigation and testing of an additional 591 of Acer's patients revealed that at least three more were infected with HIV during their dental care.[93] Of greatest concern, DNA sequence analysis of all infected patients showed close genetic relatedness to that of the dentist, significantly different from "control" HIV specimens from other HIV patients in the same area.[93] Further work on another seven patients possibly infected at Dr. Acer's practice showed that five of them had viral strains phylogenetically very close to each other and to HIV from him, but distinctly different from 35 strains from persons in the local geographic area.[94] Accordingly, investigators from CDC and the Florida Department of Health and Rehabilitive Services (DHRS) concluded that there was strong "DNA fingerprint" evidence that these patients, most of whom were without other known risk factors for HIV, had very probably been infected during procedures at Dr. Acer's dental practice.[95]

Before his death in 1990, David Acer released a statement to his patients that, "I am a gentle man and I would never intentionally expose anyone to this disease."[96] The only person to talk with him before he died, the lead medical investigator from CDC, Carol Ciesielski, was also impressed by Acer's sincere shock that anyone would think he had purposely infected any of his patients. Yet, there was still the DNA evidence: was this murder, or a remarkable accident?[97]

An investigation of another general dentist in southeastern Florida found none of the five HIV-positive of his 900 tested patients had been HIV-infected with strains similar to his.[98] That is, in one infected dentist's practice (Acer's), five of 591 patients had been infected, whereas none of 900 patients in another dental practice had been; and no clear breaks in proper sanitary procedure were known in either practice. The probability, p, that this difference could occur by chance alone is, by chi square or Fishers' exact test, much less than 0.01. Thus, many considered that while we will probably never know what happened in Dr. Acer's practice, HIV transmissions occurred there, and quite probably—in fact, almost certainly—human intention or repeated human accident was responsible.[99]

However, this was not the attitude of the journalist, Stephen Barr who, in an opinion piece in *The New York Times*,[100] asked "What if the dentist didn't do it?" Nor was it the attitude in a widely broadcast CBS *60 Minutes* piece by Mike Wallace on June 19, 1994. As Harold Jaffe, then director of the joint CDC/Florida DHRS investigation, drily commented at the time of his retirement in 2004: "... you know you're going to have a bad day when Mike Wallace from *60 Minutes* is waiting to see you." It is worth recording Jaffe's comments more fully:

> Working with a story that had been developed by the attorneys hired to defend the dentist's insurance carriers, Mr. Wallace did his best to discredit the CDC investigation by using the twisted logic that because we didn't know how this happened, it must not have happened. He also

relied heavily on the laboratory work done on contract to the insurance companies by Lionel Resnick, a Florida dermatologist, who was also an amateur molecular biologist. Soon after the program was aired, Dr. Resnick was indicted for fraud related to charging NIH [National Institutes of Health] for laboratory work...He then conveniently left Miami for the Cayman Islands. When Carol Ciesielski wrote a letter to the producer of *60 Minutes* to point out that their prime expert was a wanted criminal, she received an answer saying it didn't matter. It also apparently didn't matter that a subsequent series of independent analyses of the CDC lab data confirmed our conclusions or that the insurance carriers all settled out of court rather than going to trial.

The attitude of many of us who credit the molecular biology of this case is that television and print journalists are no more likely to concede error than most scientists. Over a decade later, dentists still take reasonable precautions not to infect or be infected by HIV, hepatitis viruses, or other pathogens. While the cause of this transmission remains a mystery, no further tragic Acer-to-Bergalis-type transmission cases have been recorded.

However, the effects of this unusual case continue to be felt. A recent survey shows that 62 percent of respondents do not think that HIV-infected dentists should be allowed to provide care.[101]

"Safe" Insemination

There has not been much controversy related to the rare transmission of HIV from blood[56, 102] or tissues and organs[103–105] that are donated or collected in the brief "window period" before an HIV-infected person will test "positive" by HIV EIAs. EIAs have become progressively more sensitive but will never detect someone who has very recently–say, within several days–become infected. As indicated above, NAT testing since 1999 has now made such infective transfusions or transplantations virtually nil. Still, better testing or screening does not solve all problems.

An ongoing epidemiologic controversy relates to the attempts to process semen from HIV-infected men in such a manner that the result can be used to safely inseminate HIV-uninfected female partners. The desire to have children despite or because of HIV-infection of the male partner has led some couples to have intercourse unprotected by condoms in the effort to have children. Drug treatment has been known to reduce the amount of HIV in semen, [106] but does not eliminate the risk to the uninfected partner or, perhaps, the offspring as well. Thus, Italian researchers described a technique whereby semen was centrifuged through a gradient that putatively eliminated HIV adherent to human sperm, and then the sperm that "swim up" from the bottom of the gradient were inseminated in 29 women. Seventeen pregnancies resulted, 10 to term; none of the inseminated women or babies had HIV infection.[107]

Again, this result was exciting for "serodiscordant" couples–the man HIV-infected, the woman not–who wanted to safely conceive. For more statistically minded researchers, however, 17 uninfected pregnancies may not be convincing given, as above, the very low transmission rates from any single male–female vaginal sex act. In the United States a CDC EIS Officer, Brian Edlin, investigated an instance of a woman who actually got infected from "processed" semen.[108] The investigation showed that her partner's semen was only centrifuged (not through a gradient and not later harvested after sperm "swim-up" procedure), and so this unfortunate woman received semen that was apparently processed in a manner to concentrate rather than eliminate HIV. Thus, this tragic instance did not clarify the safety or efficacy of the procedure described by Semprini et al.[107] Consequently, CDC demurred from issuing an opinion on the safety of the technique.

Presently, several European and a few U.S. centers offer assistance to HIV seropositive men and their seronegative partners by performing either intrauterine insemination (IUI) or in vitro fertilization. Since 1987, more than 3,600 attempts have been reported in which processed spermatozoa from HIV-seropositive men have been used to establish pregnancy in HIV-uninfected women.[109] The most recent specific investigation of 741 couples who had IUI or IVF following semen processing–with subsequent HIV PCR testing of processed specimens–shows that no female partners acquired HIV infection, over 70 percent of whom successfully became pregnant.[110] Thus, sperm washing techniques may be relatively safe and effective in offering HIV-serodiscordant couples an opportunity to have children.

References

1. Fumento, M. 1989. *The Myth of Heterosexual AIDS.* New York: Basic Books, Inc.

2. Doherty, I.A., P.A. Leone, and S.O. Aral. 2007. Social determinants of HIV infection in the deep South [letter]. *American Journal of Public Health* 97:391.

3. Reif, S., K.L. Geonnotti, and K. Whetten. 2006. HIV infection and AIDS in the Deep South. *American Journal of Public Health* 96:970–973.

4. Beltrami, J.F., S.H. Vermund, H.J. Fawal, T.D. Moon, J.C. Von Bargen, and S.D. Holmberg. 1999. HIV/AIDS in nonurban Alabama: Risk activities and access to services among HIV-infected persons. *Southern Medical Journal* 92:677–683.

5. Reif, S., K.L. Geonnotti, K. Whetten, and B.W. Pence. 2007. Social determinants of HIV infection in the Deep South [letter]. *American Journal of Public Health* 97:391–392.

6. Denizet-Lewis, B. August 3, 2003. Double lives on the Down Low. *The New York Times.*

7. Soskolne, C.L. 1984. The acquired immunodeficiency syndrome and female sexual partners of bisexual men. *Annals of Internal Medicine* 100:312.

8. Padian, N., L. Marquis, D.P. Francis, et al. 1987. Male-to-female transmission of human immunodeficiency virus. *Journal of the American Medical Association* 258:788–790.

9. Landefeld, C.S., M.M. Chren, J. Shega, T. Speroff, and E. McGuire.1988. Students; sexual behavior, knowledge, and attitudes relating to the acquired immunodeficiency syndrome. *Journal of General Internal Medicine* 3:161–165.

10. Doll, L.S., J.S. Harrison, R.L. Frey, et al. 1994. Failure to disclose HIV risk among gay and bisexual men attending sexually transmitted disease clinics. *American Journal of Preventive Medicine* 10:125–129.

11. Millett, G., D. Malebranche, B. Mason, and P. Spikes. 2005. Focusing "down low": bisexual black men, HIV risk and heterosexual transmission. *Journal of the National Medical Association* 97(7 suppl):52S–59S.

12. Wolitski, R.J., K.T. Jones, J.L. Wasserman, and J.C. Smith. 2006. Self-identification as "down low" among men who have sex with men (MSM) from 12 US cities. *AIDS Behavior* 10:519–529.

13. Holmberg, S.D., C.R. Horsburgh Jr., J.W. Ward, and H.W. Jaffe. 1989. Biologic factors in the sexual transmission of human immunodeficiency virus. *Journal of Infectious Diseases* 160:118–125.

14. Mayer, K.H., and D.J. Anderson. 1995. Heterosexual HIV transmission. *Infectious Agents and Disease* 4:273–284.

15. Padian, N.S., S.C. Shiboski, S.O. Glass, and E. Vittinghoff. 1997. Heterosexual transmission of human immunodeficiency virus (HIV) in northern California: results from a ten-year study. *American Journal of Epidemiology* 146:350–357.

16. Varghese, B., J.E. Maher, T.A. Peterman, B.M. Branson, and R.W. Steketee. 2002. Reducing the risk of sexual HIV transmission: quantifying the per-act risk for HIV on the basis of choice of partner, sex act, and condom use. *Sexually Transmitted Diseases* 29:38–43.

17. Deuchert, E., and S. Brody. 2007. Plausible and implausible parameters for mathematical modeling of nominal heterosexual HIV transmission. *Annals of Epidemiology* 17:237–244.

18. Louria, D.B., J.H. Skurnick, P. Palumbo, et al. 2000. HIV heterosexual transmission: a hypothesis about an additional potential determinant. *International Journal of Infectious Diseases* 4:110–116.

19. Peterman, T.A., R.L. Stoneburner, J.R. Allen, H.W. Jaffe, and J.W. Curran. 1988. Risk of human immunodeficiency virus transmission from heterosexual adults with transfusion-associated infections. *Journal of the American Medical Association* 259:55–58.

20. Quinn, T.C. 1995. The epidemiology of the acquired immunodeficiency syndrome in the 1990s. *Emergency Medicine Clinics of North America* 13:1–25.

21. Fowler, M.G., S.L. Melnick, and B.J. Mathieson. 1997. Women and HIV. Epidemiology and global overview. *Obstetrics and Gynecology Clinics of North America* 24:705–729.

22. Johnson, B.T., M.P. Carey, S.R. Chaudoir, and A.E. Reid. 2006 Sexual risk reduction for persons living with HIV: Research synthesis of randomized controlled trials, 1993 to 2004. *Journal of Acquired Immune Deficiency Syndromes* 41:642–650.

23. Shiboski, S.C., and N.S. Padian. 1998. Epidemiologic evidence for time variation in HIV infectivity. *Journal of Acquired Immune Deficiency Syndromes and Human Retroviruses* 19:527–535.

24. Shilts, R. 1987. *And The Band Played On: Politics, People, and the AIDS Epidemic.* New York: St. Martin's Press.

25. Padian, N.S., S.C. Shiboski, and N.P. Jewell. 1990. The effect of number of exposures on the risk of heterosexual HIV transmission. *Journal of Infectious Diseases* 161:883–887.

26. Koopman, J.S., J.A. Jacquez, G.W. Welch, et al. 1997. The role of early HIV infection in the spread of HIV through populations. *Journal of Acquired Immune Deficiency Syndromes and Human Retrovirology* 14:249–258.

27. Garnett, G.P., J. Swinton, and G. Parker. 1994. Sex acts and sex partners [letter]. *Journal of Acquired Immune Deficiency Syndromes* 7:989–990.

28. de Vicenzi, I., for the European Study Group on Heterosexual Transmission of HIV. 1994. A longitudinal study of human immunodeficiency virus transmission by heterosexual partners. *New England Journal of Medicine* 331:341–346.

29. Holmberg, S.D., J.A. Stewart, A.R. Gerber, et al. 1988. Prior herpes simplex virus type 2 infection as a risk factor for HIV infection. *Journal of the American Medical Association* 259:1048–1050.

30. Wasserheit, J.N. 1992. Epidemiological synergy. Interrelationships between human immunodeficiency virus infection and other sexually transmitted diseases. *Sexually Transmitted Diseases* 19:61–77.

31. Fleming, D.T., and J.N. Wasserheit. 1999. From epidemiological synergy to public health policy and practice: The contribution of other sexually transmitted diseases to sexual transmission of HIV infection. *Sexually Transmitted Infections* 75:3–17.

32. Rebbapragada, A., C. Wichihi, C. Pettengell, et al. 2007. Negative mucosal synergy between Herpes simplex type 2 and HIV in the female genital tract. *AIDS* 21:589–598.

33. Kingsley, L.A., J. Armstrong, A. Rahman, M. Ho, C.R. Rinaldo Jr. 1991. No association between herpes simplex virus type-2-seropositivity or anogenital lesions and HIV seroconversion among homosexual men. *Journal of Acquired Immune Deficiency Syndromes* 4:732–734.

34. Holmberg, S.D., A.R. Gerber, J.A. Stewart, R.H. Byers, and A.J. Nahmias. 1991. Herpes simplex virus type 2 and HIV seroconversion [letter]. *Journal of Acquired Immune Deficiency Syndromes* 4:732–733.

35. Hook 3rd, E.W., R.O. Cannon, A.J. Nahmias, et al. 1992. Herpes simplex virus infection as a risk factor for human immunodeficiency virus infection in heterosexuals. *Journal of Infectious Diseases* 165:251–255.

36. CDC. 1999. A cluster of HIV-positive young women, upstate New York. *Morbidity and Mortality Weekly Report* 48:413–416.

37. Robbins, K.E., P.J. Weidel, T.M. Brown, et al. 2002. Molecular analysis in support of an investigation of a cluster of HIV-1-infected women. *AIDS Research and Human Retroviruses* 18:1157–1161.

38. CDC. 2000. A cluster of HIV-infected adolescents and young adults– Mississippi, 1999. *Morbidity and Mortality Weekly Report* 49:681–684.

39. Arthur, L.O., J.W. Bess Jr., R.C. Sowder 2nd, et al. 1992. Cellular proteins bound to immunodeficiency viruses: Implications for pathogenesis and vaccines. *Science* 258:1935–1938.

40. Hader, S.L., T. Hodge, K. Buchacz, et al. 2002. Discordance at human leukocyte antigen-DRB3 and protection from human immunodeficiency virus type 1 transmission. *Journal of Infectious Diseases* 185:1729–1735.

41. Rossio, J.L., J. Bess, L.E. Henderson, P. Crasswell, and L.O. Arthur. 1995. HLA class II on HIV particles is functional in superantigen presentation to human T cells: Implications for HIV pathogenesis. *AIDS Research and Human Retroviruses* 11:1433–1439.

42. Arthur, L.O., J.W. Bess, R.G. Urban, et al. 1995. Macaques immunized with HLA-DR are protected from challenge with simian immunodeficiency virus. *Journal of Virology* 69:3117–3124.

43. Crise, B., Y. Li, C. Yuan, et al. 2005. Simian immunodeficiency virus integration preference is similar to that of human immunodeficiency virus type 1. *Journal of Virology* 79:12199–12204.

44. Lifson, J.D., J.L. Rossio, M. Piatek Jr., et al. 2004. Evaluation of the safety, immunogenicity, and protective efficacy of whole inactivated simian immunodeficiency virus (SIV) vaccines with conformationally and functionally intact envelope glycoproteins. *AIDS Research and Human Retroviruses* 20:772–787.

45. Feigal, D.W., M.H. Katz, D. Greenspan, et al. 1991. The prevalence of oral lesions in HIV-infected homosexual and bisexual men: three San Francisco epidemiological cohorts. *AIDS* 5:519–525.

46. Schechter, M.T., W.J. Boyko, B. Douglas, et al. 1986. Can HTLV-III be transmitted orally [letter]? *Lancet* 1:379.

47. Mayer, K.H., and V. DeGruttola. 1987. Human immunodeficiency virus and oral intercourse. *Annals of Internal Medicine* 107:428–429.

48. Rozenbaum, W., S. Gharakhanian, B. Cardon, E. Duval, and J.P. Coulaud. 1988. HIV transmission by oral sex [letter]. *Lancet* 1:1395.

49. Lifson, A.R., P.M. O'Malley, N.A. Hessol, S.P. Buchbinder, L. Cannon, and G.W. Rutherford. 1990. HIV seroconversion in two homosexual men after receptive oral intercourse with ejaculation: Implications for counseling concerning safe sexual practices. *American Journal of Public Health* 80:1509–1511.

50. Lane, H.C., S.D. Holmberg, and H.W. Jaffe. 1991. HIV seroconversion and oral intercourse [letter]. *American Journal of Public Health* 81:658.

51. Campo, J., M.A. Perea, J. del Romero, J. Cano, V. Hernando, and A. Bascones. 2006. Oral transmission of HIV, reality or fiction? An update. *Oral Disease* 12:219–228.

52. Centers for Disease Control and Prevention (CDC). 2003. Incorporating HIV Prevention into the Medical Care of Persons Living with HIV. Recommendations of CDC, the Health Resources Administration, the National Institutes of Health, and the HIV Medicine Association of the Infectious Diseases Society of America. *Morbidity and Mortality Weekly Report* 52(RR12):1–24.

53. Summary Report on Workgroup to Identify Opportunities for Prevention of Acquired Immune Deficiency Syndrome, January 4, 1983. CDC; Atlanta, GA; Unpublished document.

54. Barré-Sinoussi, F., J.-C. Chermann, F. Rey, et al. 1983. Isolation of a T-lymphotropic retrovirus from a patient at risk for acquired immune deficiency syndrome (AIDS). *Science* 220:868–871.

55. Curran, J.W., D.N. Lawrence, H. Jaffe, et al. 1984. Acquired immunodeficiency syndrome (AIDS) associated with transfusions. *New England Journal of Medicine* 310:69–75.

56. Lackritz, E.M., G.A. Satten, J. Aberle-Grasse, et al. 1995. Estimated risk of transmission of the human immunodeficiency virus by screened blood in the United States. *New England Journal of Medicine* 333:1721–1725.

57. Anonymous. 1995. Court upholds $405,000 award against blood banking industry. *AIDS Policy Law* 10:1, 10–11.

58. Anonymous. 1996. Blood bank trade group held liable for HIV-tainted transfusion. *AIDS Policy Law* 11:1, 10–11.

59. Anonymous. 2000. Blood bank association not liable for tainted blood. *AIDS Policy Law* 15:9.

60. Hunter, M. August 1993. Blood money: Why are French hemophiliacs dying of AIDS? Because French officials knowingly gave them tainted blood. *Discover* 70–78.

61. Institute of Medicine (IOM), Committee to Study HIV Transmission through Blood and Blood Products. 1995. *HIV and the Blood Supply: An Analysis of Crisis Decision Making.* Washington, DC: National Academy Press.

62. Keshavjee, S., S. Weiser, and A. Kleinman. 2001. Medicine betrayed: Hemophilia patients and HIV in the US. *Social Science and Medicine* 53:1081–1094.

63. Zuck, T.F. 1987. Greetings—A final look back with comment about a policy of zero-risk blood supply [editorial]. *Transfusion* 27:447–448.

64. Zuck, T.F., and M.E. Eyster. 1996. Blood safety decisions, 1982 to 1986: perceptions and misconceptions. *Transfusion* 36:928–931.

65. CDC. 2007. Blood donor screening for Chagas Disease—United States, 2006–7. *Morbidity and Mortality Weekly Report* 56:141–143.

66. Orland, J.R., B. Wang, D.J. Wright, et al. 2004. Increased mortality associated with HTLV-II infection in blood donors: A prospective cohort study. *Retrovirology* 1:4.

67. Pealer, L.N., A.A. Marfin, L.R. Petersen, et al. 2003. Transmission of West Nile virus through blood transfusion in the United States in 2002. *New England Journal of Medicine* 349:1236–1245.

68. Dodd, R.Y. 2003. Emerging infections, transfusion safety, and epidemiology [editorial]. *New England Journal of Medicine* 349:1205–1206.

69. CDC. 2005. West Nile Virus Infections in organ transplant recipients—New York and Pennsylvania, August–September, 2005. *Morbidity and Mortality Weekly Report* 54(dispatch):1–3.

70. O'Brien, T.R., J.R. George, and S.D. Holmberg. 1992. Human immunodeficiency virus type 2 infection in the United States. Epidemiology, diagnosis, and public health implications. *Journal of the American Medical Association* 267:2775–2779.

71. Onorato, I.M., T.R. O'Brien, C.A. Schable, C. Spruill, and S.D. Holmberg. 1993. Sentinel surveillance for HIV-2 infection in high-risk US populations. *American Journal of Public Health* 83:515–519.

72. Stramer, S.L., S.A. Glynn, S.H. Kleinman, et al. 2004. Detection of HIV-1 and HCV infections among antibody-negative blood donors by nucleic acid-amplification testing. *New England Journal of Medicine* 351:760–768.

73. Krombach, J., S. Kampe, B.S. Gathof, C. Diefenbach, and S.M. Kasper. 2002. Human error: The persisting risk of blood transfusion: A report of five cases. *Anesthesia and Analgesia* 94:154–156.

74. Ou, C.Y., S. Kwok, S.W. Mitchell, et al. 1988. DNA amplification for direct detection of HIV-1 in DNA of peripheral blood mononuclear cells. *Science* 239:295–297.

75. Horsburgh Jr., C.R., C.-Y. Ou, S.D. Holmberg, et al. 1989. Human immun-odeficiency virus type infections in homosexual men who remain seronegative for prolonged periods [letter]. *New England Journal of Medicine* 321:1679–1680.

76. Farzadegan, H., M.A. Polis, S.M. Wolinsky, et al. 1988. Loss of human im-munodeficiency virus type 1 (HIV-1) antibodies with evidence of viral infection in asymptomatic homosexual men. A report from the Multicenter AIDS Cohort Study. *Annals of Internal Medicine* 108:785–790.

77. Zuck, T.F. 1988. Silent sequences and the safety of blood transfusions [editorial]. *Annals of Internal Medicine* 108:895–897.

78. Gutierrez, M., V. Soriano, R. Bravo, A. Vallejo, and J. Gonzalez-Lahoz. 1994. Seroreversion in patients with end-stage HIV infection. *Vox Sanguinis* 67:238–239.

79. Holmberg, S.D., C.R. Horsburgh Jr., R.H. Byers, et al. 1988. Errors in re-porting seropositivity for infection with human immunodeficiency virus (HIV)[letter]. *Annals of Internal Medicine* 109:679–680.

80. Roy, M.J., J.J. Damato, and D.S. Burke. 1993. Absence of true seroreversion of HIV-1 antibody in seroreactive individuals. *Journal of the American Medical Association* 269:2876–2879.

81. Coyne, K.M., J.V. Parry, M. Atkins, A. Pozniak, and A. McOwan. 2007. Spon-taneous HIV-1 seroreversion in an adult male. *Sexually Transmitted Diseases* 34:627–630.

82. Imagawa, D.T., M.H. Lee, S.M Wolinsky, et al. 1989. Human immunod-eficiency virus type 1 infection in homosexual men who remain seronegative for prolonged periods. *New England Journal of Medicine* 320:1458–1462.

83. Haseltine, W.A. Silent HIV infections [editorial]. 1989. *New England Journal of Medicine* 320:1487–1489.

84. Horsburgh Jr., C.R., C.-Y. Ou, J. Jason, et al. 1989. Detection of human immunodeficiency virus infection before detection of antibody. *Lancet* 2:637–640.

85. Pan, L.Z., R. Royce, W. Winkelstein, and J.A. Levy. 1989. Human immun-odeficiency virus type 1 infection in homosexual men who remain seronegative for prolonged periods [letter]. *New England Journal of Medicine* 321:1680.

86. Bianco, C., J. Uehlinger, and H.S. Kaplan. 1989. Human immunodeficiency virus type infections in homosexual men who remain seronegative for prolonged periods [letter]. *New England Journal of Medicine* 321:1678–1679.

87. Zuck, T.F. 1989. Human immunodeficiency virus type infections in homosex-ual men who remain seronegative for prolonged periods [letter]. *New England Journal of Medicine* 321:1680–1681.

88. Pan, L.-Z., H.W. Sheppard, W. Winkelstein, and J.A.Levy. 1991. Lack of detection of human immunodeficiency virus in persistently seronegative homosexual men with high or medium risks for infection. *Journal of Infectious Diseases* 164:962–964.

89. Groopman, J.E., T. Caiazzo, M.A. Thomas, et al. 1988. Lack of evidence of prolonged human immunodeficiency virus infection before antibody seroconversion. *Blood* 71: 1752–1754.

90. Gupta, P., L. Kingsley, R. Anderson, et al. 1992. Low prevalence of HIV in high-risk seronegative homosexual men evidenced by virus culture and polymerase chain reaction. *AIDS* 6:143–149.

91. Farzadegan, H., D. Vlahov, L. Solomon, et al. 1993. Detection of human immunodeficiency virus type 1 infection by polymerase chain reaction in a cohort of seronegative intravenous drug users. *Journal of Infectious Diseases* 168:327–331.

92. Imagawa, D., and R. Detels. 1991. HIV-1 in seronegative homosexual men [letter]. *New England Journal of Medicine* 325:1250–1251.

93. CDC. 1991. Update: Transmission of HIV infection during an invasive dental procedure–Florida. *Morbidity and Mortality Weekly Report* 40:21–27, 33.

94. Ou, C.Y., C.A. Ciesielski, G. Myers, et al. 1992. Molecular epidemiology of HIV transmission in a dental practice. *Science* 256:1155–1156.

95. Ciesielski, C., D. Marianos, C.Y. Ou, et al. 1992. Transmission of human immunodeficiency virus in a dental practice. *Annals of Internal Medicine* 116:798–805.

96. Applebome, P. September 8, 1990. Dentist dies of AIDS, leaving Florida City concerned but calm. *The New York Times.*

97. Breo, D.L. 1993. The dental AIDS cases–Murder or an unsolvable mystery? *Journal of the American Medical Association* 270:2732–2734.

98. Dickinson, G.M., R.E. Morhart, N.G. Klimas, C.I. Bandea, J.M. Laracuente, and A.L. Bisno. 1993. Absence of HIV transmission from an infected dentist to his patients. An epidemiologic and DNA sequence analysis. *Journal of the American Medical Association* 269:1802–1806.

99. Ciesielski, C.A., D.W. Marianos, G. Schochetman, J.J. Witte, and H.W. Jaffe. 1994. The 1990 Florida dental investigation. The press and the science. *Annals of Internal Medicine* 121:886–888.

100. Barr, S. April 16, 1994. What if the dentist didn't do it? *The New York Times.*

101. Tuboku-Metzger, J., L. Chiarello, R.L. Sinkowitz-Cochran, A. Casano-Dickerson, and D. Cardo. 2005. Public attitudes and opinions toward physicians and dentists infected with bloodborne viruses: Results of a national survey. *American Journal of Infection Control* 33:299–303.

102. Ward, J.W., S.D. Holmberg, J.R. Allen, et al. 1988. Transmission of human immunodeficiency virus (HIV) by blood transfusions screened as negative for HIV infection. *New England Journal of Medicine* 318:473–478.

103. CDC. 1987. Human immunodeficiency virus infection transmitted from an organ donor screened for HIV antibody–North Carolina. *Morbidity and Mortality Weekly Report* 36:306–307.

104. Simonds, R.J., S.D. Holmberg, R.L. Hurwitz, et al. 1992. Transmission of human immunodeficiency virus type 1 from a seronegative organ and tissue donor. *New England Journal of Medicine* 326:726–732.

105. Simonds, R.J. 1993. HIV transmission by organ and tissue transplantation. *AIDS* 7(suppl 2):S35–S38.

106. Anderson, D.J., T.R. O'Brien, J.A. Politch, et al. 1992. Effects of disease stage and zidovudine therapy on the detection of human immunodeficiency virus type 1 in semen. *Journal of the American Medical Association* 267:2769–2774.

107. Semprini, A.E., P. Levi-Setti, M. Bozzo, et al. 1992. Insemination of processed semen of HIV-positive partners. *Lancet* 340:1317–1319.

108. CDC. 1990. HIV-1 infection and artificial insemination with processed semen. *Morbidity and Mortality Weekly Report* 39:249, 255–256.

109. Sauer, M.V. 2005. Sperm washing techniques address the fertility needs of HIV-seropositive men: A clinical review. *Reproductive Biomedicine Online* 10:135–140.

110. Savasi, V., E. Ferrazzi, C. Lanzani, M. Oneta, B. Parrilla, and T. Persico. 2007. Safety of sperm washing and ART outcome in 741 HIV-1-serodiscordant couples. *Human Reproduction* 22:772–777.

CHAPTER FIVE

Unusual and Unproven Modes of HIV Transmission

Even 10 years after the epidemic had started, AIDS phobia still pervaded the community of Belle Glade, Florida, an indigent area with many migrant Haitian workers and levels of HIV and AIDS similar to that seen in San Francisco or New York. Some high school teams refused to play there, and some Belle Glade residents suffered the indignity of watching their checks sprayed with "Lysol."[1] Some visitors wore surgical masks, and others kept their windows up in summer (in those days often in cars without air conditioning) to prevent being bitten by HIV-bearing mosquitoes. This was the height of public confusion about AIDS and in some cases it was caused by lack of information or, oddly, by being bombarded with too much contradictory information. The mid- and late-1980s were a period of intense scrutiny of HIV transmission other than by sex contact, by direct blood contact, or from mother to infant.

First, it is important to note that it is impossible to "prove a negative"–that is, that something will not occur–in this case that HIV could never, even under extreme conditions, be transmitted by unusual routes. Barring actual observation at the time of every HIV transmission, the best that can be done with highly unlikely modes of transmission is to assess the evidence that such transmission could take place and to analyze its probability. This approach has its limits, among them that the assessed risk is often vanishingly small, and the prevention of it inordinately difficult, say, if HIV were transmitted on doorknobs. However, while a statistically minded person may not be worried about a "less than one in a million" chance–which includes the probability that there is *no* actual chance–of getting HIV infection from a doorknob, this is not always perceived as such by fellow-citizens, who are convinced there will be "one" and that "one" will be them, when, in fact, they will be among the "million." (Testament to this very human, nonmathematical way of risk assessment is the popularity of state lotteries.) Such nonprobabilistic thinking was rampant during the first several years of the epidemic as tabloids and even some more credible media opined that one might get AIDS from, for example, lice or cockroaches because somewhere the risk was assessed at, say, one in a million or less.

Another general principle when evaluating any claim of an unusual mode of transmission is that HIV may rarely be recovered from any fluid or site where human white blood cells, the host cell type for HIV, may be found. Invariably, if HIV (or HTLV-IIII) was detected in the saliva, tears, urine, or body fluids other than blood or semen of HIV-infected persons, it was in minute quantities,[2] rarely detected, and unlikely to survive long when experimentally exposed to natural conditions of drying, acidity, sunlight, etc. Thus, most scientists have not taken detection of HIV in a nonblood body fluid, insect, or from the environment as evidence per se of transmission by such a route.

Finally, in discussing the limitations of recovery of HIV from anyplace other than blood, it is important to note that most early experiments used developing and not always reliable or reproducible techniques to determine the presence of HIV in body fluids, food, the environment, or insects. These techniques were often indirect assays of reverse transcriptase (RT), the enzyme that HIV uses to "read" itself from RNA to DNA, so that the virus can then insert in the human genome. These techniques are not "specific" as RT may be produced by other organisms and because cross-reactivity with these gene sequences may falsely "detect" HIV.[3]

"No Identified Risk"

Virtually the whole AIDS scientific community had, by 1983 or 1984, accepted that HIV was a sexually transmitted disease that might also be transmitted by blood contact (usually, via shared needles) or during childbirth. However, there were potent reasons to evaluate the other forms of transmission. First, there still remain some AIDS and HIV patients who deny any behavior or other risk exposure. More intensive interviewing of these shows most interviewees ultimately acknowledging some stigmatizing behavior, such as homosexual, or illegal activity, such as intravenous illicit drug use. Some only report heterosexual contact, putatively with persons whom they did not know were HIV-infected. Are these simply an irreducible fraction who will never admit or just do not remember their potential exposure to HIV? Or could other modes of transmission rarely occur? Eventually, by the end of the 1990s, facts convinced the majority of people that there were not any or many alternate ways of contracting HIV infection, but truth often percolates into the wider public at a maddeningly slow pace.

Careful and confidential re-interview of HIV or AIDS patients who initially report "no identified risk" (NIR) always shows that the majority of them can be reclassified into a standard transmission risk group. This still leaves some irreducible minimum, a single-digit percentage, who on all interviewing remain "NIR." Although we know that some adults are probably adamant in their denial—or inability to remember—sexual or blood exposure, could there be one or even a few who got infected by some unsuspected alternate route of infection? The nagging doubt persists that a flood of HIV could hide a trickle.

It is important from a public health perspective to make sure that people understand which behaviors put them at risk and conversely not to be terrorized by risks that do not exist. Also, some may not perceive a compelling reason to change known risk behavior if they are able to rationalize that they could get HIV from contact, food, or insects. In this inverted way of thinking, if one cannot protect oneself from getting AIDS from the general environment or from nonsexual sources, why bother to change sex practices?

Investigating the spread of HIV by insects, casual contact, by body fluids other than blood (saliva, sweat, or urine), or by food was a considerable time-sink for investigators in the first decade of the American HIV/AIDS epidemic. Further, at the end of even the most elegant experiments, researchers still always concluded that survival of HIV in, say, insects or on surfaces, may not match the natural situation, and retreat to positions that epidemiologic evidence for such unusual transmission simply does not exist. Still, no experiment can negate what might be called "The Public Health Official's Paradox."

This paradox is one that every health official and scientist must confront when concerned or skeptical citizens or other scientists ask if HIV absolutely cannot be transmitted by, for example, head lice. If the reply is that such transmission is not possible, the official loses credibility as an open-minded arbiter of data and perceived as reluctant to seriously investigate the (very low) possibility, and, worse, blind to a potential public health threat. However, if the official's reply that this unusual transmission route—say, by fomites or insects—may theoretically be possible, albeit under extreme and rare circumstances, some of the public will be distracted from or, worse, feel vindicated about the real and immediate threats to their health from engaging in unsafe behaviors. Some will also demand that already thin public health dollars be devoted to ineffective and unfair practices, such as by excessively strict isolation including quarantine of HIV-infected persons. This last is not a theoretical concern, as many advocated enforced quarantine of HIV patients in the 1980s,[4, 5] and Cuba actually followed such a policy.[6, 7] In fact, even 25 years into the epidemic, as new communities are first exposed to AIDS cases, there is sometimes reactive quarantine of HIV/AIDS patients, as in parts of rural China.[8]

So what is the evidence for HIV survival in the environment, insects, food, and body fluids other than blood or its components (plasma, serum), such as saliva or urine? And would this survival engender transmission of HIV? Much early work in the HIV/AIDS epidemic went into evaluating these possibilities.

Health Care Workers

Early in the AIDS epidemic there was only the example of hepatitis B virus (HBV), another blood-borne and sexually transmitted viral infection. In one review[9] it was thought that many HBV infections that occurred in health care workers with no history of nonoccupational exposure or occupational percutaneous injury might have resulted from direct or indirect blood or body fluid exposures that inoculated HBV into scratches, abrasions, burns, other lesions, or on mucosal surfaces.[10–12] Thus, early in the epidemic—and this would substantially be before hepatitis C virus had been identified (in 1988) and subsequently studied—the one epidemiologic model for human blood-borne viral transmission, hepatitis B virus, could infect people by means as simple as a splash on the conjunctiva of the eye.

However, prospective studies of health care workers indicated that the average risk of HIV transmission after a needlestick injury—that is accidental stick with needle just used on an HIV/AIDS patient (see previous chapter)—was approximately 0.3 percent (95% CI = 0.2–0.5%)[13] and after a mucous membrane exposure, approximately 0.09 percent (95% CI = 0.006–0.5%).[14]

Episodes of HIV transmission after non-intact skin, mucous membrane exposure were reported[15] by persons denying any other potential exposures to HIV: one health care worker had chapped hands, and the duration of contact with the blood of a patient experiencing a cardiac arrest may have been as long as 20 minutes; another purportedly sustained contamination of oral mucous membranes (she also had acne but did not recall having open lesions, and had sustained a scratch from a needle used to draw blood from an intravenous drug abuser of unknown HIV-infection status); and a third had a history of dermatitis involving an ear that was putatively exposed to blood of an HIV patient. In the cautious wording of the CDC *MMWR*,[9] "[T]he average risk for transmission by this route [broken skin] has not been precisely quantified but is estimated to be less than the risk for mucous membrane exposures.[16]" The report went on to comment on exposure to aerosolized plasma during plasmapheresis, as claimed by one health technician: "The risk for transmission after exposure to fluids or tissues other than HIV-infected blood also has not been quantified but is probably considerably lower than for blood exposures."[17] So, a common opinion within CDC about these three unusual cases of transmission by blood splash was summed up by one colleague who threw up his hands when it was decided to report these as: "This is science by anecdote!"

No further anecdotes of HIV transmission by splashes or contact with nonintact skin have been reported in the past 20 years, and this has led to a general attitude that if transmission by such a route can occur, this must be an exceedingly rare and evanescent event. Further, by the end of the first decade of the HIV/AIDS epidemic in the United States, it was finally clear that HIV was several fold less transmissible than HBV in the health care setting, for example, anywhere from 10 to 60 times less likely to be transmitted by needlestick.[18]

One of the most vociferous and vituperative disbelievers in the small risk to health care workers was Lorraine Day, an orthopedic surgeon at San Francisco General Hospital. In the spring of 1991 and later, Day was widely quoted in local and national newspapers such as the *Los Angeles Times* and the *New York Times*, local and national radio shows, and she appeared in widely viewed television programs such as *60 Minutes, Nightline, CNN Crossfire, Oprah Winfrey, Larry King Live*, and the *700 Club* to explain her reasons for quitting her practice over concern she was at high risk of getting infected from her patients. She published a book[19] that posited that HIV can penetrate a surgical mask and that the virus "stays alive for at least 2 feet." According to her, federal officials were purposely and markedly downplaying the risk of HIV to surgeons, and she ceased to practice surgery herself.

Ironically, CDC administered questionnaires and performed serum testing at the American Academy of Orthopaedic Surgeons meeting in March 1991 where Day made many contentious remarks.[20] Of 3,420 orthopedic surgeons who participated in the survey, only two were found to be HIV-infected; both had other, nonoccupational risks for HIV infection.[21] Still, as late as 1994, Day was still sending letters to public health officials accusing them of "mislead[ing] the public deliberately.... You must have a lot of sleepless nights. I pray for you and hope you will stop selling your soul for your pension or whatever...You have a lot of blood on your hands" (Lorraine Day, Letter to Harold Jaffe, April 14, 1994).

The Environment

In evaluating survival and transmission of HIV in the general environment or by fomites (objects that might serve as vehicles of transmission, e.g., handles, bath towels, cutting boards, etc.), one should note that the levels of infectious virus used in many investigations was much, much higher—often 1,000 or more times higher than levels of HIV found in blood[22]—and experimental conditions often do not match those found in the natural environment where variable humidity, drying, temperatures, sunlight and other factors pertain. Still, despite these caveats, this work was always considered very valuable, as long as data were interpreted and considered within the constraints of the experiment. If HIV in sufficient amounts can survive and actually be transmitted through open cuts and abrasions, or by eating or breathing it, this would clearly inform personal and public health practice. For example, disinfection of surfaces and instruments in the hospital would need to be especially rigorous.[23]

The general public clearly can easily confuse the severe and protean manifestations of AIDS—that is, its pathogenicity—with some sort of hardiness of the virus. However, almost all biologists continue to consider HIV, like other enveloped viruses, as very fragile in any environment outside the white blood or other human cells (mononuclear cells) or the warm human bloodstream. Thus, some early experiments were somewhat surprising.

Slade and others examined the survival of HIV in culture fluid, seawater, sewage, and dechlorinated tap water and found that HIV, although declining 10-fold within 1–3 days, still was detectable in these fluids for up to 11 days.[24] Although the exact nature and amount of HIV inoculum in these fluids is unclear,[23] and although this virus may have been protected from sunlight, acids, heat, or drying that would have inactivated it, clearly HIV can survive under strict experimental conditions for some considerable time in fluid.

However, the ability of HIV to survive on environmental surfaces or fomites is determined by the substance of the surface as well as ambient heat, light, and humidity. The available evidence indicates that the ability of HIV to survive on fomites is similar to that seen with other enveloped viruses,[25, 26] which are easily degraded by exposure to heat, sunlight, and acids. High concentrations of cell-free and cell-associated HIV suspended in 10 percent serum and kept at room temperature can remain infectious for several weeks; when dried on glass, virus might remain recoverable—again as determined by early and possibly falsely "positive" assays for HIV—for several days.[27] Further, the effectiveness of disinfectants used to disinfect contaminated objects and surfaces "may have been overestimated,"[23] although heat and some chemical disinfectants—for example, quarternary ammonium and phenol compounds—were still found to be efficacious. Again, these experimental conditions do not match natural ones, the amount of virus recovered would not be sufficient for transmission (nonsexually), and several experiments by CDC in the 1980s showed that once dried on any surface, HIV could not be recovered or detected by sensitive assays (Charles Schable, personal communication, January 22, 2007).

Insects

No one defends mosquitoes, bedbugs, and lice: most infectious disease epidemiologists and public health professionals still abide by Hans Zinsser's 1934 classic, *Rats, Lice and History*, that persuasively argued that insects and microbes have had more to do with human history than all the generals combined. The causes of much human misery, these hematophagous (blood-sucking) insects are apparently not even essential to their ecosystems. So, perhaps it was natural that in the early days of the AIDS epidemic intelligent people would look at the distribution of AIDS cases in West Africa, the distribution of malaria, *Aedes* and other mosquito species, and other insects, and wonder if there were some link between these. Here the "ecologic thinking" was powerful–that is, that two unpleasant phenomena occurring in the same time and place could be related causally.

Early on, several experimenters failed to demonstrate actual replication of HIV within arthropod cell lines[28]: this was important in vitro work because it indicated that insects could not provide a persistent reservoir to which humans would be frequently exposed. Thus, any transfer would have to be mechanical, carried on minute portions on the mouthparts of biting insects from one person to another. In this view, mosquitoes would act as some sort of flying tiny hypodermic needles. So, critical to this transmission would be a number of considerations: how long does HIV survive in, or perhaps on, the proboscis; and how often would a mosquito or bedbug bite an HIV-infected person and then feed on a susceptible person, and in what length of time?

Indeed, in the earliest days of the HIV/AIDS epidemic, before it was clear that many, many sexually active homosexual men must be involved, many inside and outside the AIDS community wondered if simple mechanical transfer of the agent of AIDS–that is, an insect picking up HIV by blood-feeding on one human and then transfer to another during a subsequent feeding and regurgitation–might be carried by mosquitoes. If feeding and blood regurgitation might suffice, other biting insects such as bedbugs and lice might also transfer the AIDS agent. (However, it is ironic that this theory of mechanical insect-borne blood transmission was current at roughly the same time that blood banking officials were initially dismissing the idea that the AIDS agent could be transferred through blood transfusion [see Chapter 4]).

Among almost all AIDS scientists and epidemiologists, mosquito transmission was considered unlikely even before the definitive agent of AIDS, HIV, was discovered in 1983. First, it seemed highly improbable that mosquitoes would selectively victimize west Africans, gay men in the United States and Europe, and the occasional blood-transfusion recipient exclusively, skipping the rest of us. As a colleague quipped, "What kind of mosquito only bites gay men?" So, simple epidemiologic and probabilistic thinking was powerfully against the mosquito- or bedbug- spread hypothesis. Still, many Africans were affected: could it be that some sizeable fraction were infected this way, in addition to whatever chains of transmission they might share in common with, say, gay men in San Francisco or intravenous drug users in New York?

In fact, in the earliest days of the epidemic, major and respected scientists in HIV/AIDS opined in speech or writing that insect transmission of HIV (or whatever the AIDS agent was) might occur. For example, Robert Shope, Director of Yale University's Arbovirus Unit, averred that mosquitoes were long known to transmit retroviruses and that transmission by insects would be "perfectly logical and within the realm of possibility."[29] Robert Gallo, controversial discoverer of human T-lymphocytotropic virus type III (HTLV-III, later determined to be HIV; see Chapter 2) had suggested that a similar virus, HTLV-I, linked to leukemia cases in the Caribbean and the Far East, might be spread by mosquitoes.[30]

Even after it became clear that sexual and blood-borne transmission must be the main routes of transmission, researchers continued to investigate the insect hypothesis in a series of experiments until the mid 1990s. In the earliest investigations, DNA sequences homologous—that is, chains of DNA naturally binding or annealing with one another in vitro—to HIV DNA were recovered from mosquitoes, ticks, and tsetse flies, as well as from nonbiting insects such as ant lions and cockroaches.[31, 32] Because these latter nonbiting insects should not have HIV or related immunodeficiency virus, and because of the many cell types and insects that reportedly had such gene sequences, it was thought that these results may well have been cross-reactions with other RNA viruses or even nonspecific (false positive) assays.[3]

Thus, there was some experimental validation of concern and the implications were disturbing. First, if mosquitoes (or other insects) could be the vectors of HIV, there would be no easy protection against AIDS. Mosquitoes and bedbugs are marginally controlled at best in any population exposed to these insect vectors, and carriage of a lethal infection would be more than disastrous. Even the modest possibility of some infection by this route would and did lead to feelings of hopelessness and despair by the some in the general public that anything could mitigate the AIDS epidemic, as well as obviating the sense that humans could be responsible and could address this epidemic by changing their own behaviors. The many popular references to AIDS as a new "plague" reinforced the attitude that, like the Black Death of the fourteenth century, there was little that modern people could do to avoid infection based on our limited understanding of the causes of this epidemic.

Belle Glade

Such fears peaked in 1985 in the "poverty-scarred town" of Belle Glade, Florida.[32] Already by early 1985 this town had 31 AIDS cases, including 14 intravenous drug users, five homosexual men, and nine (heterosexual) Haitians. Dubbed the "AIDS Capital of the World"–a gross exaggeration as the epidemic raged in Africa and other American cities–this rural farming community, western Palm Beach county, had many indigent and migrant farm workers from Haiti, which country was widely known for its high AIDS endemicity well before 1985. The high proportion of intravenous drug and crack-using sex workers in Belle Glade was early thought to be the reason why this area had such high AIDS prevalence; but this situation was different from other U.S. cities where it was clear that the great majority of cases to that date had been reported from gay men. CDC studies conducted in the community typically showed 2–3 percent of randomly selected residents with HIV infection,[34, 35] a rate several fold that of any other community without heavy concentration of gay men or intravenous drug users. Belle Glade was considered, in the words of one colleague, "our piece of the developing world" in the United States.

Although many infections in Belle Glade were determined to be the result of heterosexual transmission, as was the main transmission risk in Haiti itself, the possibility of mosquito-borne transmission of the AIDS agent emerged as an issue. Based on some pathologic findings, one researcher, Jane Teas, posited in a letter to the British journal *Lancet* that the AIDS agent might be a variant of African swine fever virus (ASFV),[36] an agent known to be spread by mosquitoes. (A variant had to be suggested as ASFV does not infect humans.) Although experimental work with pigs by the US Department of Agriculture's research unit on Plum Island, New York, and several other lines of evidence did not confirm the association between human or swine immunodeficiency and ASFV infection (see Chapter 2), and although AIDS patients showed no evidence of ASFV infection, as determined by the presence of antibodies to the virus in their serum,[37] concerns persisted.

There were compelling reasons for the public health community to rapidly evaluate the legitimacy of this potential vector. However, as indicated, "proving a negative" is always difficult, and refuting the possibility, no matter how remote, that mosquitoes or bedbugs could occasionally transmit HIV was more difficult than expected. Indeed, recent surveys of literate people in the developing world show the persistence of belief by a substantial minority—usually about a third—that HIV can be transmitted by mosquitoes.[38, 39] The linking of two unpleasant realities occurring in the same place at the same time is always a strong current in human attitudes.

Bedbugs, lice, and other nonflying insects were easily eliminated as frequent vectors of HIV (or some other blood-borne AIDS agent): there were simply not enough of them or frequency of different human contacts by such insects to explain the high prevalence of AIDS in Belle Glade. Yet there were other reasons to question that the most likely flying and biting insect, mosquitoes, could harbor and thereby spread HIV widely. For instance, none of 138 Belle Glade children aged 2–10 years and none of 131 senior persons aged 60-years-old or more tested positive for HIV,[34, 40] as might be expected as they would be exposed to the same biting insects as the 6 percent of HIV-seropositive people in the age range of 18–39 years. Further, as a measure of exposure to mosquitoes, blood samples in these community studies were tested for antibodies to five arboviruses. After controlling for exposure to dengue fever in Haiti, there was no correlation between arboviruses and HIV infection or AIDS.

Within a few hours, various mosquito species no longer harbor any virus no matter how intensive the HIV-rich blood fed them, and several attempts to transmit the virus to uninfected blood by interrupted feeding of these mosquito species failed.[3, 41] As the report indicated, a mosquito would have to start feeding on an HIV-infected person, be interrupted and then, within at most a few hours, feed on an uninfected person to effect transfer of the virus. Further, sufficient inoculum would be required to establish infection in the susceptible second host.[3] Mosquitoes will digest any HIV along with the blood meal, but, again, only the tiny amount of residual blood from a previous victim that remains on a mosquito's mouthparts could be regurgitated or exposed to the next victim.

True, HIV could be cultured from bedbugs up to four hours after engorging blood,[41, 42] but the abnormally high levels of HIV for the feeding—10^4–10^5 tissue culture units (TCUs)—were over 100 times higher than HIV levels seen in human blood.[22] Later work showed that under experimental conditions bedbugs could retain HIV up to 8 days after concentrated blood meals; however, "mechanical transmission of HIV by bedbugs could not be demonstrated in an in vitro model."[43]

Does this mean that mosquitoes or bedbugs cannot transmit HIV? One can calculate the probability of such transfer by estimating the likelihood of, say, a mosquito biting an HIV-infected person, being interrupted in that blood meal, immediately finding an uninfected person to bite with regurgitation (blood on mouthparts) to the uninfected person, and likelihood of productive infection with of such a small inoculum of HIV. By multiplying each of these conditional probabilities, Charles Bailey, then Chief of the Department of Arboviral Entomology, U.S. Army Medical Research Institute, Ft. Detrick, Maryland estimated the likelihood of such transfer of HIV at one in 10 million or less (including the possibility of no transmission).[3]

However, it seems no argument is ever completely resolved. Even as late as 1993, investigators found that HIV could be detected in blood-meal regurgitants of the African soft tick for up to 10 days and that these insects, in the authors' conclusion "could contribute somewhat to HIV-1 transmission in areas of Central Africa where prevalence is high."[44]

Saliva and Biting

Many researchers thought the public focus and fear about being bitten by an AIDS patient reflected a subtle demonizing of such patients; however, more to the point, the real risk of biting is for the person doing the biting, because as their teeth and mouth are exposed to the bitten person's blood, this is a far more likely route of HIV transmission than being the person bitten. A bitten person is exposed to very small amounts of HIV, if any, in saliva, whereas a biter may be exposed to high levels of virus in the blood. However, there does not appear to have been any case reporting probable transmission to someone who has bitten, not been bitten by, an HIV-infected individual.

HIV has been very rarely recovered from saliva.[45, 46] Further, elements in saliva inhibit HIV infectivity;[47−49] these factors may include IgA antibodies, lysozyme, defensins, secretory leukocyte protease inhibitor, and some types of mucins.[50, 51] But does this mean that human bites may not transmit HIV to the bitten by infected saliva? A high enough concentration of virus in saliva exposed to the blood of the susceptible person may lead to transmission under special circumstances. Indeed, there have been a few such reports over the years, but for all of these, there is no surefire way of confirming that the investigated bite exposure was really the only contact the bitten individual had to HIV. The cases reported have had problems.

A young child in Germany died from AIDS and his only known exposure was a bite on his forearm from his younger brother 6 months earlier[52]; however, an incubation period of only 6 months from putative infection to death−normally, it takes over 10 years just from HIV infection (at birth) till AIDS, not death, for a child born to an infected mother−would be highly unusual, especially given the low inoculum of virus in saliva. Also, the skin of the bitten child had not reportedly been broken. A second brief report involved a women who was bitten on her leg during a fight with her HIV-infected drug-abusing sister in 1985: she was found to be HIV-seropositive 2 years later and denied any other HIV risk.[53] A third instance, a 47-year-old Slovenian man bit his 53-year-old neighbor during a seizure, the latter becoming HIV-antibody-test positive 54 days later, despite starting zidovudine (AZT) prophylaxis 10 hours after the incident.[54] Another involved an HIV-positive man who during a grand mal seizure bit the hand of his 59-year-old widowed mother, who denied sexual intercourse or other risk behavior in the 10 years previous, and who subsequent to the bite was "positive" on a sensitive/less sensitive immunoassay of her blood 40 days after the bite.[55] (This so-called "detuned" assay is a test that shows recent infection if the sensitive test is "positive" and the less sensitive test has not yet turned "positive."[56] Still, the sensitive/less sensitive assay has proven imperfect,[57, 58] even in expert hands, in discriminating recent from old infections.) Finally, there was a report about a Trinidadan 3-year-old child, whose mother tested HIV-antibody-negative, but whose HIV-infected father, who had bleeding gums, had reportedly bitten the child in 2000 on her middle finger, causing bleeding at the site; the child was found to be HIV-seropositive more than 4 years later.[59] There was no way of determining if the father had had sex or blood contact with the child, as he had died before the child was found to be HIV-infected.

In some of the cases of possible bite transmission above, when these were observed, the biter was usually described as having poor dentition and bad gingivitis, with observable blood in his saliva. There was also the single case reported referable to kissing, in which the saliva of the HIV-infected man who had bad dental disease frequently had observable blood in his saliva.[60] In this and the blood-stained saliva in the bites described above, the reports are more credible as blood-to-blood (mucous membrane) transmission may have occurred.

However, against these intriguing but inconclusive anecdotes, no prospective study has documented HIV-seroconversion (from "negative" to "positive") in any American health care worker bitten by an HIV patient in hospital. Tereskerz and colleagues looked at 10,125 incidents in 50 hospitals between 1993 and 1995; none of 50 bites of health care workers by HIV patients resulted in infection of them.[61] Extrapolating, these investigators estimated that 622 such bites occurred yearly in US hospitals, without any report yet of HIV infection in a bitten health worker, despite standard procedures to test such bitten workers (95% upper confidence limit, binomial exact test, 0.00825 transmissions per 100 person-years).

Food

One of the most tenacious misconceptions early in the HIV/AIDS epidemic was that the virus would survive well and long on surfaces or in food, and then be transmitted orally by eating or by touching the mouth with a contaminated hand. From the middle to late 1980s, CDC was asked to evaluate whether virus could be or had been introduced to foods. For example, in one of these unadvertised set of experiments, CDC had to investigate an anonymous threat from an AIDS patient who claimed he had injected tomatoes in a Chicago supermarket with his own blood. Accordingly, CDC was rapidly called on to investigate the likelihood that tomatoes so injected could indeed harbor the virus. Theoretically, it seemed to the researchers highly unlikely that this would be an efficient mode of transmission.

Although it might seem to some of the public that because it is an infection of such protean and severe manifestations HIV would easily survive a wide range of environmental conditions, to the contrary, investigators had early on found that HIV was generally unable to withstand conditions very different from those of the human bloodstream. Stability experiments demonstrated that HIV infectivity (ability to infect cells) declined within seconds when the virus was placed on surfaces such as metal, glass, plastic, and wood—particularly if the fluid in which the HIV resided dried on the experimental surface. Thus, HIV has not been recovered from natural and artificial surfaces, that have characteristics of temperature, salinity, humidity, and acidity (pH) outside the narrow range found in human blood (white blood cells, CD4+ cells) or serum. Further, several experiments at CDC by the HIV Diagnostic Serology Section, according to Charles Schable, its then Chief, showed that "HIV survived poorly in both high and low pH levels" and "deteriorated very quickly in a non-blood environment and rapidly lost its ability to infect WBC [while blood cells]" (Schable, personal communication, January 16, 2007). This was definitely the case with tomatoes and tomato products that have a pH around 3.5–4.9, that is, at least 100 times more acidic than human blood. Further cooking would rapidly inactivate any HIV in food. Finally, even if HIV survived in food, as above, saliva contains elements that inactivate HIV, and the levels of gastric acid (pH less than 3.0, and may even drop to 1.0 on an empty stomach) will immediately disrupt any HIV virions that survive to reach the stomach.

The rationale for these experiments with food was double-edged: on one hand, the public's and a few scientists' concerns needed to be met; on the other, though, "the time spent doing these experiments set back the timetable for other more fruitful endeavors in the laboratory" (Schable, personal communication, January 22, 2007). The general concern about transmission of HIV in food has not surfaced as a scientific or epidemiologic issue in the last 15 or more years.

Sweat, Tears, and Urine

On December 5, 2004, Senate Majority Leader Bill Frist, MD, was asked in an interview with George Stephanopolous on ABC's *This Week* if he really thought HIV could be transmitted through tears or sweat. Rather than a simple "no," Senator Frist replied that he "didn't know" if such transmission could occur as it "would be very hard. . . . I mean, you can get virus in tears and sweat but in terms of the degree of infecting somebody, it would be very hard." However, what is the evidence that HIV can be transmitted from perspiration, especially during contact sports?

When the enormously popular Magic Johnson announced in November 1991 that he was HIV-infected, the impact was tidal, well beyond its effect on American professional basketball (see Figure 1.2). His revelation of many female partners—he denied homosexual contact or intravenous drug abuse— finally drove home to many that HIV could be acquired heterosexually. Editorials bemoaned that his sports ability, fame, and personal attractiveness did not protect him from a fatal infection; then president George H.W. Bush immediately invited him to join his National Commission on AIDS; and both adults and children learned that even sports heroes can get AIDS. Yet as much as Johnson's courage was critical in finally getting Americans to understand the potential for heterosexual AIDS, the intervening years have dulled the force of this wave in the general public.[62] As indicated in Chapter 3, public apathy has increased concomitant with the increases in heterosexual HIV infections in the South, especially in African-Americans.

A darker underside to Johnson's admission was evident when he announced his intention to return to the Los Angeles Lakers a year later, only to call it off when some players in the NBA expressed fear of HIV exposure. This concern about getting HIV from contact sports percolated into the many amateur playing fields of football, basketball, baseball, and other sports. Still, Dr. Frist notwithstanding, HIV has not actually been recovered from eccrine sweat,[63] and according to one calculation the chance of a professional football player becoming infected with HIV on the field must be less than 1 in 85 million.[64]

It is true that HIV has rarely been isolated from the tears of one of seven HIV-infected persons[65] and the urine of one of five samples, and in low titers.[2] Again, any body fluid that may have white blood cells secreted in it may occasionally have detectable HIV with modern sensitive tests. However, a review in 1988 of HIV in these fluids did not find any who became HIV-infected after exposure to them[22]; nor have there been any case reports of HIV transmission by such body fluids in the intervening years.

Household Transmission

After all the experimental considerations, it still remains that a negative cannot absolutely be disproved. The Discussion sections of almost any of the articles referenced above seek to put parameters or limits on the probability of HIV transmission by any "alternate" route: one will usually read the careful, equivocating statement that the study described could not absolutely dismiss that transmission by an alternate route might occur under extreme conditions. So, what is the epidemiologic evidence of the spread of HIV whether by fomites, food, insects or nonblood exposure? Studies of nonsexual, nonparenteral (e.g., needle-sharing) contacts of HIV/AIDS patients have been critical to understanding the magnitude of risk from alternate or unproven modes of transmission; these were sometimes called "horizontal" transmission studies.

Many household transmission studies were undertaken in the 1980s.[66–68] The nonsexual household contacts of documented HIV/AIDS patients–who had casual and kissing contact and even shared razors, eating utensils, toothbrushes, and bathroom facilities with them–were carefully investigated by extensive interview and testing for HIV. An early review of 11 studies in the United States and Europe showed no (unexplained) HIV infections in over 700 nonsexual household contacts of HIV patients, especially contacts of HIV-infected children, who would not be expected to transmit to others by sexual or other means.[22] Further, European studies showed that none of an additional 699 children born to HIV-infected mothers but who were themselves HIV-negative remained so over the next 2 years despite continuing personal contact with their HIV mothers. While this also does not disprove that "horizontal" transmission between family members might occur, these studies did allow some statistical statement that even if not zero, the risk of household transmission is less than 4 per 100,000 (95% upper confidence limit by exact binomial test = 0.00367 per 100 tested persons).

Researchers could find only one instance of HIV-seroconversion in 8,596 person-years of observation of about 4,000 HIV-uninfected children in Ugandan households followed between 1989 and 1993, and the one infection detected was thought to be caused by infected breast milk (see Chapter 4). This implies an HIV infection rate of 0.12/1000 person-years of observation (py) [95% confidence that HIV transmission in these children in their households less than 0.35 per 1000 py]. If the one case detected did not represent "casual" household transmission, the chance of HIV infection from such household exposure is even less than 1 per 100,000 exposed household members.

The net result of these household studies were reassuring, and after the early 1990s no further such large studies were undertaken, nor were such claims of "casual" transmission credited in the mainstream popular media. As stated at the head of this chapter, we cannot prove a "negative," but it is informative that, with at most one exception, in prospective studies all identified HIV-infected children under a few years old have acquired HIV from birth to an infected mother or from infected breast milk.

However, there have been a few case reports that have made researchers rethink the possibility of "casual" transmission within households. In one case described in CDC's *Morbidity and Mortality Weekly Report* regarding two young HIV-infected hemophilic brothers, laboratory typing of the virus and epidemiologic investigation indicated strongly that that one brother indeed infected the other, but "several opportunities occurred for intravenous or percutaneous exposure to the [infecting] brother's blood."[69] Likewise, a report a year later described a unique virus shared by two children born to different HIV-1 infected mothers but living in the same household for 3 years and sharing the same virus (with resistance to the drug zidovudine).[70] This, too, was thought to be transmission from one child to the other "probably through unrecognized exposure to blood," but the fact that the second child no longer had HIV by antibody test 6 months later and thereafter[71] made the research community end up dismissing the report. In any case, over the last 12 years, no further instances of horizontal or "casual" transmission between two children have been reported in the medical literature.

For many of the individual case reports above, HIV/AIDS investigators were skeptical from the beginning and spent much time considering the data and its implications. Despite the inevitable irritation that a researcher may feel if a substantial portion of his or her activity for a long duration is dedicated to correcting "mis-science," there is some comfort that ultimately a correctly informed public is better able to protect itself. In all the studies above, mainly done by government and academic researchers, one impetus has always been to put the real risk of HIV infection in correct perspective.

The public should not be fatalistic because they think they can acquire HIV from several or unavoidable routes of transmission, nor should they be complacent that continued unprotected sexual activity or sharing needles, even in a low prevalence area, is safe. Indeed, current surveys even of minority adolescents[72] show reasonably good understanding of how HIV is and is not transmitted, but, as the example of Senator Frist shows, some misconceptions can persist even in highly educated people. Finally, as a caution, in areas now undergoing the most rapid increases in HIV and AIDS incidence in this country[73] and abroad, misperceptions persist. Surveyed individuals in countries such as Nigeria,[74] China,[75] or India[76] continue to show a distressingly high percentage with misunderstandings about how HIV is or is not transmitted.

References

1. Rimer, S. 1990. November 14, 1990. Spotlight fades on AIDS in town, but the disease and stigma remain. *The New York Times.*

2. Levy, J.A., L.S. Kaminsky, W.J. Morrow, et al. 1985. Infection by the retrovirus associated with the acquired immunodeficiency syndrome. *Annals of Internal Medicine* 103:694–699.

3. Office of Technology Assessment, U.S. Congress. *AIDS-Related Issues: Do Insects Transmit AIDS?* Government Printing Office, 1987.

4. Burris, S. 1985. Fear itself: AIDS, herpes and public health decisions. *Yale Law and Policy Review* 3:479–518.

5. Musto, D.F. 1986. Quarantine and the problem of AIDS. *Milbank Quarterly* 54(suppl 1):97–117.

6. Hansen, H., and N. Groce. 2001. From quarantine to condoms: shifting policies and problems of HIV control in Cuba. *Medical Anthropology* 19:259–292.

7. Hansen, H., and N. Groce. 2003. Human immunodeficiency virus and quarantine in Cuba. *Journal of the American Medical Association* 290:2875.

8. Anonymous. 2005. China: Alleged quarantine of HIV-positive people in several provinces. *HIV/AIDS Policy and Law Review* 10: 35, 37.

9. CDC. 2001. Report: Updated U.S. Public Health Service Guidelines for the Management of Occupational Exposures to HBV, HCV, and HIV and Recommendations for Postexposure Prophylaxis. *Morbidity and Mortality Weekly Report* 50(RR11): 1–42.

10. Francis, D.P., M.S. Favero, and J.E. Maynard. 1981. Transmission of hepatitis B virus. *Seminars in Liver Disease* 1:27–32.

11. Favero, M.S., J.E. Maynard, N.J. Petersen, et al. 1973. Hepatitis B antigen on environmental surfaces [letter]. *Lancet* 2:1455.

12. Lauer, J.L., N.A. VanDrunen, J.W. Washburn, and H.H. Balfour Jr. 1979. Transmission of hepatitis B virus in clinical laboratory areas. *Journal of Infectious Diseases* 140:513–516.

13. Bell, D.M. 1997. Occupational risk of human immunodeficiency virus infection in healthcare workers: An overview. *American Journal of Medicine* 102(suppl 5B):9–15.

14. Ippolito, G., V. Puro, G. De Carli, and the Italian Study Group on Occupational Risk of HIV Infection. 1993. The risk of occupational human immunodeficiency virus in health care workers. *Archives of Internal Medicine* 153:1451–1458.

15. CDC. 1987. Epidemiologic notes and reports update: Human immunodeficiency virus infections in health-care workers exposed to blood of infected patients. *Morbidity and Mortality Weekly Report* 36:285–289.

16. Fahey, B.J., D.E. Koziol, S.M. Banks, and D.K. Henderson. 1991. Frequency of nonparenteral occupational exposures to blood and body fluids before and after universal precautions training. *American Journal of Medicine* 90:145–153.

17. Henderson, D.K., B.J. Fahey, M. Willy, et al. 1990. Risk for occupational transmission of human immunodeficiency virus type 1 (HIV-1) associated with clinical exposures: A prospective evaluation. *Annals of Internal Medicine* 113:740–746.

18. Allen, J.R. 1988. Health care workers and the risk of HIV transmission. *Hastings Center Report* 18:S2–S5.

19. Day, L. 1991. *AIDS: What the Government Isn't Telling You.* Palm Desert, CA: Rockford Press.

20. Cal, A.M. March 9, 1991. Some surgeons quit over fear of AIDS, orthopedists meeting in Anaheim told. *Los Angeles Times.*

21. Tokars, J.I., M.E. Chamberland, C.A. Schable, et al. 1992. A survey of occupational blood contact and HIV infection among orthopedic surgeons. The American Academy of Orthopaedic Surgeons Serosurvey Study Committee. *Journal of the American Medical Association* 268:489–494.

22. Lifson, A.R. 1988. Do alternate modes for transmission of human immunodeficiency virus exist [review]? *Journal of the American Medical Association* 259:1353–1356.

23. Sattar, S.A., and V.S. Springthorpe. 1991. Survival and disinfectant inactivation of the human immunodeficiency virus: A critical review. *Reviews of Infectious Diseases* 13:430–437.

24. Slade, J.S., E.B. Pike, R.P. Eglin, J.S. Colbourne, and J.B. Kurtz. 1989. The survival of human immunodeficiency virus in water, sewage and sea water. *Water Science and Technology* 21:55–59.

25. Hall, C.B., R.G. Douglas Jr., and J.M. Geiman. 1980. Possible transmission by fomites of respiratory syncytial virus. *Journal of Infectious Diseases* 141:98–102.

26. Bean, B., B.M. Moore, B. Sterner, L.R. Peterson, D.N. Gerding, and H.H. Balfour Jr. 1982. Survival of influenza viruses on environmental surfaces. *Journal of Infectious Diseases* 146:47–52.

27. van Bueren, J., R.A. Simpson, P. Jacobs, and B.D. Cookson. 1994. Survival of human immunodeficiency virus in suspension and dried onto surfaces. *Journal of Clinical Microbiology* 32:571–574.

28. Srinivasan, A., D. York, and C. Bohan. 1987. Lack of HIV replication in arthropod cells [letter]. *Lancet* 1:1094–1095.

29. Leishman, K. September 1987. AIDS and insects. *The Atlantic Monthly* 260:56–72.

30. Gallo, R.C. 1986. The first human retrovirus. *Scientific American* 255:88–98

31. Becker, J.L., U. Hazan, M.T. Nugeyre, et al. 1986. [Infection of insect cells by the HIV virus, an agent of AIDS, and a demonstration of insects of African origin infected by this virus] (French). *Comptes rendus de l'Académie des sciences. Série III, Sciences de la vie* 303:303–306.

32. Chermann, J.C., J.L. Becker, U. Hazan, et al. 1987. HIV related sequences in insects from central Africa [abstract]. Presented at the Third International Conference on AIDS, Washington, DC, June 1, 1987.

33. Nordheimer, J. May 2, 1985. Poverty-scarred town now stricken by AIDS. *The New York Times.*

34. Castro, K.G., S. Lieb, H.W. Jaffe, et al. 1988. Transmission of HIV in Belle Glade, Florida: lessons for other communities in the United States. *Science* 239:193–197.

35. Ellerbrock, T.V., S. Chamblee, T.J. Bush, et al. 2004. Human immunodeficiency virus infection in a rural community in the United States. *American Journal of Epidemiology* 160:582–588.

36. Teas, J. 1983. Could AIDS agent be a new variant of African swine fever virus [letter]? *Lancet* 1:923.

37. Colaert, J., J. Desmyter, J. Goudsmit, N. Clumeck, and C. Terpstra. 1983. African swine fever virus not found in AIDS patients [letter]. *Lancet* 1:1098.

38. Bishop, G.D. 1996. Singaporean beliefs about HIV and AIDS. *Singapore Medical Journal* 37:617–621.

39. Bockarie, M.J., and R. Paru. 1996. Can mosquitoes transmit AIDS? *Papua New Guinea Medical Journal* 39:205–207.

40. CDC. 1986. Acquired immunodeficiency virus (AIDS) in western Palm Beach County, Florida. *Morbidity and Mortality Weekly Report* 35:609–612.

41. Jupp, P.G., and S.F. Lyons. 1987. Experimental assessment of bedbugs (*Cimex lectularis* and *Cimex hemipterous*) and mosquitoes (*Aedes aegypti formosus*) as vectors of human immunodeficiency virus. *AIDS* 1:171–174.

42. Lyons, S.F., P.G. Jupp, and B.D. Schoub. 1986. Survival of HIV in the common bedbug [letter]. *Lancet* 2:45.

43. Webb, P.A., C.M. Happ, G.O. Maupin, B.J.B. Johnson, C.-Y. Ou, and T.P. Monath. 1989. Potential for insect transmission of HIV: Experimental exposure of *Cimes hemipterus* and *Toxorhynchites amboinensis* to human immunodeficiency virus. *Journal of Infectious Diseases* 160:970–977.

44. Humphery-Smith, I., G. Donker, A. Turzo, C. Chastel, and H. Schmidt-Mayerova. 1993. Evaluation of mechanical transmission of HIV by the African soft tick, *Ornithodoros moubata. AIDS* 7:341–347.

45. Groopman, J.E., S.Z. Salahuddin, M.G. Sarngadharan, et al. 1984. HTLV-III in saliva of people with AIDS-related complex and healthy homosexual men at risk for AIDS. *Science* 226: 447–449.

46. Ho, D.D., R.E. Byington, R.T. Schooley, T. Flynn, T.R. Rota, and M.S. Hirsch. 1985. Infrequency of isolation of HTLV-III from saliva in AIDS. *New England Journal of Medicine* 313:1606.

47. Archibald, D.W., and G.A. Cole. 1990. In vitro inhibition of HIV-1 infectivity by human salivas. *AIDS Research and Human Retroviruses* 6:1425–1432.

48. Fox, P.C., A. Wolff, C.K. Yeh, J.C. Atkinson, and B.J. Baum. 1989. Salivary inhibition of HIV-1 infectivity: Functional properties and distribution in men, women, and children. *Journal of the American Dental Association* 118:709–711.

49. Fultz, P.N. 1986. Components of saliva inactivate human immunodeficiency virus [letter]. *Lancet* 2:1215.

50. Campo, J., M.A. Perea, J. del Romero, J. Cano, V. Hernando, and A. Bascones. 2006. Oral transmission of HIV, reality or fiction? An update. *Oral Disease* 12:219–228.

51. Habte, H.H., A.S. Mall, C. de Beer, Z.E. Lotz, and D. Kahn. 2006. The role of crude human saliva and purified salivary MUC5B and MUC7 mucins in the inhibition of Human Immunodeficiency Virus type 1 in an inhibition assay [letter]. *Virology Journal* 3:99.

52. Wahn,V., H.H. Kramer, T. Voit, H.T. Brüster, B. Scrampical, and A. Scheid. 1986. Horizontal transmission of HIV infection between two siblings [letter]. *Lancet* 2:694.

53. Anonymous. 1987. Transmission of HIV by human bite [letter]. *Lancet* 2:522.

54. Vidmar, J., M. Poljak, J. Tomazic, K. Seme, and I. Klavs. 1996. Transmission of HIV-1 by human bite [letter]. *Lancet* 347:1762–1763.

55. Andreo, S.M., L.A. Barra, L.J. Costa, M.C. Sucupira, I.E. Souza, and R.S. Diaz. 2004. HIV type 1 transmission by human bite. *AIDS Research and Human Retroviruses* 20:349–350.

56. Janssen, R.S., G.A. Satten, S.L. Stramer, et al. 1999. New testing strategy to detect early HIV-1 infection for use in incidence estimates and for clinical and prevention purposes. *Journal of the American Medical Association* 281:42–48.

57. Kothe, D., R.H. Byers, S.P. Caudill, et al. 2003. Performance characteristics of a new less sensitive HIV-1 enzyme immunoassay for use in estimating HIV seroincidence. *Journal of Acquired Immune Deficiency Syndromes* 33:625–634.

58. Parekh, B.S., D.J. Hu, S. Vanichseni, et al. 2001. Evaluation of a sensitive/less-sensitive testing algorithm using 3A11-LS assay for detecting recent HIV seroconversion among individuals with HIV-1 subtype B or E infection in Thailand. *AIDS Research and Human Retroviruses* 17:453–458.

59. Bartholomew, C.F., and A.M. Jones. 2006. Human bites: A rare risk factor for HIV transmission. *AIDS* 20:631–632.

60. CDC. 1997. Transmission of HIV possibly associated with exposure of mucous membrane to contaminated blood. *Morbidity and Mortality Weekly Report* 46:620–623.

61. Tereskerz, P.M., M. Bentley, and J. Jagger. 1996. Risk of HIV-1 infection after human bites. *Lancet* 348:1512.

62. Brown, W.J., and M.D. Basil. 1995. Media celebrities and public health: responses to 'Magic' Johnson's disclosure and its impact on AIDS risk and high-risk behaviors. *Health Communication* 7:345–370.

63. Wormser, G.P., S. Bittker, G. Forseter, et al. 1992. Absence of infectious human immunodeficiency virus type 1 in "natural" eccrine sweat. *Journal of Infectious Diseases* 165:155–158.

64. Anonymous. 1995. Study finds extremely low risk of HIV infection in football. *AIDS Policy and Law* 10:12.

65. Fujikawa, L.S., S.Z. Salhuddin, A.G. Palestine, H. Masur, R.B. Nussenblatt, and R.C. Gallo. 1985. Isolation of human T-lymphotropic virus type III from the tears of a patient with the acquired immunodeficiency syndrome [letter]. *Lancet* 2:529–530.

66. Rogers, M.F., C.R. White, R. Sanders, et al. 1990. Lack of transmission of human immunodeficiency virus from infected children to their household contacts. *Pediatrics* 85:210–214.

67. Friedland, G.H., B.R. Saltzman, M.F. Rogers, et al. 1986. Lack of transmission of HTLV-III/LAV infection to household contacts of patients with AIDS or AIDS-related complex with oral candidiasis. *New England Journal of Medicine* 314:344–349.

68. Kaplan, J.E., J.M. Oleske, J.P. Getchell, et al. 1985. Evidence against transmission of human T-lymphotropic virus/lymphadenopathy-associated virus (HTLV-III/LAV) in families of children with the acquired immunodeficiency syndrome. *Pediatric Infectious Diseases* 4:468–471.

69. CDC. 1992. HIV transmission between two adolescent brothers with hemophilia. *Morbidity and Mortality Weekly Report* 41:228–231.

70. Fitzgibbon, J.E., S.Gaur, L.D. Frenkel, F. Laraque, B.R. Edlin, and D.T. Dubin. 1993. Transmission from one child to another of human immunodeficiency virus type 1 with a zidovudine-resistance mutation. *New England Journal of Medicine* 329:1835–1841.

71. Gaur, S., L.D. Frenkel, D.T. Dubin, and F. Laraque. 1994. Reply: Transmission of HIV-1 from one child to another [letter]. *New England Journal of Medicine* 330:1314.

72. Cohall, A., J. Kassotis, R. Parks, R. Vaughan, H. Bannister, and M. Northridge. 2001. Adolescents in the age of AIDS: myths, misconceptions, and misunderstandings regarding sexually transmitted diseases. *Journal of the National Medical Association* 93:64–69.

73. Hancock, T., B.I. Mikhail, A. Santos, A. Nguyen, H. Nguyen, and D. Bright. 1999. A comparison of HIV/AIDS knowledge among high school freshman and senior students. *Journal of Community Health Nursing* 16:151–163.

74. Iliyasu, Z., I.S. Abubakar, M. Kabir, and M.H. Aliyu. 2006. Knowledge of HIV/AIDS and attitude towards voluntary counseling and testing among adults. *Journal of the National Medical Association* 98:1917–1922.

75. Derlega, V.J., X. Yang, and H. Luo. 2006. Misconceptions about HIV transmission, stigma and willingness to take sexual risks in southwestern China. *International Journal of STD and AIDS* 17:406–409.

76. Kalasagar, M., B. Sivapathasundharam, and T.B. Einstein. 2006. AIDS awareness in Indian metropolitan slum dwellers: A KAP (knowledge, attitude, practice) study. *Indian Journal of Dental Research* 17:66–69.

CHAPTER SIX

Issues in Prevention

Despite the fact that we understand the agent of AIDS, how it is transmitted, and the risk factors for acquiring it—and despite many successes[1]—most would admit that HIV prevention efforts have been difficult and only partially successful. Behavioral interventions for HIV must change the most intimate and compulsive of human sexual or addictive behaviors, behaviors often modulated by the effect of drugs, alcohol, or money.

It is extremely difficult, if even possible, to get a truly contemporaneous estimate of current HIV incidence (Chapter 3) and, thereby, the effectiveness of various prevention programs. AIDS cases reflect HIV infections acquired years previous, and HIV reports also usually reflect infections acquired years before. As described in Chapter 3, new methodologies for detecting recent HIV infection among those testing positive—such as sensitive/less sensitive testing (STARHS[2]) or use of HIV RNA testing[3]—may pick up only a few "new" infections among many tested. The small numbers of new infections detected and unknown sensitivity and specificity of these testing methods to detect early HIV infection means that the confidence intervals on any estimated HIV incidence rate are quite large. Thus, aside from specific studies of specific groups, we are often left looking at current AIDS rates to assess effectiveness of prevention efforts a decade ago. Also, because of the widespread use of highly active antiretroviral therapy (HAART) since 1996, it has become essentially impossible to do back-calculation, because AIDS trends no longer reflect the natural history of the disease.[4]

HIV Testing

Fully one quarter of HIV-infected Americans are thought to be unaware of their HIV status,[5, 6] although up to 80 percent have had the opportunity for such testing in health-care settings such as emergency rooms.[7, 8] From a medical perspective, earlier detection of HIV would allow clinicians to provide better therapy earlier.[9] All treatment guidelines recommend treatment be started before the HIV patient's CD4+ lymphocyte count has declined to under 200 cells/mm.[3, 10] Also, from a public health perspective, persons unaware they are infected are estimated to be threefold more likely than people aware they are infected to spread HIV to others,[11] so HIV "screening" or testing of persons at risk of infection must be a cornerstone of HIV prevention.[12, 13] However, mandated testing of any persons at risk of HIV infection has not been adopted in the United States.

"AIDS exceptionalism," the treatment of HIV infection as distinct from other diseases and conditions, has been controversial throughout the AIDS epidemic. People are not tested for HIV at the discretion of their doctor in the same manner they would be tested or scanned for any other disease. Since the introduction of a commercial EIA test for HIV, specific, written and informed consent must be obtained before an American citizen is tested for HIV. The reasons for "AIDS exceptionalism" have been based on political and social concerns about identifying and stigmatizing already marginalized groups—gay men, injection drug users, women who trade sex. For example, name-based reporting and identification of persons testing HIV-positive in Colorado after 1986 initially led to several fold drops in gay men voluntarily getting tested.[14]

Part of the controversy stems from conventional approaches to controlling infectious diseases that were developed in the nineteenth century and to which public health and policy tend to revert. These measures include: mandatory testing and identification of infected person's and measures such as quarantine or isolation. Indeed, the initial reaction to AIDS in some quarters was to advocate procedures that were used for acute, self-limited infectious disease outbreaks. Nonetheless, it was clear to many that given the potentially tens or hundreds of thousands of U.S. AIDS patients anticipated even by the early 1980s quarantine was not at all a practical option.[15]

Mandatory testing has remained attractive to some, as they argue that 10–15 percent of HIV-infected persons would not have learned of their HIV status unless they were mandated to receive an HIV test to get health insurance or to enter the armed services.[16] Thus, legislative bills requiring premarital mandatory HIV testing were first considered in the late 1980s. Only two states, Illinois and Louisiana, enacted and enforced them; but Louisiana repealed its testing statute 7 months after it became effective; and Illinois repealed its statute 20 months after it became effective. During the period that the Illinois statute was in effect, less than 0.02 percent of those tested were found to be HIV-seropositive.[17] Two other states, Missouri and Texas, adopted conditional, mandatory premarital HIV testing statutes. Missouri has retained its statute but does not actively enforce it, and Texas repealed its statute in 1991. Thus, many states now require that parties applying for a marital license must be offered an HIV test and/or must be provided with information on AIDS and tests available.

The short life spans of the Louisiana and Illinois mandatory testing statutes are attributable to the constitutional and public policy problems with the legislation. Laws mandating HIV testing may violate an individual's constitutional right to due process or equal protection under the Fourteenth Amendment and unreasonable search and seizure (blood drawing) under the Fourth Amendment.[17] And, from a scientific or public health and policy viewpoint, such mandatory testing will detect very few previously unknown infections, will drive persons worried about their HIV status "underground" (or to other states to be married), and does not necessarily lead to behavior changes in sexual risk and probability of spreading HIV to others. Beyond the constitutional and ethical issues, one economic evaluation indicated that under likely conditions the cost per case of HIV infection prevented would be between $70,000 and $127,000.[18] So, for legislative, ethical, constitutional, economic and, not least, public health reasons, mandatory testing of U.S. citizens has not been used in prevention efforts.

Beyond constitutional issues, there have been many personal barriers to getting tested. People often cannot or do not want to articulate to their doctor or interviewer the real reasons they avoid or decline offered testing. When they do provide reasons, these include optimistic denial of HIV risks, assumption that their doctor would perform it without asking permission, not receiving information about HIV, fear of discrimination, and general issues of mistrust and fear of the medical or political establishment.[19–21] Not often included on surveys are the fear of how such knowledge will necessitate changing one's sexual and social life; how asymptomatic infection with a chronic and potentially lethal virus may not be a particular concern in lives already stressed by other life events such as home eviction, imprisonment of self or family members, unemployment, and other more immediately pressing issues; or general laziness or procrastination in dealing with a medical problem that at the time does not present any symptoms. Regarding the last, people are generally unlikely to admit to such human frailty.

While many people who avoid HIV testing are poor, minority, or foreign-born, all U.S. populations have members who will avoid getting tested. For example, in our initial CDC cohort studies of homosexual and bisexual men in San Francisco, Chicago, and Denver,[22] up to 15 percent of the San Francisco cohort in 1986 and 1987 wanted to be part of the study, but refused to receive their HIV test results. (Oddly, many nonetheless wanted to know their CD4+ cell count, which if low, was a strong indicator of HIV infection.) These gay men were generally white, had been well educated—almost 90 percent had a high school diploma or more—and had middle-class incomes. A similar situation pertained to the NIAID's Multicenter AIDS Cohort Study (MACS) in its first years.[23] Anecdotally, we know that many felt that that since there was no treatment—until zidovudine (AZT) became available in 1987—an HIV-positive test result was tantamount to a death sentence. The psychologic stress from having a positive test result was a serious concern of many.[23]

Although by 1990 all members of the CDC cohort were either persuaded by the study staff or because of illness knew their HIV status, there were still some cohort-participants who delayed getting tested until they had AIDS-defining conditions.[24] Thus, it is not surprising to many HIV epidemiologists and public health personnel that even in an era of HAART (that is, effective combination therapy or "drug cocktail" for HIV), about 40–50 percent of all infected persons, especially injection drug users and men and women infected heterosexually, nonetheless do not get tested for HIV until they are sick. Such persons typically find out they are HIV-infected at the time or within a year of their initial AIDS symptoms and diagnosis.[25,26] Anxiety about having an HIV diagnosis, denial of their risk for HIV, misperceptions about the efficacy of modern therapy, and fear of legal or social repercussions are some reasons offered for such delay.[27]

Required testing for health or life insurance, military induction, and immigration still accounts for about 13–15 percent of adults who become aware of their HIV seropositive status.[26] Further, aliens visiting the United States must also be tested for HIV since 1987,[28] a legislation of dubious value as an infected visitor is not any more likely than an American to infect anyone or to affect the 40,000 incident HIV infections acquired in this country yearly. In fact, the symbolic and practical implications of this politically motivated legislation led the International AIDS Society to cease holding the International AIDS Conference in the United States after 1987.

Given that mandatory testing of most American populations had so many problems, the public health community has offered voluntary HIV testing under two different rubrics, "routine" testing and "anonymous" testing. In general, before 2006 U.S. guidelines for testing have recommended "routine" and "confidential" HIV counseling and testing for persons at high risk for HIV and for those in acute-settings in which HIV prevalence is greater than

1 percent.[29] That is, all patients at putative risk of HIV infection, whether in hospital, clinic, or emergency room, should be actively encouraged to get HIV tested, and such testing necessitates pre- and posttest counseling.

In particular, the one kind of transmission that was both preventable and within the health care setting was transmission from HIV-infected mother-to-infant, which could be prevented with prophylactic drug therapy. In 1998, the Institute of Medicine (IOM) recommended the testing of all pregnant women in the United States, calling for a shift from stringent consent to an informed right of refusal,[30] so-called "opt-out" testing. A year later, the American Academy of Pediatrics and the American College of Obstetricians and Gynecologists jointly endorsed universal opt-out screening for pregnant women. When the CDC considered these recommendations in 2001, it endorsed universal screening of pregnant women.[31] But, while calling for a simplified pretest process counseling, it did not explicitly recommend an opt-out approach that does testing unless specifically declined by the patient.

Still, such routine encouragement of HIV testing has been accepted by 93 percent of parturient women, and mother-to-child transmission (MTCT) of HIV is now thought to account for fewer than 50 infections per year.[32] Prenatal screening of pregnant women, along with screening the blood supply, have been singular successes in preventing HIV transmission in the United States.

If presented as a standard or routine procedure, permission is more likely to be acceptable to populations of particular concern, such as inner-city African American women.[21] However, the unpleasant truth is that people who accept "voluntary" testing are more likely to accept such testing when the care provider believes in it and presents it in a subtly coercive way, that is, without explaining and ensuring "explicit informed consent"[33] and the patient has low general health knowledge.[34]

"Anonymous" testing offers a way to get tested without having one's name or other identifying information recorded in a national database. This is distinct from "name-based" reporting of positive HIV test results as has been enforced in Colorado and Arizona for the past 20 years, and is now also mandated in 31 states. Some important jurisdictions are leery of name-based reporting, such as in California, where some researchers cite test-taker concerns[35] while others do not find a deterrent effect or avoidance of HIV testing because of name-based (but confidential) reporting.[36] The theory is that fear of having one's name in such a database is a major reason people who need it do not get HIV tests; however, surveys do not find this fear a major reason for test avoidance.[37]

Underlying the controversy is that anonymous testing is frustrating to public health personnel, as patients cannot be contacted or followed; indeed, about 37 percent of persons tested at publicly funded confidential testing sites—approximately 10 percent of all those tested for HIV in the United States—especially young African Americans,[38,39] and about half of all adolescents who get anonymously tested don't return to get their HIV test results;[40] and so there is no way to inform them if they are HIV-seropositive. Nor can patients who are not HIV-infected but who do not return be adequately counseled posttesting. Thus, some States have eliminated anonymous testing in their publicly funded clinics, but this has not seemed to affect overall testing rates.[41] However, it is fair to say that there has remained a lack of consensus among researchers and policymakers about voluntary vs. mandatory HIV testing even in constrained environments such as prisons,[42] where consent is still obtained. The largest survey of anonymous HIV testing, the Multistate Evaluation of Surveillance of HIV (MESH) Study[43] concluded that, whatever its problems, anonymous testing contributed to early HIV testing and medical care.

One type of anonymous testing, home-testing kits, have been available since the mid-1990s. Public health officials have especially not liked this method of testing as it is likely to be done without pre- and posttest counseling. Still, it was approved for use by the FDA in 1996. Some felt based on preliminary testing from those provided with such kits that these would be a "safe and effective alternative" to conventional testing.[44] However, several years later, only about 1 percent of all persons tested for HIV had cited using home test kits.[45] In fact, there was such a distinct lack of public interest in these tests that Johnson & Johnson, maker of one of the two kits offered, discontinued its production of "Confide" kits in August 1997.[46] The concern that many would get tested outside the medical or public health system, and not receive appropriate counseling and referral to HIV care, has not materialized.

Another important advance has been the introduction of "rapid" saliva or finger-stick tests for HIV that allow the practitioner to give results of HIV testing to a patient within minutes rather than many days later. While many patients find such testing stressful—that is, very anxiety-provoking to know they will receive test results rapidly[47]—these tests are increasingly used as an initial screening tactic in sites where HIV prevalence in the community is high, such as inner-city emergency rooms and STD clinics.

An example of how widespread testing may increasingly affect the U.S. HIV epidemic is the practice of gay men in San Francisco and elsewhere to "serosort." Recently appreciated and described by public health researchers, serosorting is the practice of only having sex with men of the same serostatus— that is, HIV-antibody-seropositive with seropositive men, and seronegative men with seronegative men.[48] Serosorting is being increasingly adopted, rather than condom use, by young gay men,[49–51] but its effectiveness is limited by at least two factors. The first is that, while it may decrease HIV transmission, gay men in San Francisco have experienced ongoing syphilis and other sexually transmitted infections, often in HIV-seropositive men who "serosort" and have sex with each other.[52] Thus, one "cost" of this method of reducing the HIV epidemic is an increase in other diseases, that may be especially difficult to treat and control in HIV-infected persons. Another problem is that, while knowledge of one's own HIV serostatus remains high, usually above 90 percent, in surveys of men who have sex with men in California, one must trust that partners are telling the truth about their serostatus. These two factors limit the effectiveness of serosorting.

After all the data and controversy supporting or not supporting mandatory or voluntary testing–whether confidential and name-based vs. anonymous– the fact still remains that many who are HIV-infected, especially heterosexual men and women, do not know it and are spreading HIV to others. Again, it appears that 80 percent of these are seen in healthcare venues well before they are diagnosed with HIV or AIDS. In an era in which HAART can substantially improve the longevity and quality of life of HIV-infected persons–often with only one, two, or a few pills a day–early identification of HIV-infected persons has become ever more a medical and public health necessity.

Despite success in some areas, because the incidence of HIV infection is thought to have remained at about 40,000 new infections each year for the last 10 or more years,[53–55] and given new technologies such as rapid tests, the pendulum of opinion has swung to stressing ever more routine HIV testing in clinical settings.[56] The era of "AIDS exceptionalism" seems to be coming to a close.[57]

A seminal event has been CDC's most recently revised recommendations for HIV testing (September 2006), in which the concept of "opt-out" testing is being studied and encouraged.[54] Under the "opt-out" strategy, HIV testing is included as part of the patient's overall consent to receive care at an emergency room, clinic, or in-hospital ward, with the proviso that patients still retain the right to decline testing. "Opt-out" testing will not be implemented widely immediately, as most states have statutes from the 1980s requiring pre-test counseling and explicit and separate informed consent for HIV testing. However, in situations in which such "opt-out" testing has been adopted, especially for prenatal HIV testing of women, this has resulted in a dramatic increase in the number of pregnant women being tested for HIV.[58] We have moved from an era in which fear and relative therapeutic powerlessness had to be balanced against respect for autonomy and privacy rights–that is, away from policies and practices that would only drive the epidemic further underground–to an era in which patients need to be more strongly encouraged to be tested for their own and the greater public's benefit.

The Person at Risk, or the Person Known to Be HIV-Infected?

The consideration of best testing strategies segues, again, to why public health personnel want to identify HIV-infected persons. One clear evolution in the HIV epidemic has been a shift in focus from the person at risk of HIV to the HIV-infected person who poses that risk.[56] At the beginning of the U.S. epidemic, much effort went into the provision of information to citizens on how to protect themselves from infection. Establishment of CDC's National AIDS information line (1983) and the National AIDS Clearinghouse (1987) were important steps in trying to provide objective information to the public. The nationwide mailing of the brochure *Understanding AIDS* (1988), a brochure fostered by then Surgeon General Koop, was historic in that this was the first public health mailing delivered to every U.S. residential mailing address.[59] This symbolic mailing was criticized as some thought that the millions of dollars required for the mailing effort might be better directed to targeted prevention programs, although public officials publicly skirted stating so directly.[60]

Such behavioral intervention programs rest on the assumption that persons will be more willing to change their behavior to protect themselves than to protect others. There is a general agreement that providing correct and clearly enunciated risk information to persons at risk of HIV infection forms the first bulwark in preventing HIV transmission. As seen from the trends in AIDS cases in Figure 3.2, gay men realized their risk and adjusted their behavior early in the epidemic. An extensive meta-analysis of behavioral interventions for reducing sexual risk behavior in them presents overwhelming evidence that risk reduction programs are effective in men who have sex with men.[61] Similarly, prevention interventions have also reduced the risky sex behaviors of injection drug users.[62] Many behavioral intervention programs for those at risk have been implemented and investigated; more than 50 interventions for populations at risk have been packaged for use in local HIV prevention programs.[56, 63] Prevention efforts have been effective, but not completely so and not always demonstrably so.

What has been somewhat less appreciated is that each advance in diagnosis and treatment has engendered changes in the sexual strategies of some people in reaction to complex, somewhat conflicting and shifting information. For example, it has been thought for some time that HIV-infected persons with high viral loads and low CD4+ cells counts are more likely to transmit virus to their sex partners (see Chapter 4).[64–66] Conversely, HAART ther-apy reduces viral load in blood and genital secretions, so may be important as a way of combating further HIV transmission.[66, 67] In truth, antiretro-viral therapy does diminish but does eliminate HIV in semen.[68, 69] Also, drug-resistant strains of virus, engendered by HAART, may also leave viral strains at a "fitness cost" in terms of their replicative capacity.[70] So, in sum, HAART-takers may have more drug-resistant HIV strains that are possibly less likely to transmit HIV.[71] Use of HAART by infected persons in the San Francisco gay community putatively reduced their infectiousness,[72] and re-searchers in Amsterdam likewise reported declining trend in transmission of drug-resistant HIV-1.[73] However, drug-resistant viruses and other organisms frequently have adaptive mechanisms[74] which may ultimately help them compensate a temporarily reduced replication rate. There is also no denying that the more frequent acquisition of drug-resistant strains of HIV by newly infected persons poses a major medical and public health problem.

This scientific murkiness as to whether HAART therapy by both lowering HIV viral load in treated persons and also increasing drug-resistant strains is a net gain, a net loss, or a "wash" in terms of our ability to decrease HIV trans-mission is further complicated by the behaviors of persons taking HAART. Even in the pre-HAART era, and although an undocumented observation, we know that in some of our studies that some HIV-infected homosexual[67, 75] and heterosexual men[76, 77] viewed high CD4+ cell counts and low viral loads, as provided to them during these studies, as indices of their diminished infec-tiousness to their partners. More recently there may have been increases in risky sexual behaviors by persons starting HAART.[78–82] For example, stud-ies in Alabama showed that effective therapy with protease inhibitor drugs led to decreased use of condoms in HIV-infected gay men.[83] Others have likewise found that response to HAART was associated with increasing risk behaviors in injection drug users.[84]

Thus, the benefit of modern antiretroviral therapy and attendant increases in immunologic competence and decreased shedding and transmission of HIV[66, 67, 69] must be balanced against potentially increased risk behavior by those receiving or anticipating better HIV treatments.[37] Again, it is not clear how much such behavior occurs in those taking HAART,[78] and how much it diminishes the possible advantages of HAART in reducing viral infectiousness.

Another factor limiting prevention effectiveness is so-termed "recidivism" in risk behavior. Sustaining safe sex behaviors often lapses in men who have sex with men, as does avoidance of drugs and sustaining safe injection practices in drug users.[85] In released prisoners, "recidivism" also refers to poor adherence to HIV therapeutic drugs, relapse to criminal behavior, and reincarceration.[86, 87] In contrast to data from one-time cross-sectional studies of people's behavior, following them over time shows considerable instability in risk reduction.[85] Further, some groups such as adolescents, urban minorities, and African Americans living in the rural and small-city South have traditionally been difficult to convince in the first place of the possibility of infection and the need for behavioral changes to avoid it.

Again, the immutable fact has been that the estimated number of new HIV infections–40,000 per year–had not substantially changed since 1992, and new thinking was needed to further reduce this unacceptable condition. The continuing high incidence of HIV in the United States; behavioral recidivism among those at risk; the replenishment of transmission risk groups with new members who did not recognize their risk for infection; the availability of effective therapies for HIV after 1995 and the need to get HIV-infected people to adhere to them; the preliminary data suggesting that HIV-infected patients who were treated were less infectious to their partners; the availability of rapid tests to identify HIV-infected persons (rather than lose many who do not return to get their results); and the greater use of "opt-out" testing to identify more people with HIV infection: all these were among the important factors that led many thoughtful public health personnel to the conclusion that more focus needed to be placed on changing behavior of those who were identified as already HIV-infected. In 1999, a review of 55 state and city applications to CDC for HIV prevention programs showed that only 18 (33%) were focused in part or mainly on HIV-infected persons as the target population.[88]

Thus, in 2001, CDC introduced the Serostatus Approach to Fighting the HIV Epidemic (SAFE), which represented a new or additional paradigm in combating the epidemic.[88] In contrast to the great majority of previous prevention programs aimed at reducing risk of infection in susceptible persons, SAFE provided a framework for improving the health of already HIV-infected persons and preventing their transmission to others. Briefly put, the objectives of SAFE are to (1) increase the number of HIV-infected persons who know they are infected; (2) increase the use of health care and preventive services by them and by the estimated 5 million Americans at most risk of HIV; (3) increase high-quality care and treatment; (4) increase adherence to antiretroviral therapy by infected persons; and (5) increase the number of individuals with HIV who adopt and sustain HIV risk reduction behavior. In 2003, CDC also described the Advancing HIV Prevention (AHP) Initiative,[89] which adopted prevention with persons living with HIV as an important focus of a comprehensive approach to HIV prevention.

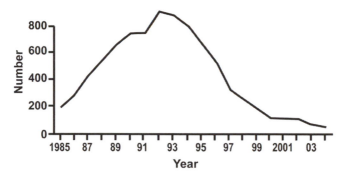

Figure 6.1 Estimated number of cases of perinatally acquired AIDS, by year of diagnosis—United States, 1985–2004. From reference 90: data adjusted for reporting delays and for estimated proportional redistribution of cases reported without an identified risk factor.

Preventing Mother-to-Infant Spread

Prevention of MTCT has been one of the signal successes of fighting the AIDS epidemic. In an appropriately titled "Achievements in Public Health,"[90] CDC has recently documented the decline in perinatal AIDS cases and HIV transmission over the past 20 years. Figure 6.1 shows these dramatic declines in reported AIDS cases.

In the United States, considering the size and composition of typical working groups,[54, 90] it appears that there are now more perinatal AIDS experts than there are perinatal AIDS cases.

In general, an infected woman who is not identified as such and without prenatal antiretroviral treatment has a 25–30 percent chance of transmitting to her infant. (Early in the HIV/AIDS epidemic, infant infection was hard to determine for the first several months after birth as, while most newborns would not acquire HIV, all do acquire maternal HIV antibodies that would show as EIA antibody-test positive. This problem has been ameliorated but not completely eliminated with the use of HIV RNA tests.) With antiretroviral therapy—even single monotherapy with zidovudine in the 1990s[91]—this rate of transmission was reduced to a few percentage of newborns of HIV-infected mothers. In the United States, HAART (combinations of a protease inhibitor or a non-nucleoside RTI plus two nucleoside RTIs) has reduced MTCT to less than 2 percent. Neonatal antiretroviral prophylaxis is given as well, usually within fewer than 12 hours after birth.

Despite such gains in the United States, substantial challenges and controversies remain in reducing MTCT worldwide.[92] Some of these, such as extending prenatal identification of HIV-infected mothers and getting them appropriate drug therapy, especially in the developing world, are laudable goals shared by everyone. Others, such as whether breast milk can transmit HIV, have been pretty much settled in the affirmative. Initially, this was questioned as HIV is not transmitted in foods and there are many salivary factors in the mouth and gastric juices in the stomach to inactivate the virus. However, newborns lack their own immunoglobulins and salivary components and have much lower gastric acidity than adults. By the end of the 1980s, transmission of HIV after birth, presumably via breast milk, had already been seen in at least a handful of cases.[93] Accordingly, when possible, bottle-feeding of infants by HIV-infected mothers is recommended.

In resource-limited areas such as sub-Saharan Africa less intensive regimens with zidovudine, lamivudine, and nevirapine as single drugs or in combination still substantially reduce MTCT. A major debate now is about the use of non-nucleoside reverse transcriptase inhibitors (RTIs), specifically nevaripine, for prophylaxis of mother-to-child spread during childbirth. Single-dose nevirapine is safe, inexpensive, and effective for prevention of MTCT in the developing world.[94] However, in the early 2000s, nevirapine was denounced as a "poison" by South Africa's Minister of Health, Manto Tshabalala-Msimang.[95] The reasons given for this startling declaration were that the U.S. Food and Drug Agency had not approved nevirapine for this use (for parturient mothers); some thought that this was in keeping with South Africa's official resistance to acknowledging HIV as the cause of AIDS and the moral imperative, and expense, of dealing with it.[95] In 2000, President Mbeki avowed his skepticism of the link between HIV and AIDS, despite hosting the International AIDS Conference in Durban that very year.

It is true that nevirapine use engenders viral drug resistance both to itself and to other members of the same class of drugs, that is, other non-nucleoside drugs such as efavirenz, used widely as part of initial HAART in developed countries and increasingly in others. K103N-containing human immunodeficiency virus (HIV)-1 mutations are selected in some women who receive single-dose nevirapine for prevention of HIV-1 mother-to-infant transmission. Even after a single dose of nevirapine, K103N-carrying variants (resistant mutants) can be detected 6–8 weeks later in over 40 percent of women.[96] Such drug resistance may compromise the efficacy of nevirapine for subsequent pregnancies of the women, for infants born to mothers who received nevirapine (requiring resistance testing before their treatment)[97] and, more generally, use of non-nucleoside RTIs widely in the general population. However, while resistant strains can persist at low levels in the absence of antiretroviral drug exposure in persons infected with resistant strains, in those who discontinue non-nucleoside RTI therapy, these resistant strains usually wane over a period of several months.[98, 99]

At the time of this writing, this controversy is not resolved, although some think that such resistance is counterbalanced by the safety, low cost, and efficacy of single-dose nevirapine in resource-constrained settings. However, given the political furor over this issue, this problem will probably only be resolved by more widespread provision of multidrug therapy (without nevirapine) in the developing world as is currently available in the developed countries.

Needle and Syringe Exchange; Condom Provision

Provision of clean needles to addicts and condoms to sexually active adults and adolescents has been hampered by the attitude that giving people the means to protect themselves from HIV and other sexually transmitted diseases encourages them to have sex or to inject drugs. While this attitude has prevailed in some political circles, in fact, the data do not support such claims.

Injection drug use is thought to account for about 25–33 percent of all new HIV cases, and almost all hepatitis C virus (HCV) infections, in the United States; looked at the other way, over 20 percent of injection drug users on the East Coast have HIV infection, and 70 percent or more nationally have hepatitis C.[100] (Why the HIV infection prevalence in injection drug users on the West Coast has remained under 5 percent but on the East Coast over 20 percent has remained a mystery.[101]). Sharing HIV contaminated needles is the most efficient manner of transmission, so needle and syringe exchange programs (NSEPs), which have been informally run as early as the 1970s, are thought to be useful for the over one million injection drug users in the United States in the 1990s. Most public health officials have felt that state laws criminalizing possession of injection equipment have actually fueled continued spread among needle and syringe exchanging drug users.

There were about 140 operational NSEPs in the United States in the mid-1990s.[102] This number may be compared with, for example, the 3,000 NSEPs at the same time in Australia. In the United States, the Republican House and Senate felt that NSEPs condoned or, worse, actually stimulated drug use.

In the mid-1990s there was little conclusive information about the impact of NSEPs in the United States, which is a reason CDC started the seven-city Collaborative Injection Drug User Study (CIDUS) in 1993.[103] Although NSEPs were widely used in other developed countries, CIDUS and other U.S. studies ultimately showed that access to such programs did not foster increased drug use but did indeed reduce transmission of blood-borne viruses such as HIV and HCV in this country.[103–107] Nonetheless, despite meetings and consensus even among government doctors and public health officials as to the utility of NSEPs, in April 1998 the U.S. House of Representatives passed legislation (H.R. 3717) on a "fast track" to permanently ban federal funding for needle exchange programs in the United States.[108] President Bill Clinton's administration refused to lift the ban, even though then Health and Human Services Secretary Donna Shalala cited reports that led her to believe NSEPs did not, in fact, encourage more injection drug use.[109] Thus, while CDC and NIH were funding studies that were showing that NSEPs not only did not increase drug use but effectively reduced HIV and HCV transmission (whereas provision of bleach for disinfection of needles was probably not efficacious),[110] the legislative and Chief Executive arms of the government had passed legislation that precluded the use of these data for rational funding for preventing HIV and HCV in injection drug users. That is, even sympathetic legislators had found NSEPs too controversial or risky to support[111]; and the controversy was eventually trumped by political concerns rather than scientific data.

Currently, there are still only about 150 NSEPs in this country, half of whom are supported by local and not-for-profit organizations, and usually located in cities with strong political activism, such as a local ACT-UP chapter, rather than necessarily cities with the most need.[112]

The same attitude toward provision of sterile needles and syringes to drug addicts—that it encourages drug use—has been applied to providing condoms or sex education to teenagers and others—as some think that such encourages sexual activity. The evidence that condom use would protect against HIV, STDs, and unwanted pregnancies has been dismissed by the current George W. Bush Administration in favor of abstinence-only programs. Technically, this is presented as the "ABC" approach to combating sexual transmission of HIV: Abstinence; Being Monogamous; and Condoms. Under the Bush administration, this is widely and cynically known in the public health community as a program of "Anything But Condoms."

What is the evidence for "abstinence only"? The Abstinence Clearinghouse (www.abstinence.net) lists 15 studies that purportedly show the effectiveness of abstinence programs, eight of which have been published in peer-reviewed journals. In the most prominent of these, the 10 percent of boys and 16 percent of girls who reported having taken a pledge to remain a virgin were at "significantly lower risk of early age of sexual debut."[113] This descriptive and exploratory study—that was mainly about suicide and substance use prevention—did not specify the length of this delay in sexual debut, was not a comparison of taking the "virginity pledge" with any other intervention, and did not adjust analysis for other collinear factors affecting the minority taking a virginity pledge, such as whether they had better relationships at home and school, or were simply more religious and abstemious regardless of the virginity pledge.[113] Also, such reports and their interpretations elide over the fact that no one questions teaching sexual abstinence to the young, only using it as the sole policy to reduce HIV, STDs, and unwanted pregnancies, eschewing sex-education programs.

Nonetheless, abstinence-only programs have received from the federal government at least $158 million per year, $1.5 billion over the past decade. Compared with 1995, more teenagers were receiving abstinence-only education in 2002, and fewer received instruction about birth control methods; only 62 percent of adolescent women and 54 percent of adolescent men had received instruction about birth-control methods before their first sex.[114] (Seventy-seven percent of Americans have had first sexual intercourse before age 20.)

In 1999, CDC published a fact sheet with messages to encourage sexually active people to use condoms to prevent HIV and other STIs. In 2001, under pressure from anticondom activists within the Bush Administration, CDC removed that document, replacing it a year later with a different fact sheet. While there are many nuanced differences between the two fact sheets, the 2002 fact sheet shows a bias within the administration toward promoting abstinence over condom use, even for those who are sexually active.

For example, in December 2002, about 20 high-level health officials were summoned by Claude Allen, then Deputy Secretary at the Department of Health and Human Services–he was indicted 3 years later for felonious shoplifting–to a "workshop" on HIV risk avoidance. This was known facetiously by some of the participants as an "abstinence boot camp" where they spent an entire day learning of the importance of stressing premarital sexual abstinence. When asked how abstinence would apply to gay men who cannot have marital sex, the reply was that it didn't matter, they should be abstinent, presumably forever. Contractors told these high-level health officials or researchers about the studies they were doing or planned to do on this subject, and these doctors had to listen to what one dubbed a "professional virgin."

So, what has been the effect of the $1.5 billion spent federal government on programs to foster abstinence-until-marriage? The idée fixe by some that AIDS in America could be effectively countered by teaching teenagers not to have sex before marriage was strongly contradicted in April 2007 by the preliminary release of Congressionally funded and mandated study results by Mathematica Policy Research, Inc., which showed that high school students who participated in sexual abstinence programs were just as likely to have sex a few years later as those who did not.[115] Supporters of abstinence-only teaching sometimes point to the recent decline in pregnancy rates in recent years, but researchers have found that, in fact, 86 percent of the decline can be attributed to greater and more effective use of condoms.[116]

In summary, "best-evidence" scientific analyses continue to stress the importance of provision of condoms and clean needles and syringes to reduce the HIV epidemic in the United States.[1] However, as of the time of this writing, use of neither is supported by the U.S. federal government. Some political debates may not be resolved by facts.

Circumcision

One major current and very interesting debate has been about the effectiveness of circumcision or a lack of foreskin as protective against HIV acquisition by men. To date, this has mainly been a debate about controlling HIV in Africa, but many see wider implications. It has long been thought that the friable, easily abraded, foreskin, might allow easier transmission of HIV than for penises that do not have a prepuce. Further, the foreskin is rich in HIV target cells (e.g., CD4+ cells, macrophages, Langerhans', and other cells). The biologic plausibility seemed to gain some credence when the earliest ecological analyses from Africa showed geographic concordance between areas in Africa that commonly practiced circumcision of men and low HIV prevalence.[117] However, as noted, ecologic arguments–this one essentially geographic–are considered the weakest evidence. Compared to uncircumcised men, circumcised men probably had many religious and cultural as well as geographic differences. Small distances in Africa can imply major cultural and sexual behavior differences, and underlying background prevalence of HIV in the community has a major effect on one's likelihood of acquiring it. So, one would like to see a comparison of uncircumcised and circumcised men in one geographic area, with similar sex behavior, and essentially similar risk of acquiring HIV.

Indeed, as the "next step up" from ecological analyses, several cross-sectional studies in the early 1990s also came to a similar conclusion: analysis of 18 cross-sectional studies from six countries showed various mixed results, but concluded an overall statistically significant association between male circumcision and protection from HIV infection.[118] A revisiting of the whole issue in 1999 found that when data from 29 studies were pooled, circumcised men were actually at a greater risk of acquisition and transmission of HIV.[119] However, in a contemporaneous analysis stratifying rather than "pooling" the various studies, others found that an intact foreskin increased an (African) man's risk of HIV infection by roughly 50 percent.[120]

Advocating even a minor surgical procedure as a way to combat AIDS has been viewed with some skepticism and reluctance, especially when the different analyses of similar data come to contradictory conclusions. Which men would submit to circumcision; what would be the soft tissue infection rate; more important, would newly circumcised men inappropriately consider themselves relatively immune to HIV infection and so increase their HIV sexual risk behaviors? These and many questions continue to worry the more cautious, and there was always the comfortable defense that lacking a randomized prospective study we should not advocate circumcising adult African (or any) men as a way to combat HIV transmission.

However, now, researchers in Rakai, Uganda, in collaboration with Johns Hopkins University[121] and in Kisumu, Kenya, in association with the University of Illinois at Chicago[122] have recently published randomized controlled trials of male circumcision as a procedure to prevent HIV acquisition. Such prospective studies, that randomize comparable men from the same locality and with the same background and behaviors to either receive or not receive circumcision represents probably the strongest study design of this difficult issue. In both studies, male circumcision reduced HIV incidence by half in men so treated; this protective effect was not affected by sex behaviors following the intervention (circumcision) time, which were essentially the same in both the circumcised and uncircumcised men. Both studies, finding such strong treatment effects, were terminated at 24 months.

We are now in an interesting circumstance: should we ramp up circumcision for African and other men, perhaps in the United States and other developed countries as well? Many are understandably anxious[123]: will circumcised men inappropriately think they are immune to HIV infections and so continue risk behaviors? Yet others are convinced that safe and acceptable adult male circumcision has been and can continue to be practiced in developing countries as one method to prevent HIV transmission.[124] At the time of this writing, it seems that the latter camp has the facts on their side.[125]

References

1. Lyles, C.M, L.S. Kay, N. Crepaz, et al. 2007. Best-evidence interventions: Findings from a systematic review of HIV behavioral interventions for US populations at high risk, 2000–2004. *American Journal of Public Health* 97:133–143.

2. Janssen, R.S., G.A. Satten, S.L. Stramer, et al. 1998. New testing strategy to detect early HIV-1 infection for use in incidence estimates and for clinical and prevention purposes. *Journal of the American Medical Association* 280:42–48.

3. Pilcher, C.D., S.F. Fiscus, T.Q. Nguyen, et al. 2005. Detection of acute infections during HIV testing in North Carolina. *New England Journal of Medicine* 352:1873–1883.

4. Rosenberg, P. S. 2001. HIV in the late 1990s: What we don't know may hurt us. *American Journal of Public Health* 91:1016–1017.

5. Glynn, M., and P. Rhodes. 2005. Estimated HIV prevalence in the United States at the end of 2003 [abstract]. Presented at the National HIV Prevention Conference, June 12–15, Atlanta, Georgia.

6. Fleming, P.L., P.M. Wortley, J.M. Karon, K.M. DeCock, and R.S. Janssen. 2000. Tracking the HIV epidemic: Current issues, future challenges. *American Journal of Public Health* 90:1037–1041.

7. CDC. 2006. Missed opportunities for earlier diagnosis of HIV infection–South Carolina, 1997–2005. *Morbidity and Mortality Weekly Report* 55:1269–1272.

8. Klein, D., L.B. Hurley, D. Merrill, and C.P. Quesenberry Jr. 2003. Review of medical encounters in the 5 years before a diagnosis of HIV-1 infection: Implications for early detection. *Journal of Acquired Immune Deficiency Syndromes* 32:143–152.

9. Palella, F.J., M. Deloria-Knoll, J.S. Chmiel, et al. 2003. Survival benefit of initiating antiretroviral therapy in HIV-infected persons in different CD4+ cell strata. *Annals of Internal Medicine* 138:620–626.

10. U.S. Department of Health and Human Services (U.S. DHHS). Office of AIDS Research Advisory Council (OARAC) Guidelines for the Use of Antiretroviral Agents in HIV-infected Adults and Adolescents. October 10, 2006. Available at http://aidsinfo.nih.gov/contentfiles/AdultandAdolescentGL.pdf.

11. Marks, G., N. Crepaz, and R.S. Janssen. 2006. Estimating sexual transmission of HIV from persons aware and unaware that they are infected with the virus in the USA. *AIDS* 20:1447–1450.

12. Sabatier, R., and E. Cecil. 1988. HIV: A testing dilemma. *AIDS Watch* 2:4–5.

13. Paltiel, A.D., M.C. Weinstein, A.D. Kimmel, et al. 2005. Expanded screening for HIV in the United States–An analysis of cost-effectiveness. *New England Journal of Medicine* 352:586–595.

14. Byron, P. May 27, 1986. This is not only a test. The hidden risks of antibody screening. *The Village Voice* 31:29–30.

15. Bayer, R. 1992. As the second decade of AIDS begins: An international perspective on the ethics of the epidemic. *AIDS* 6:527–532.

16. Field, M.A. 1990. Testing for AIDS: Uses and abuses. *American Journal of Law and Medicine* 16:33–106.

17. Lisko, E.A. February 26, 1999. Mandatory premarital HIV testing. Available at http://www.law.uh.edu/healthlaw/perspectives/HIVAIDS/990226Premarital. html.

18. McKay, N.L., and K.M. Phillips. 1991. An economic evaluation of mandatory premarital testing for HIV. *Inquiry* 28:236–248.

19. Daniels, P., and Y. Wimberly. 2004. HIV testing rates among African Americans: Why are they not increasing? *Journal of the National Medical Association* 96:1107–1108.

20. Aynalem, G., P. Mendoza, T. Frederick, and L. Mascola. 2004. Who and why? HIV-testing refusal during pregnancy: Implications for pediatric HIV epidemic disparity. *AIDS and Behavior* 8:25–31.

21. Sobo, E.J. 1994. Attitudes toward HIV testing among impoverished inner-city African-American women. *Medical Anthropology* 16:17–38.

22. Holmberg, S.D., S.P. Buchbinder, L.J. Conley, et al. 1995. The spectrum of medical conditions and symptoms before acquired immunodeficiency syndrome in homosexual and bisexual men infected with the human immunodeficiency virus. *American Journal of Epidemiology* 141:395–404.

23. Lyter, D.W., R.O. Valdiserri, L.A. Kingsley, W.P. Amoroso, and C.R. Rinaldo Jr. 1987. The HIV antibody test: Why gay and bisexual men want or do not want their results. *Public Health Reports* 102:468–474.

24. Holmberg, S.D., L.J. Conley, S.P. Buchbinder, et al. 1993. Use of therapeutic and prophylactic drugs for AIDS by homosexual and bisexual men in three US cities. *AIDS* 7:699–704.

25. Wortley, P.M., S.Y. Chu, T. Diaz, et al. 1995. HIV testing patterns: where, why, and when were persons with AIDS tested for HIV? *AIDS* 9:487–492.

26. Inungu, J.N., C. Quist-Adade, E.M. Beach, T. Cook, and M. Lamerato. 2005. Shift in the reasons why adults seek HIV testing in the United States: Policy implications. *AIDS Reader* 15:35–38, 42.

27. Schwarcz, S., J. Stockman, V. Delgado, and S. Sheer. 2004. Does name-based HIV reporting deter high-risk persons from HIV testing? Results from San Francisco. *Journal of Acquired Immune Deficiency Syndromes* 35:93–96.

28. U.S. Department of Health and Human Services (U.S. DHHS). 1987. Medical examination of aliens (AIDS); final rule. *Federal Register* 52:21532–21533.

29. CDC. 2001. Revised guidelines for HIV counseling, testing, and referral. *Morbidity and Mortality Weekly Report* 50(RR-19):1–62.

30. Stoto, M.A., D.A. Alimario, and M.C. McCormick (eds.). 1999. *Reducing the Odds: Preventing Perinatal Transmission of HIV in the United States.* Washington, DC: National Academy Press.

31. CDC. 2002. HIV testing among pregnant women–United States and Canada, 1998–2001. *Morbidity and Mortality Weekly Report* 51:1013–1016.

32. Working Group on Antiretroviral Therapy and Medical Management of HIV-infected Children. October 26, 2006. *Guidelines for the Use of Antiretroviral Agents in Pediatric HIV Infection.* Bethesda, MD: U.S. Department of Health and Human Services.

33. Irwin, K.L., R.O. Valdiserri, and S.D. Holmberg. 1996. The acceptability of voluntary HIV antibody testing in the United States: A decade of lessons learned [review]. *AIDS* 10:1707–1717.

34. Barragan, M., G. Hicks, M.V. Williams, C. Franco-Paredes, W. Duffus, and C. el Rio. 2005. Low health literacy is associated with HIV test acceptance. *Journal of General Internal Medicine* 20:422–425.

35. Charlebois, E.D., A. Maiorana, M. McLaughlin, et al. 2005. Potential deterrent effect of name-based HIV infection surveillance. *Journal of Acquired Immune Deficiency Syndromes* 43:249–250.

36. Hecht, F.M., M.A. Chesney, J.S. Lehman, et al. 2000. Does HIV reporting by name deter testing? MESH Study Group. *AIDS* 14:1801–1808.

37. Schwarcz, S., S. Scheer, W. MacFarland, et al. 2007. Prevalence of HIV infection and predictors of high-risk transmission sexual risk behavior among men who have sex with men. *American Journal of Public Health* 97:1067–1075.

38. Valdiserri, R.O., M. Moore, A.R. Gerber, C.H.J. Campbell, B.A. Dillon, and G.R. West. 1993. A study of clients returning for counseling after HIV testing: Implications for improving rates of return. *Public Health Reports* 108:12–18.

39. Kamb, M.L., M. Fishbein, J.M. Douglas Jr., et al. 1998. Efficacy of risk-reduction counseling to prevent human immunodeficiency virus and sexually transmitted diseases: a randomized controlled trial. Project RESPECT Study Group. *Journal of the American Medical Association* 280:1161–1167.

40. Lazebnik, R., T. Hermida, R. Szubski, S. Dieterich-Colón, and S.F. Grey. 2001. The proportion and characteristics of adolescents who return for anonymous HIV test results. *Sexually Transmitted Diseases* 28:401–404.

41. Castrucci, B.C., D.E. Williams, and E. Foust. 2002. The elimination of anonymous HIV testing: A case study in North Carolina. *Journal of Public Health Management and Practice* 8:30–37.

42. Amankwaa, A.A., L.C. Amankwaa, and C.O. Ochie Sr. 1999. Revisiting the debate of voluntary versus mandatory HIV/AIDS testing in U.S. prisons. *Journal of the Health and Human Services Administration* 22:220–236.

43. Bindman, A.B., D. Osmond, F.M. Hecht, et al. 1998. Multistate evaluation of anonymous HIV testing and access to medical care. Multistate Evaluation of Surveillance of HIV (MESH) Study Group. *Journal of the American Medical Association* 280:1416–1420.

44. Frank, A.P., M.G. Wandell, M.D. Headings, M.A. Conant, G.E. Woody, and C. Michel. 1997. Anonymous HIV testing using home collection and telemedicine counseling. A multicenter evaluation. *Archives of Internal Medicine* 157:309–314.

45. Colfax, G.N., J.S. Lehman, A.B. Bindman, et al. 2002. What happened to home HIV test collection kits? Intent to use kits, actual use, and barriers to use among persons at risk for HIV infection. *AIDS Care* 14:675–682.

46. Anonymous. 1997. Home test kit for HIV fails to capture public's interest. *AIDS Policy and Law* 12:14.

47. Smith, L.V., E.T. Rudy, M. Javanbakht, et al. 2006. Client satisfaction with rapid HIV testing: comparison between an urban sexually transmitted disease clinic and a community-based testing center. *AIDS Patient Care and STDs* 20:693–700.

48. Cairns, G. February 2006. New directions in HIV prevention: Serosorting and universal testing. *International Association of Physicians in AIDS Care (IAPAC) Monthly* 12:42–45.

49. Xia, O., E. Molitor, D.H. Osmond, et al. 2006. Knowledge of sexual partner's HIV status and serosorting practices in a California population-based sample of men who have sex with men. *AIDS* 20:2081–2089.

50. Patel, P., M.M. Taylor, J.A. Montoya, M.E. Hamburger, P.R. Kerndt, and S.D. Holmberg. 2006. Circuit parties: Sexual behaviors and HIV disclosure practices among men who have sex with men at the White Party, Palm Springs, California, 2003. *AIDS Care* 18:1046–1049.

51. Osmond, D.H., L.M. Pollack, J.P. Paul and J.A. Catania. 2007. Changes in prevalence of HIV infection and sexual risk behavior in men who have sex with men: San Francisco, 1997–2002. *American Journal of Public Health* 97: 2007 Apr 26; [Epub ahead of print]

52. Truong, H.M., T. Kellogg, J.D. Klausner, et al. Increases in sexually transmitted infections and sexual risk behavior without a concurrent increase in HIV incidence among men who have sex with men in San Francisco: A suggestion of HIV serosorting? *Sexually Transmitted Infections* 82:461–466.

53. Holmberg, S.D. 1996. The estimated prevalence and incidence of HIV in 96 large US metropolitan areas. *American Journal of Public Health* 86:642–654.

54. Branson, B.M., H.H. Handsfield, M.A. Lampe, et al.. 2006. Revised Recommendations for HIV Testing of Adults, Adolescents, and Pregnant Women in Health-care Settings. *Morbidity and Mortality Weekly Report* 55(RR-14):1–26. Available at http://www.cdc.gov/mmwr/pdf/rr/rr5514.pdf.

55. CDC. 1999. Guidelines for National Human Immunodeficiency Virus Case-surveillance, including Monitoring for Human Immunodeficiency Virus Infection and Acquired Immunodeficiency Syndrome. *Morbidity and Mortality Weekly Report* 48(RR-13):1–29.

56. Wolitski, R.J., K.D. Henry, C.M. Lyles, et al. 2006. Evolution of HIV/AIDS Prevention– United States 1981–2006. *Morbidity and Mortality Weekly Report* 55:597–603.

57. Bayer, R., and A.L. Fairchild. 2006. Changing the paradigm for HIV testing– The end of exceptionalism [perspective]. *New England Journal of Medicine* 355:647–649.

58. Jayaraman, G.C., J.K. Preiksaitis, and B. Larke. 2003. Mandatory reporting of HIV infection and opt-out prenatal screening for HIV infection: Effect on testing rates. *Canadian Medical Association Journal* 168:679–682.

59. Mason, J.O., G.R. Noble, B.K. Lindsay, et al. 1988. Current CDC efforts to prevent and control human immunodeficiency virus infection and AIDS in the United States through information and education. *Public Health Reports* 103:255–263.

60. Allen, J.R., and J.W. Curran. 1988. Prevention of AIDS and HIV infection: Needs and priorities for epidemiologic research. *American Journal of Public Health* 78:381–386.

61. Herbst, J.H., R.T. Sherba, N. Crepaz, et al. 2005. A meta-analytic review of HIV behavioral interventions for reducing sexual risk behavior of men who have sex with men. *Journal of the Acquired Immune Deficiency Syndromes* 39:228–241.

62. Semaan, S., D.C. Des Jarlais, E. Sogolow, et al. 2002. A meta-analysis of the effect of HIV prevention interventions on the sex behaviors of drug users in the United States, *Journal of Acquired Immune Deficiency Syndromes* 30(suppl 1):S73–S93.

63. Neumann, M.S., and E.D. Sogolow. 2000. Replicating effective programs: HIV/AIDS prevention technology transfer. *AIDS Education and Prevention* 12(5 suppl):S35–S48.

64. O'Brien, T.R., M.P. Busch, E. Donegan, et al. 1994. Heterosexual transmission of human immunodeficiency virus type 1 from transfusion recipients to their sex partners. *Journal of Acquired Immune Deficiency Syndromes* 7:705–710.

65. Hisada, M. T.R. O'Brien, P.S. Rosenberg, and J.J. Goedert. 2000. Virus load and risk of heterosexual transmission of human immunodeficiency virus and hepatitis C virus by men with hemophilia. The Multicenter Hemophilia Cohort Study. *Journal of Infectious Diseases* 181:1475–1478.

66. Quinn, T.C., M.J. Wawer, N. Sewankambo, et al. 2000. Viral load and heterosexual transmission of human immunodeficiency virus type 1. Rakai Project Study Group. *New England Journal of Medicine* 342:921–929.

67. Politch, J.A., K.H. Mayer, A.F. Abbott, and D.J. Anderson. 1994. The effects of disease progression and zidovudine therapy on semen quality in human immunodeficiency virus type 1 seropositive men. *Fertility and Sterility* 61:922–928.

68. Hosseinipour, M., M.S. Cohen, P.L. Vernazza, and A.D. Kashuba. 2002. Can antiretroviral therapy be used to prevent sexual transmission of human immunodeficiency virus type 1? *Clinical Infectious Diseases* 34:1391–1395.

69. Mayer, K.H., S. Boswell, R. Goldstein, et al. 1999. Persistence of human immunodeficiency virus in semen after adding indinavir to combination antiretroviral therapy. *Clinical Infectious Diseases* 28:1252–1259.

70. Cong, M.E., W. Heneine, and J.G. Garcia-Lerma. 2007. The fitness cost of mutations associated with human immunodeficiency virus type 1 drug resistance is modulated by mutational interactions. *Journal of Virology* 81:3037–3041.

71. Leigh Brown, A.J., S.D. Frost, W.C. Mathews, et al. 2003. Transmission fitness of drug-resistant human immunodeficiency virus and the prevalence of resistance in the antiretroviral-treated population. *Journal of Infectious Diseases* 187:683–686.

72. Porco, T.C., J.N. Martin, K.A. Page-Shafer, et al. 2004. Decline in HIV infectivity following the introduction of highly active antiretroviral therapy. *AIDS* 18:81–88.

73. Bezemer, D., S. Jurriaans, M. Prins, et al. 2004. Declining trend in transmission of drug-resistant HIV-1 in Amsterdam. *AIDS* 18:1571–1577.

74. Maisnier-Patin, S., and D.I. Andersson. 2004. Adaptation to the deleterious effects of antimicrobial drug resistance mutations by compensatory evolution. *Research in Microbiology* 155:360–369.

75. Mimiaga, M.J., H. Goldhammer, C. Belanoff, A.M. Tetu, and K.H. Mayer. 2007. Men who have sex with men: Perceptions about sexual risk, HIV and sexually transmitted disease testing, and provider communication. *Sexually Transmitted Diseases* 34:113–119.

76. Padian, N.S., T.R. O'Brien, Y. Chang, S. Glass, and D.P. Francis. 1993. Prevention of heterosexual transmission of human immunodeficiency virus through couple counseling. *Journal of Acquired Immune Deficiency Syndromes* 6:1043–1049.

77. VanDevanter, N., A.S. Thacker, G. Bass, and M. Arnold. 1999. Heterosexual couples confronting the challenges of HIV infection. *AIDS Care* 11:181–193.

78. Crepaz, N., T.A. Hart, and G. Marks. 2004. Highly active antiretroviral therapy and sexual risk behavior. A meta-analytic review. *Journal of the American Medical Association* 292:224–236.

79. Chen, S.Y., S. Gibbon, M.H. Katz, et al. 2002. Continuing increases in sexual risk behavior and sexually transmitted infections among men who have sex with men: San Francisco, Calif.; 1999–2001. *American Journal of Public Health* 92:1387–1388.

80. Dukers, N.H.T.M., J. Goudsmit, J.B.F. de Wit, et al. 2001. Sexual risk behavior relates to the virological and immunological improvements during highly active antiretroviral therapy in HIV-1 infection. *AIDS* 15:369–378.

81. Katz, M.H., S.K. Schwarcz, T.A. Kellogg, et al. 2002. Impact of highly active antiretroviral treatment on HIV seroincidence among men who have sex with men: San Francisco. *American Journal of Public Health* 92:388–394.

82. Sheer, S., P.L. Chu, J.D. Klausner, et al. 2001. Effect of highly active antiretroviral therapy on diagnoses of sexually transmitted diseases in people with AIDS. *Lancet* 357:432–435.

83. DiClemente, R.J., E. Funkhouser, G. Wingood, H. Fawal, S.D. Holmberg, and S.H. Vermund. 2002. Protease inhibitor combination therapy and decreased condom use among gay men. *Southern Medical Journal* 95:421–425.

84. Tun, W., S.J. Grange, D. Vlahov, S.A. Strathdee, and D.D. Celentano. 2004. Increase in sexual risk behavior associated with immunologic response to highly active antiretroviral therapy among HIV-infected injection drug users. *Clinical Infectious Diseases* 38:1167–1174.

85. Becker, M.H., and J.G. Joseph. 1988. AIDS and behavioral change to reduce risk: A review. *American Journal of Public Health* 78:394–410.

86. Springer, S.A., E. Pesanti, J. Hodges, T. Macura, G. Doros, and F.L. Altice. 2004. Effectiveness of antiretroviral therapy among HIV infected prisoners: reincarceration and the lack of sustained benefit after release to the community. *Clinical Infectious Diseases* 15:1754–1760.

87. Vigilante, K.C., M.M. Flynn, P.C. Affleck, et al. 1999. Reduction in recidivism of incarcerated women through primary care, peer counseling, and discharge planning. *Journal of Women's Health* 8:409–415.

88. Janssen, R.S., D.R. Holtgrave, R.O. Valdiserri, M. Shepherd, and H.D. Gayle. 2001. The serostatus approach to fighting the HIV epidemic: Prevention strategies for infected individuals. *American Journal of Public Health* 91: 1019–1024

89. CDC. 2003. Advancing HIV prevention: new strategies for a changing epidemic—United States, 2003. *Morbidity and Mortality Weekly Report* 52:329–332.

90. CDC. 2006. Achievements in Public Health: Reduction in prenatal transmission of HIV infection—United States, 1985–2005. *Morbidity and Mortality Weekly Report* 55:592–597.

91. Connor, E.M., R.S. Sperling, R. Gelber, et al. 1994. Reduction of maternal-infant transmission of human immunodeficiency virus type 1 with zidovudine treatment. Pediatric AIDS Clinical Trails Group Protocol 076 Study Group. *New England Journal of Medicine* 331:1173–1180.

92. Abrams, E.J. 2004. Prevention of mother-to-child transmission of HIV-successes, controversies and critical questions. *AIDS Reviews* 6:131–143

93. Ryder, R.W., and S.E. Hassig. 1988. The epidemiology of prenatal transmission of HIV. *AIDS* 2(suppl 1):S83–S89.

94. Guay, L.A., P. Musoke, T. Fleming, et al. 1999. Intrapartum and neonatal single-dose nevirapine compared with zidovudine for prevention of mother-to-infant transmission of HIV-1 in Kampala, Uganda. HIV NET-012 randomised trial. *Lancet* 354:795–802.

95. Garrett, L. July 8, 2002. Rage over 'Poison' as AIDS treatment, South African's fears disputed by Others. *Newsday*.

96. Flys, T.S., D. Donnell, A. Mwatha, et al. 2007. Persistence of K103N-containing HIV-1 variants after single-dose nevirapine for prevention of HIV-1 mother-to-child transmission. *Journal of Infectious Diseases* 195:711–715.

97. Persaud, D., P. Palumbo, C. Ziemniak, et al. 2007. Early archiving and pre-dominance of nonnucleoside reverse transcriptase inhibitor-resistant HIV-1 among recently infected infants born in the United States. *Journal of Infectious Diseases* 195:1402–1410.

98. Little, S.J., K. Dawson, N.S. Hellman, D.D. Richman, and S.D.W. Frost. 2003. Persistence of transmitted drug-resistant virus among subjects with primary HIV infection deferring antiretroviral therapy. *Antiviral Therapy* (Suppl) 8:S129.

99. Palmer, S., V. Boltz, F. Madarelli, et al. 2006. Selection and persistence of non-nucleoside reverse transcriptase inhibitor-resistant HIV-1 in patients starting and stopping non-nucleoside therapy. *AIDS* 20:701–710.

100. National Institutes of Health (NIH). 2002. Consensus Development Conference Statement on the Management of Hepatitis C. Conference held June 10–12, 2002.

101. Garfein, R.S., E.R. Monterroso, T.C. Tong, et al. 2004. Comparison of HIV infection risk behaviors among injection drug users from East and West Coast US cities. *Journal of Urban Health* 81:260–267.

102. Gostin, L.O., Z. Lazzarini, T.S. Jones, and K. Flaherty. 1997. Prevention of HIV/AIDS and other blood-borne diseases among injection drug users. A national survey on the regulation of syringes and needles. *Journal of the American Medical Association* 277:53–62.

103. Monterroso, E.R., M.E. Hamburger, D. Vlahov, et al. 2000. Prevention of HIV infection in street-recruited injection drug users. *Journal of Acquired Immune Deficiency Syndromes* 25:63–70.

104. Office of Technology Assessment (OTA), U.S. Congress. 1990. The Effectiveness of Drug Abuse Treatment: Implications for Controlling HIV/AIDS Infection. Washington, DC: OTA, Publication 052-003-0120-3.

105. Des Jarlais, D., M. Marmor, D. Paone, et al. 1996. HIV incidence among injection drug users in New York City syringe exchange programmes. *Lancet* 348:987–991.

106. Des Jarlais, D., S.R. Friedman, T. Perlis, et al. 1999. Risk behavior and HIV infection among new drug injectors in the era of AIDS in New York City. *Journal of Acquired Immune Deficiency Syndromes* 20:67–72.

107. Gibson, D.R., N.M. Flynn, and D. Perales. 2001. Effectiveness of syringe exchange programs in reducing HIV risk behavior and HIV seroconversion among injecting drug users. *AIDS* 15:1329–1341.

108. Anonymous. May 15, 1998. House approves ban on Federal aid for needle exchanges. *AIDS Policy and Law* 13:1, 11.

109. Anonymous. May 1, 1998. Clinton refuses to fund needle-exchange programs. *AIDS Policy and Law* 13:1, 6–7.

110. Vlahov, D., and B. Junge. 1998. The role of needle exchange programs in HIV prevention. *Public Health Reports* 113(suppl 1):75–80.

111. Kim, B. June 13, 1997. Needle-exchange programs: A prickly debate. *AIDS Policy and Law* 12:6–8.

112. Tempalski, B., P.L. Flom, S.R. Friedman, et al. 2007. Social and political factors predicting the presence of syringe exchange programs in 96 US metropolitan areas. *American Journal of Public Health* 97:437–447.

113. Resnick, M.D., P.S. Bearman, R.W. Blum, et al. 1997. Protecting adolescents from harm. Findings from the National Longitudinal Study on Adolescent Health. *Journal of the American Medical Association* 278:823–832.

114. Lindberg, L.D., J.S. Santelli, and S. Singh. 2006. Changes in formal sex education: 1995–2002. *Perspectives on Sexual and Reproductive Health* 38:182–189.

115. Trenholm, C., B. Devaney, K. Fortson, L. Quay, J. Wheeler, and M. Clark. April 2007. Impacts of Four Title V, Section 510 Abstinence Programs. Final Report. Princeton, N.J.;Mathematica Policy Research, Inc.

116. Santelli, J.S., L.D. Lindberg, L.B. Finer, and S. Singh. 2007. Explaining recent declines in adolescent pregnancy in the United States: The contribution of abstinence and improved contraceptive use. *American Journal of Public Health* 97:150–156.

117. Moses, S., J.E. Bradley, N.J.D. Nagelkerke, A.R. Ronald, J.O. Ndinya-Achola, and F.A. Plummer. 1990. Geographic patterns of male circumcision practices in Africa: Association with HIV seroprevalence. *International Journal of Epidemiology* 19:693–697.

118. Moses, S., F.A. Plummer, J.E. Bradley, J.O. Ndinya-Achola, N.J. Nagelkerke, and A.R. Ronald. 1994. The association between lack of male circumcision and risk for HIV infection: A review of the epidemiological data. *Sexually Transmitted Diseases* 21:201–210.

119. Van Howe, R.S. 1999. Circumcision and HIV infection: Review of the literature and meta-analysis. *International Journal of STD and AIDS* 10:8–16.

120. O'Farrell, N., and M. Egger. 2000. Circumcision in men and the prevention of HIV infection: A 'meta-analysis' revisited. *International Journal of STDs and AIDS* 11:137–142.

121. Gray, R.H., G. Kigozi, D. Serwadda, et al. 2007. Male circumcision for HIV prevention in men in Rakai, Uganda: A randomized trial. *Lancet* 369:617–619.

122. Bailey, R.C., S. Moses, C.B. Parker, et al. 2007. Male circumcision for HIV prevention in young men in Kisumu, Kenya: A randomized controlled trial. *Lancet* 369:617–619.

123. Muula, A.S. 2007. Male circumcision to prevent HIV transmission and acquisition: What else do we need to know? *AIDS and Behavior* 11:357–363.

124. Kreiger, J.N., R.C. Bailey, J.C. Opeya, et al. 2007. Adult male circumcision outcomes: experience in a developing country setting. *Urologia Internationalis* 78:235–240.

125. Moszynski, P. 2007. Experts recommend circumcision to combat male HIV infections in Africa. *British Medical Journal* 334:712–713.

CHAPTER SEVEN

Early Drugs and Biomedical Interventions

The road to zidovudine (AZT) and subsequent antiretroviral drugs was originally paved with many attempts at treatment[1] that have now largely been forgotten. In 1986, there were an estimated 17,000 (known) AIDS patients but only about 4,000 of them could be enrolled in drug trials.[2] Many were desperate, and were willing to try anything that might have antiviral properties. Almost all of these drugs are now largely forgotten or abandoned as antiretroviral therapy: peptide T, dextran sulfate, AL721, HPA-23, dideoxyadenosine, suramin, and ampligen. Others such as foscarnet (phosphonoformate), interferon alpha, interleukin-2, and ribavirin were found to be useful for other viral conditions. These were all widely tried in the 1980s, and even in the early 1990s, after zidovudine became available, all these were still being used by a fraction of HIV-infected homosexual and bisexual men in major U.S. cities.[3] Several men were trying alternative therapies either because they were afraid of or had experienced toxic side effects from zidovudine, and were now taking peptide T, AL721, ozone, "compound Q" (Chinese cucumber root derivative), DNCB (usually used as a skin test for anergy), etc. Meanwhile, small studies were trying to quickly evaluate these and many other drugs that had shown promise in the laboratory. However, the story of almost all of these drugs was that they were promising in vitro, but disappointing in vivo.

The "Pre-Zidovudine" Drugs

In the mid-1980s there were essentially no treatment options for HIV, and even after zidovudine was introduced in 1987, there was a skepticism. As per

Paul O'Malley (personal communication, June 14, 2007), lead Disease Control Investigator for the CDC-funded cohort of gay men at the San Francisco Department of Health:

> The best the medical establishment had to offer at that time was a drug that proved to be a failure. I remember that individuals were desperate to try anything that might work. For example, I remember one cohort member who was on high dose vitamin C therapy, wanting us to spread the word to others that it was curative. I think 1984–6 was a special time of fear and anxiety. It was more than just the pre-AZT therapy period. The scope of this epidemic and its implications had finally reached home. In 1981–1983, the knowledge of this new disease was not widespread. Most gay men did not personally know someone suffering with this disease—that had all changed by early 1987.

Among the experimental drugs that men in San Francisco and elsewhere were taking was Peptide T, a modified octapeptide (d-ala-Peptide-T-amide) segment of the HIV envelope gp120. It was thought that chemical might block entry of HIV into white blood cells by competitively binding to CCR-5 receptor molecule on white blood cells (CD4+ cells),[4] and initial pilot studies of its intranasal administration were promising. Phase 1 testing of this drug given to 14 AIDS patients over 12 weeks showed some modest cognitive and motor function improvement in patients with moderate neuropsychologic impairment; the study-subjects also gained an average of 2 kg (4.4 lbs) and reported an increased sense of well-being.[5] However, while there was some early enthusiasm for its use, it became clear to most that this drug was not preventing HIV disease progression to AIDS or death. In the mid-1990s, placebo-controlled prospective studies of intranasal peptide T found that while this drug appeared safe, there was no apparent benefit on many measures of cognitive and neuropsychological functioning.[6] Nor was it more effective than placebo in preventing the pain of distal neuropathy.[7] Still, this drug has been found to bind to CCR-5 receptors on CD4+ cells, so might competitively—but not completely—block entry of HIV into cells and lead to increases in CD4+ cell counts in some patients.[8] However, while peptide T drug could conceivably be resurrected as an adjunctive rather than a primary therapy, given the various and more potent antiretroviral drugs currently available, this seems unlikely.

Foscarnet (phosphonoformate) has been known to inhibit reverse transcriptase (of avian retroviruses, initially) even before 1980.[9] Further, it was early known to have in vitro effectiveness against herpes group viruses (herpes, cytomegalovirus, Epstein-Barr virus, and others)[10] by inhibiting

DNA polymerase. It is FDA-approved as effective treatment for severe cytomegalovirus (CMV) infection,[11, 12] especially for CMV retinitis, a major opportunistic infection in AIDS, and for systemic CMV infections in therapeutically immunosuppressed patients (such as following transplantation). Other drugs for CMV infections can have problems: CMV may develop resistance to acyclovir; gancyclovir has marked myelosuppressive effects leading to anemia and neutropenia; and cidofovir has toxic effects on the kidneys. So, foscarnet remains an effective alternate therapy for CMV. Foscarnet is not without its own problems, as it was early recognized as a highly nephrotoxic drug that induces acute tubular necrosis.[13] However, dosage reduction and adequate hydration mitigate this toxic effect.[14] The putative survival benefits seen in these patients when receiving foscarnet and zidovudine (possibly linked to synergy between zidovudine and foscarnet or the inherent anti-HIV activity of foscarnet), offer potentially important advantages for foscarnet over ganciclovir and other drugs in the treatment of patients with both HIV and CMV infection.[15]

Given the murky role of herpes group viruses in AIDS (Chapter 2), and its effects against reverse transcriptase, many early HIV patients personally experimented with foscarnet as an antiretroviral treatment. What has been the experience of using this drug specifically to treat HIV? Shortly after the approval of zidovudine (AZT) in 1987 as the first antiretroviral drug, it was clear that this drug alone would not cure HIV/AIDS. So, the thought was that zidovudine could be combined with other experimental HIV drugs, and that two or more drugs would act synergistically against HIV.[16] Since phosphonoformate significantly inhibits HIV replication, some researchers observed a significant decline in HIV plasma RNA (viral load) levels in small groups of patients for whom foscarnet was added to zidovudine therapy.[17] However, this decrease in HIV RNA was from mean 5.82 log RNA/ml to 5.30 log RNA/ml, so, while statistically significant, this is not substantial and leaves patients with higher-than-acceptable levels of HIV. Also, treatment of CMV with foscarnet is associated with rebound of CMV after discontinuation of the drug (although foscarnet operates by a different mechanism in HIV than CMV). Finally, and not least important, the cost of a year's treatment with foscarnet was estimated in 1992 at about U.S. $20,000, well outside the purse of most AIDS or HIV patients.[18] Probably all these considerations, and the availability of highly active antiretroviral therapy (protease inhibitors and non-nucleoside reverse transcriptase inhibitors) after 1995, have all combined to leave foscarnet as an anti-HIV drug of more historical than current interest.

AL 721, a lipid mixture from egg yolks that purportedly increased cell membrane fluidity leading to better mitogen responsiveness, was also tried by some early HIV patients. Even by the time zidovudine became available, it was questioned whether there was any altered membrane fluidity from this exogenous source of phospholipids and triglycerides; still, AL 721 enhanced mitogen responses in vitro.[19] Might better mitogen responsiveness, indicating better T-lymphocyte responsiveness, be helpful in mitigating HIV infection? Already by 1990, there were anecdotal reports that HIV patients taking AL 721 were not apparently doing any better clinically than those who were not taking this experimental agent.[20] But the "death blow" to AL 721 came from an open-label trial of the drug at varying doses fed to 40 HIV-infected men for 8 weeks: although some men transiently gained weight and improved serum triglyceride and cholesterol levels while taking AL 721, the trial found no evidence to support using AL 721 as an antiretroviral agent.[21] No one has proposed its use for treating HIV since 1990.

Dextran sulfate may interfere with an early step of the virus replicative cycle (adsorption), and was also taken by some patients before reverse transcriptase inhibitor (RTI) drugs, such as zidovudine or didanosine (ddI), became available. The mechanism of action of dextran, a collection of high molecular weight polyanions, is still not entirely clear, but may relate to an interaction between dextran and the V3 region of gp120 of the HIV membrane, that binds to target cell CD4 and other receptors;[22] or, dextran may induce internalization of CD4, removing it as a binding site for HIV.[23] In any case, few patients were still taking it by the early 1990s,[3] and in vitro studies suggested that pairing it with dideoxynucleoside RTIs (such as zidovudine) gave inconsistent and confusing results when used against then newly emergent drug-resistant strains of virus.[24] It has not been proposed as an antiretroviral agent in many years.

HPA-23 (ammonium-5-tungsto-2-antimoniate, antimoniotungstate) was known to inhibit rabies virus in the laboratory and, as one of the few antiviral agents known in the early 1980s, was quickly evaluated by French HIV researchers. These demonstrated that HPA-23 was a potent inhibitor of DNA polymerase alpha,[25] and it was tried with some promising results in four HIV/AIDS patients.[26] Indeed, an open-label trial of the drug in 69 U.S. AIDS patients showed that the drug was reasonably well tolerated at low doses, but, even in this safety study, "no improvement in the clinical status of the patients was observed during 8 weeks of therapy."[27] This lack of results was confirmed by French researchers as well who found that their 12 patients given HPA-23 showed persistent or even increased HIV p24 antigenemia (indicative of active HIV replication), and nine developed thrombocytopenia.[28] No further clinical trials of this drug for HIV were performed.

Similarly, toxicity quickly scuttled extended trials of the nucleoside reverse transcriptase inhibitor (NRTI), F-dideoxyadenosine (F-ddA, lodenosine). Like other NRTIs such as zidovudine (AZT) and later didanosine (ddI) and didedoxycytidine (ddC), these nucleoside congeners are taken up as the HIV-reverse transcriptase chain is being elongated, and inhibit further elongation and production of the complete enzyme. Dideoxyadenosine (Iodenosine) was known to be an effective NRTI in the laboratory by 1991,[29–31] and in the mid-1990s there was hope that this would be a more potent antiretroviral drug than zidovudine.[32] However, when a phase II trial of Iodenosine in 176 participants resulted in one death and several with liver and kidney damage, this trial and any further investigation of this drug were stopped.[33]

Several antimicrobial drugs, known to be effective for other viruses and parasites, were also intensively and briefly studied as potential antiretroviral agents. Notable among these was ribavirin, used in the 1980s as an aerosol for the treatment of respiratory syncytial virus, a serious infection of infants; it is currently approved for use in influenza and for herpes viruses. This drug inhibits inosine monophosphate dehydrogenase and thereby decreases the pool of guanosine triphosphate available for mRNA priming and elongation. This action does inhibit HIV replication, but it also inhibits zidovudine phosphorylation, a necessary step for zidovudine activity; thus, it would not "boost" the antiretroviral activity of zidovudine and could not be used in combination with it.

As had been seen for other drugs, there was a prominently published report of favorable outcomes (delays in progression to AIDS) in 10 patients receiving ribavirin 600 mg daily.[34] However, in a contemporaneous multi-center, double-blind, placebo-controlled trials including 215 patients, no clinical or immune improvement was observed,[35] and the initial negative findings of this study were reported early at conferences.[36, 37] Ribavirin reduced (transiently) the hazard ratio of progression to AIDS by 43 percent but this was not statistically significant ($p = 0.19$); there was no measurable improvement in immunologic or virologic parameters; and many had a decline in hematocrit, although this was reversible once the drug was discontinued.

The research community at this point felt that ribavirin was, at best, equivocal in its utility as an antiretroviral drug and focused their attentions on zalcitabine (ddC) and didanosine (ddI), nucleoside RTIs nearing approval by FDA for use in substitution or in conjunction with zidovudine (see Appendix). However, after presenting their preliminary results at conferences over the preceding two years, Richard Roberts and his colleagues at New York Hospital published in 1990 results of their study that purported to show that 53 patients randomized to receive 800 mg ribavirin daily (but not those in the arm receiving 600 mg daily) had a significantly prolonged period to AIDS over 24 weeks compared to 56 subjects who received placebo.[38] Although this was a double-blind, randomized, placebo-controlled study, it was flawed in many regards and highlights some of the problems even with this widely respected study design. The main problem was that relatively few patients were followed for a very brief period, so aberrant or odd results had a substantial impact on the reported findings. Indeed, in this study, placebo-takers (the comparison or control group) had a surprisingly high rate of progression to AIDS within the 24 weeks,[39] suggesting that the placebo-takers were much later in their HIV infection and not truly comparable to the ribavirin-treated patients (ascertainment bias). Further, it turned out that people who had already developed AIDS–the outcome measure–were randomized to treatment arms, although they were later removed from analysis. Finally, immunologic and virologic measures did not significantly improve in those taking ribavirin. These problems highlight how statistical testing itself cannot solve problems with study design problems or bad luck in not obtaining comparable groups for comparison and not knowing it.

Suramin, a drug used for the parasitic infections causing trypanosomiasis and onchocerciasis, was also found to inhibit reverse transcriptase and block infectivity of HIV in vitro.[40] It was found to be safe in phase I studies in a few volunteers,[41] but five men taking suramin from 19 to up to 37 weeks had the same HIV antigenemia as five untreated men.[42] A larger study of 98 men taking suramin at different doses showed no clinical or immunologic improvement, many with reversible suramin-induced neutropenia, thrombocytopenia and liver and kidney enzyme abnormalities.[43] Suramin was essentially abandoned as a drug of interest after 1988.

Immunomodulating treatments were also tried in the period before and just following the introduction of zidovudine in 1987. Notable among these was interferon-alpha, natural production of which is induced in the human body by exposure to viruses or tumor cells; in turn, interferon induces production of enzymes that seem to interfere with transcription-translation of mRNA, protein synthesis, assembly, and release of HIV virions. However, as early as 1983, it was recognized that men with AIDS had natural killer cells with much diminished production of interferon-alpha in response to viruses.[44, 45] So, it was reasonable to think that injected interferon-alpha could enhance protection from HIV,[46] and from the common HIV-associated tumor, Kaposi's sarcoma (KS).[47] In regards the activity of interferon against KS, several initial studies indicated that high-dose (not low-dose) interferon alpha resulted in significant antitumor regression in many, but this was mainly in persons with already well established immune function (i.e., higher CD4+ cell counts).[48–52] Because of these and other reports, interferon alpha was approved by the FDA for AIDS-related KS as early as 1988.

If interferon was effective for tumors, what was its effect on HIV itself? Also, were people who were receiving both interferon and zidovudine responding to the interferon or to the NRTI? These were difficult issues to tease out. Regarding the first, an early volunteer study of 17 asymptomatic patients with high CD4+ cell counts (greater than 400 cells/mm^3) who received interferon-alpha showed sustained CD4 counts in them, whereas 17 placebo controls had slight declines in these counts, and five developed AIDS.[53] However, in a much larger study, there was no apparent benefit to adding interferon alpha to zidovudine in the treatment of 559 adult Ugandans with HIV infection.[54] Even in the treatment of KS, at least one study from the Netherlands found that addition of interferon to zidovudine seemed to add no additional benefit (beyond zidovudine) in the treatment of AIDS-associated KS.[52] Both these questions became moot as ever more effective antiretroviral therapies were shown to effectively increase CD4+ cells and to induce regression of KS. Currently, relatively few patients are receiving interferon for KS, and even fewer if any are receiving it as an antiretroviral drug. However, (pegylated) interferon alfa is currently a critical drug in the treatment of hepatitis C and B viruses.

This was not the only research into interferon alpha for AIDS or AIDS-associated KS in the 1990s, and it was certainly not the most public. In 1990, researchers reported in the *East African Medical Journal* that the use of an oral low-dose of interferon alpha (Kemron) was efficacious in a 10-week trial in 204 HIV patients in Nairobi, Kenya: Karnofsky scores, reflecting physical functionality, improved, and 18 (8.8%) reportedly even "seroreverted" in HIV assays.[55] This report rapidly became public at meetings and conferences, but was greeted with great skepticism by researchers: injected doses of interferon 10,000-fold higher than delivered by oral Kemron had not been effective as antiretroviral treatment; and "seroreversion" had not been demonstrated in any other patient treated (or not) with antiretroviral drugs such as zidovudine.

Nonetheless, because of worldwide attention to this report, the claims of Davey Koech and Arthur Obel[55] required further investigation. German researchers found no harm but also no benefit to Kemron in a double-blind randomized placebo-controlled trial of 60 patients.[56] Several other small studies were also not able to substantiate the claims from the Kenyan investigators.[57] However, the backlash against Western experts and their medicine extended not only to African HIV patients who would buy expensive Kemron on the black market but also to African Americans, activists, and doctors who clamored for at least one American clinical trial, even if some of them, too, were skeptical. Indeed, NIH started a trial in the mid 1990s, but this was terminated due to a lack of voluntary participation and a high dropout rate of those who did.[58] Professor Obel, one of the Kenyan scientists who reported and extolled Kemron (and the other alternative medicine "Pearl Omega") and who also claimed that condoms imported from Europe were infected with HIV, was ultimately sued by Kenyan patients on whom Kemron was originally and unsuccessfully tested.[59]

Experimental Antiretroviral Therapies Now Largely Abandoned

These are only some of the drugs that were posited in the 1980s and early 1990s as potential therapies for HIV and AIDS[1]; many others did not make it to definitive clinical trials. In general, these follow a script of promise in vitro and sometimes in small phase I safety studies, but no or equivocal effectiveness when tested in phase I or II clinical trials. These drugs include known antiviral agents such as interferon beta, which has been tried recently and unsuccessfully for the AIDS-defining condition progressive multifocal leukoencephalopathy[60] and ampligen (mismatched, double-stranded RNA) that acts synergistically with zidovudine on HIV strains in vitro,[61] but had equivocal efficacy at best in phase I studies in humans.[62] So-called ABPP (2-amino-5-bromo-6-phenyl-3(H)-pyrimidine) is a natural product that induces interferon production, but also caused orthostatic hypotension, vomiting, and leg cramps in initial volunteers.[1] Avarol, a natural quinone derived from a marine sponge which, like over 150 other sponge products, showed anti-HIV activity in the laboratory[63] never made it out of inconclusive phase I HIV clinical trials.

In addition to agents with known specific antiviral properties, nonspecific immunomodulators have also been investigated. Prominent among these was interleukin-2 (IL-2) that stimulates the expression of T cells, B cells and natural killer cells, that are important in delaying the progression of HIV disease.[64] Patients taking highly active antiretroviral therapy (HAART) and recombinant IL-2 may have higher CD4 cell counts, lower HIV-RNA burdens, and somewhat improved clinical outcomes than those on HAART alone. However, very few patients taking both HAART and IL-2 have so far been observed particularly for long periods of time.[65, 66] Our own analysis of HIV Outpatient Study patients followed for 7 years showed that those taking IL-2 in addition to HAART had improved quantitative measures of immune function—namely, higher CD4+ cells—but no clearly improved clinical benefit.[67] This agent is still undergoing investigation.

However, other immunomodulators have been evaluated, but eventually discarded and no longer in clinical trials for HIV therapy. Interferon-gamma showed no benefit when administered to AIDS patients;[68] granulocyte-macrophage colony-stimulating factor (GM-CSF), used widely for immune reconstitution in cancer patients, was avoided once it was suspected of possibly activating HIV production;[69] although it may be that GM-CSF is actually inhibitory and may be used as an adjunct to HAART for HIV,[70] its toxicity and high cost have generally precluded its wide evaluation in anti-HIV therapy. Other immunomodulators have usually shown either equivocal or no clear clinical benefit, difficult route of delivery (e.g., requiring intravenous administration), limiting toxicity, or some combination of these problems when tried among small numbers of volunteers[1]: methionine-enkephalin, an opiod pentapetide that stimulates natural killer cells; thymopentin, a synthetic peptide that stimulates production of thymocytes (T-lymphocytes, CD4+, and CD8+ cells); Imreg-1 and Imreg-2, immunomodulating polypetides that stimulate interferon and interleukin-2 by CD4+ cells; isoprinosine that stimulates killer cell and macrophage activity; imuthiol (sodium diethyldithiocarbamate), a metal-chelating agent that somehow induces T-cell maturation and differentiation; and carrisyn, an aloe derivative polysaccharide that stimulates fibroblasts, monocytes and macrophages.

Clearly, there were many agents with antiviral or immunomodulating effects in vitro that failed to improve the potency or to synergistically enhance zidovudine when tried in the 1980s and early 1990s. To these must be added the many alternative and herbal medications that were tried before, with or instead of the first FDA-approved antivirals (zidovudine, zalcitabine, and didanosine, all approved between 1987 and 1992 [Appendix]) and outside controlled clinical trials of other experimental agents. These include, but were not limited to "natural" medicines: "compound Q," St. John's wart, and amygdalin were all tried by desperate AIDS patients in the early days of the epidemic.

To all these experimental oral and injected drugs must be added the story of heat-treatment or hyperthermia of HIV. Whole-body hyperthermia (WBHT) is based on the idea that pathogens and tumor cells do not survive temperatures above 108° F (42°C) and has been used to try to treat syphilis in the past and currently as experimental adjunctive or salvage therapy for some cancers. HIV is also heat-sensitive, an important principle in heat treatment (eradication) of HIV from antihemophilic factor.[71] The term "whole-body" is somewhat of a misnomer, as blood is pumped from the body of an anesthetized patient, heated to 108°F, and returned to the patient's body in continuous cycles over many hours: this is more properly "extracorporeal" heat-treatment and is directed to blood alone.

The first two AIDS patients were treated in Atlanta in 1990 by Drs. Kenneth Alonso and Wlliam Logan and were widely reported to have undergone dramatic clinical improvement after the therapy; the first patient who had failed zidovudine and interferon alpha treatment was reported to have disappearance of skin lesions diagnosed as KS after WBHT. However, federal investigators led by Lawrence Deyton, chief of the Community

Clinical Research Branch for the NIH's AIDS Program, concluded a few months later that this patient never had KS.[72, 73] By the time Logan and Alonso investigating hyperthermia published their report in 1991,[74] they had parted ways, but the controversy about WBHT as a potential treatment for AIDS was a public topic and vigorously debated in the AIDS community.

The Gay Men's Health Crisis urged NIH in August 1990 to assess and develop WBHT, although Dr. Alonso had by that time treated a patient in Mexico City who died the day following treatment.[75] On the other side of this public controversy were the vast majority of HIV clinicians who questioned the plausibility of this approach. Probably the fact causing the most skepticism of WBHT was that HIV is widely distributed through tissues and organs in the body and also sequestered in lymph tissue: it seemed highly improbable that heat treatment of blood alone would affect the wider reservoir of HIV. There was also the potential risk from the procedure, such as from blood clotting and heart failure, and the high cost ($40,000).

Nevertheless, under pressure, FDA approved a safety and feasibility study in six gay men in July 1994; the results of this study[76, 77] showed that while there seemed to be some small improvement in Karnofsky score and weight maintenance, any effects on plasma HIV RNA (viral load) and CD4+ cell counts were transient, as might be expected from the presence of a wide and persistent reservoir of HIV in the body. By the mid-1990s highly active antiretroviral regimens with protease inhibitor and non-nucleoside RTIs were available, so there was no further interest in this potentially dangerous, expensive, and unsubstantiated therapy for HIV.

Zidovudine

The report of the first phase II double-blind, placebo-controlled trial of zidovudine (azidothymidine, AZT, ZDV)[78] in 1987 was hailed initially, and then quickly became controversial for the next several years. One hundred forty-five subjects received the drug and 137 received placebo, but the study was terminated at 24 weeks when a data monitoring board who had access to the unblinded data saw that 19 placebo-recipients, but only one zidovudine-recipient, had died during the brief study. Only 27 (9.7%) of all participants had been observed for 24 weeks, the remainder for only 8–16 weeks. Normally, these would not have been enough observations to recommend drug approval; but the universal fatality of HIV infection, the activism of the gay community, and the many needing treatment led to rapid approval by the U.S. FDA and its use,[79] especially in patients who were moribund. In later months and years, many questioned the real long-term efficacy and the toxicities of zidovudine, and, in reaction, much research was dedicated to vindicating or even extolling its use. In retrospect, this initial antiretroviral drug may not have deserved either extreme attitude.

Regarding its efficacy, a follow-up study by Margaret Fischl and her colleagues who first reported the good results from the truncated clinical trial of zidovudine reported the survival rates in 127 zidovudine recipients from this original treatment group, many of whom had advanced disease: only 57.6 percent were surviving after 21 months.[80] While this was modestly better than would be expected with no treatment, it was still not very encouraging. Nonetheless, many scientists were convinced that this drug would or was turning the AIDS epidemic around; for example, some thought that zidovudine use explained the beginnings of observed decrease in AIDS incidence in gay men[81, 82] (see Chapter 3).

Other scientists, though, were concerned about the toxicity—namely, anemia and neutropenia (low red and white blood cells)—in up to a quarter of the men taking zidovudine in the initial study.[83] Indeed, within months of this initial report, other researchers were reporting that the immunologic and clinical benefits of zidovudine were transient, and that "disappointing results were partly related to the hematological toxicity of the drug, which led to interruption of treatment in many patients."[84] While it also became evident that hematologic toxicity and other adverse events decreased with its use over time[80] and with a reduced dosage[84] (up to 250 mg every 4 hours to 1500 mg per day in initial studies, whereas currently the usual dosage is 500–600 mg per day), still there was a widespread public perception by many that zidovudine was not only ineffective, it was "poison." For example, a Google search for "AZT," "zidovudine," and "poison" will yield hundreds of entries, many in popular books and articles.

Also, many clinicians (and patients) were trading personal notes, observations, and anecdotes at HIV/AIDS and other scientific conferences and concluding that, even reducing the dose to 500 mg per day rather than the 1200 or 1500 mg per day used in early studies and correcting or letting initial anemia correct itself, zidovudine was still, at best, modestly effective in those who already had AIDS.[85] This led to the question whether, like other drugs tried in the 1980s, zidovudine might have more effectiveness if used earlier in HIV infection, to prevent the development of AIDS, rather than reserving it for those who were moribund, with low CD4+ cell count.

It is important to note at this point that the debate was never about the benefit of zidovudine, or whether HIV patients should receive it, especially those who were in extremis: these issues were not in question.[86] Rather, the controversy was about the about the absolute effect of the medical benefit individually and the impact on HIV/AIDS epidemiology nationally.

One group of scientists was convinced that zidovudine was a more potent drug, especially if administered before the patient had AIDS; they believed that zidovudine was having a discernable impact on AIDS case incidence (as measured nationally at CDC). In regards the medical efficacy of zidovudine, Neil Graham and other investigators from NIAID's Multicenter AIDS Cohort Study (MACS) of thousands of HIV-infected and uninfected gay men presented a series of articles that tended to emphasize the positive aspects of zidovudine. Their prominent 1991 and 1992 articles in the *New England Journal of Medicine* and *Lancet* purported to show that early treatment with zidovudine and *Pneumocysitis carinii* pneumonia (PCP) prophylaxis—with trimethoprim-sulfamethoxazole (Bactrim, Septra) or inhaled pentamidine— improved survival and retarded the progression of HIV disease.[87, 88] This was not unreasonable, as, with several experimental drugs listed above, results seemed to be better when given to HIV patients who were not already CD4+ cell depleted (e.g., had not progressed to under 200 or 100 cells/mm^3); for example, several had proposed that interferon alpha was most efficacious if given to patients with high CD4+ counts, earlier in HIV infection.[49, 50, 53]

In the MACS observational study of the effects of zidovudine with PCP prophylaxis, adjusting for the effects of PCP prophylaxis indicated that the "treatment effect" of zidovudine in prolonging survival was strongest early in the observation but was no longer statistically significant 24 months after zidovudine initiation.[88] This suggested that the benefit of zidovudine was modest and time-limited. Also, the analysis of the MACS observational data was discordant with an earlier experimental study in which Veterans' Administration HIV patients were randomized to receive or not receive (high-dose) zidovudine.[89, 90] In that experimental study design, zidovudine therapy either "late" or "early" in HIV infection (at various CD4+ cell counts) lended only limited survival benefit. Also, another observational cohort study of patients in AIDS Clinical Trial Group (ACTG 019) reported that earlier use of zidovudine in asymptomatic disease was, again, of transient benefit and no more likely than later use of zidovudine to retard disease progression.[91]

The concept that early zidovudine could delay the development of AIDS and so effect the course of the U.S. AIDS epidemic was promoted by mathematical modelers, especially Mitch Gail[81] and Phil Rosenberg[82] of the National Cancer Institute. They advocated greater use of zidovudine for asymptomatic patients. Other researchers questioned whether, given a 9–11 year incubation period, infection of gay men in the early 1980s[92] would have resulted in the observed peak and then decline of AIDS cases in the early 1990s anyway; whether the limited use of zidovudine in the mid- and late 1980s by so few asymptomatic HIV patients would be enough to make any discernible difference in the thousands of AIDS patients being diagnosed; [3]

and whether, given the problems with toxicity and development of drug resistance—and the limited effectiveness of zidovudine—whether it was wise to advocate widespread use of zidovudine for persons who were not sick. In retrospect, examining the actual incidence of AIDS over the past 25 years in Figure 1.1, it does not appear that zidovudine use in 1987 had any discernible impact on AIDS incidence in gay men at that time.

A second study by the MACS investigators of zidovudine plus 600–800 mg per day of acyclovir also purportedly showed a prolongation of survival.[93] This study indicated a 44 percent reduction in death with the use of acyclovir after an AIDS diagnosis; but this might be expected as acyclovir treats disseminated herpes viruses, including herpes simplex 1 and 2 (cold sores and genital herpes), varicella-zoster (shingles, chicken pox), and the Epstein-Barr virus (mononucleosis), any of which might exacerbate or hasten HIV disease. It might also modestly retard HIV progression in those with coinfections earlier in HIV disease, when host immune function is less impaired. Indeed, this modest treatment effect—a decrease in mortality of about 7 percent per 6-monthly visit—was observed with acyclovir given before an AIDS diagnosis.[93] However, this set of analyses was not constructed and did not address the effect of zidovudine alone on survival or delay of development of AIDS, and so imputations about how much addition of acyclovir improved zidovudine efficacy were not possible.

We also looked at this issue in 490 HIV-infected men in cohort studies in San Francisco and elsewhere between 1988 and 1993.[94] Rather than start observing HIV patients at some unknown point in their HIV infection, and then trying to control for stage of disease by, for example, incorporating CD4+ cell counts in an adjusted Cox proportional hazards model,[88] we had data on a subset of homosexual and bisexual men whose date of actual HIV infection could be approximated because these had an HIV-negative test followed within months by an HIV-positive assay. We could also specify that men had taken zidovudine at least 6 months, so we were not hampered by not knowing who had ceased to take zidovudine because of toxicity. In these men who were well characterized by their dates of HIV infection and in whom we could look at AIDS diagnosis (rather than a surrogate endpoint), we found that 48 men who took zidovudine for 6 months before an AIDS diagnosis developed AIDS at 106.6 months after HIV infection, whereas 40 men who did never took zidovudine developed AIDS within a mean of 97.1 months, that is, 9.5 months earlier.[94]

Yet this analysis showed us that ours and others' analyses of observational data were unavoidably limited by opposite and competing biases. The average (San Francisco) gay man in our study who was infected around 1981 or 1982[92] and survived without AIDS to be given zidovudine after its approval in 1987 or later already had "extra" months of incubation compared with untreated men (onset confounding). Thereafter, men who were taking zidovudine were probably sicker—for example with "pre-AIDS" or AIDS-related complex symptoms such as lymphadenopathy, fever, and weight loss—and at increased likelihood (hazard) of developing AIDS soon, thereby decreasing their incubation time (selection bias). Analyses including Cox proportional hazards model using time-dependent covariates could control for one bias or the other, but not both. Still, all analyses, whether controlled for one problem or the other, kept indicating a modest delay of only several months in developing AIDS in those taking zidovudine compared to those not. This was similar to the several months delay in death in those treated with zidovudine once they already had AIDS.[80]

Two developments essentially ended the debate regarding early vs. late treatment with zidovudine. The first was the preliminary report of the much anticipated "Concorde" trial.[95] The Concorde study was designed in 1988 as a European, multicenter, randomized double-blind, and placebo-controlled study specifically of immediate vs. deferred treatment for HIV patients without symptoms. Analysis of the 1,762 study-subjects so randomized into each of the two treatment arms found no significant difference in either immediate or deferred zidovudine arms in terms of survival or disease progression. While some questioned whether in the preliminary analysis the numbers of patients followed were large enough[96] or the duration of follow-up long enough,[97] subsequent and final analyses of Concorde and the similar Opal study data showed limited benefit and no difference between zidovudine started early or late.[98] Thus, by 1994, most clinicians and researchers had concluded that early zidovudine provided limited and transient efficacy in prolonging survival.[99]

After Zidovudine

The other major developments that effectively ended or mitigated the debates about zidovudine were initial clinical trials of didanosine (ddI) and zalcitabine (ddC), reported at conferences, and leading to rapid FDA approval in 1991 and 1992, respectively (see Appendix). These drugs supplanted or supplemented zidovudine rapidly after their introduction. Didanosine was clearly efficacious for patients intolerant of or failing zidovudine therapy,[100, 101] and zalcitabine[102] for use in combination with zidovudine. These two drugs were better tolerated than zidovudine that had undergone its clinical trials at what, in retrospect, was too high a dosage; they also appeared to have better effect on CD4+ cell counts and viral loads and so, putatively, treatment of and survival with HIV infection.

By the start of the HIV Outpatient Study (HOPS) in 1993, an observational cohort study, the first 1,018 HIV patients enrolled were taking the following: 457 (45%) were on monotherapy, 65 percent of these on zidovudine monotherapy; 299 (29%) were taking two or more nucleoside RTI drugs; and 262 (26%) were taking no antiretroviral therapy (James Richardson, personal communication, May 30, 2007).

Graham and other MACS investigators suggested that combination therapy—adding didanosine or zalcitabine to failing regimens of zidovudine was no better or worse than stopping zidovudine and providing sequential therapy with the newer nucleoside RTIs.[103] However, before real controversy could develop, two large randomized trials—ACTG 175 and Delta—had convinced most that initiating therapy with two drugs—zidovudine with either didanosine or zalcitabine—was better than zidovudine monotherapy.[104, 105] This is not to indicate that combination therapy was without its own problems seen early on,[106] such as didanosine-related pancreatic toxicity. However, by the time of the introduction of new classes of antimicrobials—the protease inhibitor drugs and non-nucleoside reverse transcriptase inhibitors—most clinicians and patients were gravitating toward initial combination therapy rather than sequential monotherapy.

Marty Hirsch and his colleagues at Harvard's Massachusetts General Hospital argued early for the use of combination therapy as they cited laboratory and limited clinical data to indicate that sequential or "alternating" therapy led to decreased antiretroviral drug efficacy and accelerated development of resistance.[107, 108] At AIDS and other scientific conferences, Hirsch pointed to the in vitro additive or synergistic effect of using two, or even all three, of the then available nucleoside RTIs—zidovudine, didanosine, and zalcitabine. In addition to better efficacy than would be seen with any of these drugs alone, combination therapy also allowed the use of drugs at lower doses than used in monotherapy, putatively decreasing drug toxicity. Combination regimens might also delay the emergence of multiply resistant regimens.

For a brief period in early 1993, it even seemed that there was a "Eureka" moment as a medical student in Hirsch's group at Massachusetts General Hospital in Boston reported initial in vitro results of the use of the two nucleoside RTIs, zidovudine, and didanosine with the addition of either of the non-nucleoside RTIs, nevirapine, or the experimental drug, pyridinone.[109] Yang-Kang Chow's concept of "convergent" combination therapy was that, rather than using drugs with different targets in the replicative cycle of HIV, the three drugs would all target HIV reverse transcriptase. In theory, an HIV strain that developed resistance to all three drugs would be rare and would lose its replicative capacity.[110, 111] Treatment in vitro with the two nucleoside RTIs plus a non-nucleoside RTI putatively fostered multidrug resistant and nonreplicating or poorly replicating HIV-1. That is, HIV paid an adaptive "price" for developing multiple drug resistance in terms of its ability to replicate; further, elimination of reverse transcription by convergent combination therapy might also limit multidrug resistance.[111] While the authors urged caution in interpreting whether this would be a "cure" in vivo, once given to humans with many quasi-species of HIV, the implications were not lost on anyone.[109]

Unfortunately, this exciting breakthrough in the February 18, 1993, issue of *Nature* had to be retracted in print by August.[112] Chow and his colleagues found four previously unnoticed and unintended mutations—not related to the antiviral drugs used—in reverse transcriptase on further sequencing; these mutations could explain why the viruses derived from the clones used by Chow et al were not viable, and would explain the discrepancy between their report and the 1993 reports of Larder et al.[113] and Emini et al.[114] These latter investigators found that HIV resistant to the drugs used by Chow et al. still retained viability—that is, these induced mutations were not lethal to the virus. An anonymous editorial in the August 5 issue of *Nature*, the week before the retraction was published, summed it up well:

> Whatever the outcome, the history of this article illustrates a problem now all too common in AIDS research but also in other fields. The paper by Chow *et al.* was carefully reviewed, and it was agreed that the results would be useful in planning strategies to manage AIDS. Such reports should obviously be published with speed so that beneficial knowledge may be more quickly shared. But, by the same test, retractions should also be speedy and full-throated. Publicity does not help; the scientific community is tolerant of admissions of honest error, but honest errors seem more grievous if they follow wide publicity. Sadly, there is no escape from that.[115]

However, one irony of the episode was that the combination that Chow et al. used—that is, of a non-nucleoside RTI such as neviripine and two nucleoside RTIs such as zidovudine and didanosine—was recognized within the next few years as a potent HIV treatment nonetheless, one of the first highly active antiretroviral therapies (HAART).[116, 117] With the ability to add drugs of other classes—protease inhibitor drugs and non-nucleoside RTIs, initially nevirapine, and efavirenz—to nucleoside RTIs, potent "drug cocktails" (as the newspapers dubbed them) could be given to HIV patients. Combination therapy and those who advocated it were indeed vindicated; but, despite the ability to now treat HIV patients effectively, HAART had its own problems and controversies.

References

1. Clumeck, N., and P. Hermans. 1988. Antiviral drugs other than zidovudine and immunomodulating therapies in human immunodeficiency virus infection. *American Journal of Medicine* 85:165–172.

2. Eckholm, E. July 13, 1986. Ideas and trends: Should the rules be bent in an epidemic? *New York Times.*

3. Holmberg, S.D., L.J. Conley, S.P. Buchbinder, et al. 1993. Use of therapeutic and prophylactic drugs for AIDS by homosexual and bisexual men in three US cities. *AIDS* 7:699–704.

4. Ruff, M.R., L.M. Melendez-Guerrero, Q.E. Yank, et al. 2001. Peptide T inhibits HIV-1 infection mediated by the chemokine receptor-5 (CCR-5). *Antiretroviral Research* 52:63–75.

5. Bridge, T.P., P.N. Heseltine, E.S. Parker, et al. 1991. Results of extended peptide T administration in AIDS and ARC patients. *Psychopharmacology Bulletin* 27:237–245.

6. Heseltine, P.N., K. Goodkin, J.H. Atkinson, et al. 1998. Randomized double-blind placebo-controlled trial of peptide T for HIV-associated cognitive impairment. *Archives of Neurology* 55:41–51.

7. Simpson, D.M., D. Dorfman, R.K. Olney, et al. 1996. Peptide T in the treatment of painful distal neuropathy associated with AIDS: results of a placebo-controlled trial. The Peptide T Neuropathy Study Group. *Neurology* 47:1254–1259.

8. Polianova, M.T., F.W. Ruscetti, C.B. Pert, et al. 2003. Antiviral and immunological benefits in HIV patients receiving intranasal peptide T (DAPTA). *Peptides* 24:1093–1098.

9. Sundquist, B., and B. Oberg. 1979. Phosphonoformate inhibits reverse transcriptase. *Journal of General Virology* 45:273–281.

10. Cheng, Y.C., S. Grill, D. Derse, J.Y. Chen, S.J. Caradonna, and K. Connor. 1981. Mode of action of phosphonoformate as an anti-herpes simplex virus agent. *Biochimica et Biophysica Acta* 652:90–98.

11. Tyms, A.S., D.L. Taylor, and J.M. Parkin. 1989. Cytomegalovirus and the acquired immunodeficiency syndrome. *Journal of Antimicrobial Chemotherapy* 23(suppl A):89–110.

12. Anonymous. 1997. Foscavir receives new indication. *AIDS Alert* 12:71.

13. Deray, G., F. Martinez, C. Katalama, et al. 1989. Foscarnet nephrotoxicity: Mechanism, incidence and prevention. *American Journal of Nephrology* 9:316–321.

14. Chrisp, P., and S.P. Clissold. 1991. Foscarnet. A review of its antiviral activity, pharmacokinetic properties and therapeutic use in immunocompromised patients with cytomegalovirus retinitis. *Drugs* 41:104–129.

15. Wagstaff, A.J., and H.M. Bryson. 1994. Foscarnet. A reappraisal of its antiviral activity, pharmacokinetic properties and therapeutic use in immunocompromised patients with viral infections. *Drugs* 48:199–226.

16. Tartaglione, T.A., and A.C. Collier. 1987. Development of antiviral agents for the treatment of human immunodeficiency virus infection. *Clinical Pharmacology* 6:927–940.

17. Kaiser, L., L. Perrin, B. Hirschel, et al. 1995. Foscarnet decreases human immunodeficiency virus RNA. *Journal of Infectious Diseases* 172:225–227.

18. Altman, L.K. July 23, 1992. Cost of treating AIDS patients is soaring. *New York Times.*

19. Traill, K.N., F. Offner, U. Winter, F. Paltauf, and G. Wick. 1988. Lipid requirements of human T lymphocytes stimulated with mitogen in serum-free medium. Membrane "fluidity" changes are an artefact of lipid (AL721) uptake by monocytes. *Immunobiology* 176:450–464.

20. Peters, B.S., J.M. Bennett, D.J. Jeffries, K. Knox, A. Kocsis, and A.J. Pinching. 1990. Ineffectiveness of AL721 in HIV disease [letter]. *Lancet* 355:545–546.

21. Mildvan, D., J. Buzas, D. Armstrong, et al. 1991. An open-label, dose-ranging trial of AL 721 in patients with persistent generalized lymphadenopathy and AIDS-related complex. *Journal of Acquired Immune Deficiency Syndromes* 4:945–951.

22. Callahan, L.N., M. Phelan, M. Mallinson, and M.A. Norcross. 1991. Dextran sulfate blocks antibody binding to the principal neutralizing domain of human immunodeficiency virus type 1 without interfering with gp 120-CD4 interactions. *Journal of Virology* 65:1543–1550.

23. Thiele, B., and F. Steinbach. 1994. Dextran sulfate induces a PKC and actin independent internalization of CD4. *Immunology Letters* 42:105–110.

24. Busso, M.E., and L. Resnick. 1990. Anti-human immunodeficiency virus effects of dextran sulfate are strain dependent and synergistic or antagonistic when dextrasn sulfate is given in combination with dideoxynucleosides. *Antimicrobial Agents and Chemotherapy* 34:1991–1995.

25. Ono, K., H. Nakane, T. Matsumoto, F. Barré-Sinoussi, and J.C. Chermann. 1984. Inhibition of DNA polymerase alpha activity by ammonium 21-tungsto-9-antimoniate (HPA23). *Nucleic Acids Symposium Series* 15:169–172.

26. Rozenbaum, W., D. Dormont, B. Spire, et al. 1985. Antimoniotungstate (HPA 23) treatment of three patients with AIDS and one with prodrome [letter]. *Lancet* 1:450–451.

27. Moskovitz, B.L. 1988. Clinical trial of tolerance of HPA-23 in patients with acquired immune deficiency syndrome. *Antimicrobial Agents and Chemotherapy* 32:1300–1303.

28. Burgard, M., P. Sansonetti, D. Vittecoq, et al. 1989. Lack of HPA-23 antiviral activity in HIV-infected patients without AIDS. *AIDS* 3:665–668.

29. Agarwal, R.P., M.E. Busso, A.M. Mian, and L. Resnick. 1989. Uptake of 2',3'-dideoxyadenosine in human immunodeficiency virus-infected and noninfected human cells. *AIDS Research and Human Retroviruses* 5:541–550.

30. Cao, W., E.E. Sikorski, B.A. Fuchs, M.L. Stern, M.I. Luster, and A.E. Munson. 1990. The B lymphocyte is the immune cell target for 2',3'-dideoxyadenosine. *Toxicology and Applied Pharmacology* 105:492–502.

31. Luster, M.I., G.J. Rosenthal, W. Cao, et al. 1991. Experimental studies of the hematologic and immune system toxicity of nucleoside derivatives used against HIV infection. *International Journal of Immunopharmacology* 13(suppl 1):99–107.

32. Gallant, J.E. 1999. New antiretroviral agents. *Hopkins HIV Report* 11:3,12.

33. Highleyman, L. 1999. Lodenosine trials stopped due to safety concerns. *BETA Bulletin of Experimental Treatments for AIDS* 12:4.

34. Crumpacker, C., W. Heagy, G. Bubley, et al. 1987. Ribavirin treatment of the acquired immunodeficiency syndrome (AIDS) and the acquired-immunodeficiency-syndrome-related complex (ARC). A phase 1 study shows transient clinical improvement with suppression of the human immunodeficiency virus and enhanced lymphocyte proliferation. *Annals of Internal Medicine* 107:664–674.

35. The Ribavirin ARC Study Group. 1993. Multicenter clinical trial of oral ribavirin in symptomatic HIV-infected patients. *Journal of Acquired Immune Deficiency Syndromes* 6:32–41.

36. Vernon, A., and R.S. Schulof. 1987. Serum HIV core antigen in symptomatic ARC patients taking oral ribavirin or placebo [abstract]. *Proceedings of the 3rd International Conference on AIDS*, Washington, DC, June 1–5, 1987:58.

37. Spector, S.A., C. Kennedy, J.A. McCutchan, et al. 1989. The antiviral effect of zidovudine and ribavirin in clinical trials and the use of p24 antigen levels as a virologic marker. *Journal of Infectious Diseases* 159:822–828.

38. Roberts, R.B., G.M. Dickinson, P.N. Heseltine, et al. 1990. A multicenter clinical trial of oral ribavirin in HIV-infected patients with lymphadenopathy. The Ribavirin-LAS Collaborative Group. *Journal of Acquired Immune Deficiency Syndromes* 3:884–892.

39. Bodsworth, N., and D.A. Cooper. 1990. Ribavirin: A role in HIV infection [editorial commentary]? *Journal of Acquired Immune Deficiency Syndromes* 3:893–895.

40. Mitsuya, H., S. Matsushita, B. Yarchoan, and S. Broder. 1984. Protection of T cells against infectivity and cytopathic effect of HTLV-III in vitro. *Princess Takamatsu Symposium* 15:277–288.

41. Collins, J.M., R.W. Klecker Jr., R. Yarchoan, et al. 1986. Clinical pharmacokinetics of suramin in patients with HTLV-III/LAV infection. *Journal of Clinical Pharmacology* 26:22–26.

42. Schattenkerk, E., J.K., S.A. Danner, J.M. Lange, et al. 1988. Persistence of human immunodeficiency virus antigenemia in patients with the acquired immunodeficiency syndrome treated with a reverse transcriptase inhibitor, suramin. Ten patient case-control study. *Archives of Internal Medicine* 148:209–211.

43. Cheson, B.D., A.M. Levine, D. Mildvan, et al. 1987. Suramin therapy in AIDS and related disorders. Report of the US Suramin Working Group. *Journal of the American Medical Association* 258:1347–1351.

44. Lopez, C., P.A. Fitzgerald, and F.P. Siegal. 1983. Severe acquired immune deficiency syndrome in male homosexuals: Diminished capacity to make interferon-alpha in vitro associated with severe opportunistic infections. *Journal of Infectious Diseases* 148:962–966.

45. Abb, J., M. Kochen, and F. Deinhardt. 1984. Interferon production in male homosexuals with the acquired immune deficiency syndrome (AIDS) or generalized lymphadenopathy. *Infection* 12:240–242.

46. Hirsch, M.S., and J.C. Kaplan. 1985. Prospects of therapy for infections with human T-lymphotropic virus type III. *Annals of Internal Medicine* 103:750–755.

47. Volberding, P.A., and R. Mitsuyasu. 1985. Recombinant interferon alpha in the treatment of acquired immune deficiency syndrome-related Kaposi's sarcoma. *Seminars in Oncology* 12 (4 suppl 5):2–6.

48. Rozenbaum, W., S. Gharakhanian, M.S. Navarette, R. De Sahb, B. Cardon, and C. Rouzioux. 1990. Long-term follow-up of 120 patients with AIDS-related Kaposi's sarcoma treated with interferon alpha-2a. *Journal of Investigative Dermatology* 95(6 suppl):161S–165S.

49. Krown, S.E., F.X. Real, S. Vadhan-Raj, et al. 1986. Kaposi's sarcoma and the acquired immune deficiency syndrome. Treatment with recombinant interferon alpha and analysis of prognostic factors. *Cancer* 57(8 suppl):1662–1665.

50. Krown, S.E., J.W. Gold, D. Niedzwiecki, et al. 1990. Interferon-alpha with zidovudine: Safety, tolerance, and clinical and virologic effects in patients with Kaposi

sarcoma associated with the acquired immunodeficiency syndrome (AIDS). *Annals of Internal Medicine* 112:812–821.

51. de Wit, R., J.K. Schattenkerk, C.A. Boucher, P.J. Bakker, K.H. Veenhof, and S.A. Danner. 1988. Clinical and virologic effects of high-dose recombinant interferon-alpha in disseminated AIDS-related Kaposi's sarcoma. *Lancet* 2:1214–1217.

52. de Wit, R., S.A. Danner, P.J. Bakker, J.M. Lange, J.K. Eeftinck Schattenkerk, and C.H. Veenhof. 1991. Combined zidovudine and interferon-alpha treatment in patients with AIDS-associated Kaposi's sarcoma. *Journal of Internal Medicine* 229: 35–40.

53. Lane, H.C., V. Davey, J.A. Kovacs, et al. 1990. Interferon-alpha in patients with asymptomatic human immunodeficiency virus (HIV) infection. A randomized, placebo-controlled trial. *Annals of Internal Medicine* 112:805–811.

54. Katabira, E.T., N.K. Sewankambo, R.D. Mugerwa, et al. 1998. Lack of efficacy of low dose oral interferon alfa in symptomatic HIV-1 infection: A randomized, double blind, placebo controlled trial. *Sexually Transmitted Diseases* 74:265–270.

55. Koech, D.K., and A.O. Obel. 1990. Efficacy of Kemron (low dose oral natural human interferon alpha) in the management of HIV-1 infection and acquired immune deficiency syndrome (AIDS). *East African Medical Journal* 67(7 suppl 2): SS64–SS70.

56. Kaiser, G., H. Jaeger, J. Birkmann, J. Poppinger, J.M. Cummins, and W.M. Gallmeier. 1992. Low-dose oral natural human interferon-alpha in 29 patients with HIV-1 infection: a double-blind, randomized, placebo-controlled trial. *AIDS* 6:563–569.

57. Roberts, J. 1992. About turn in US on interferon alpha. *British Medical Journal* 305:1243–1244.

58. Highleyman, L. September 1997. Kemron trial stopped. *Bulletin of Experimental Treatments for AIDS*, p. .

59. Dodd, R. 1996. Patients sue the "AIDS-cure" Kenyan scientist. *Lancet* 347:1688.

60. Nath, A., A. Venkataramana, D.S. Reich, I. Cortese, and E.O. Major. 2006. Progression of progressive multifocal leukoencephalopathy despite treatment with beta-interferon. *Neurology* 66:149–150.

61. O'Marro, S.D., J.A. Armstrong, C. Asuncion, L. Gueverra, and M. Ho. 1992. The effect of combinations of ampligen and zidovudine or dideoxyinosine against human immunodeficiency viruses in vitro. *Antiviral Research* 17:169–177.

62. Armstrong, J.A., D. McMahon, X.L. Huang, et al. 1992. A phase I study of ampligen in human immunodeficiency virus-infected subjects. *Journal of Infectious Diseases* 166:717–722.

63. Tziveleka, L.A., C. Vagias, and V. Roussis. 2003. Natural products with anti-HIV activity from marine organisms. *Current Topics in Medicinal Chemistry* 3:1512–1535.

64. Ullum, H., A. Cozzi Lepri, H. Aladdin, et al. 1999. Natural immunity and HIV disease progression. *AIDS* 13:557–563.

65. Emery, S., W.B. Capra, D.A. Cooper, et al. 2000. Pooled analysis of 3 randomized, controlled trials of interleukin-2 therapy in adult human immunodeficiency virus type 1 disease. *Journal of Infectious Diseases* 182:428–434.

66. Davey Jr., R.T., R.L. Murphy, F.M. Graziano, et al. 2000. Immunologic and virologic effects of subcutaneous interleukin 2 in combination with antiretroviral

therapy: A randomized controlled trial. *Journal of the American Medical Association* 284:183–189.

67. Lichtenstein, K.A., C. Armon, A.C. Moorman, K.C. Wood, and S.D. Holmberg. 2004. A 7-year longitudinal analysis of IL-2 in patients treated with highly active antiretroviral therapy. *AIDS* 18:2346–2348.

68. Murray, H.W., D. Scavuzzo, J. Jacobs, et al. 1987. *In vitro* and *in vivo* activation of human mononuclear phagocytes by interferon-γ. *Journal of Immunology* 138:2457–2462.

69. Barnes, D.M. 1987. Cytokines alter AIDS virus production. *Science* 236:1626–1627.

70. Kedzierska, K., S.H. Crowe, S. Turville, and A.L. Cunningham. 2003. The influence of cytokines, chemokines and their receptors on HIV-1 replication in monocytes and macrophages. *Reviews in Medical Virology* 13:39–56.

71. McDougal, J.S., L.S. Martin, S.P. Cort, et al. 1985. Thermal inactivation of acquired immunodeficiency virus human T lymphotropic virus III/lymphadenopathy associated virus with special reference to antihemophilic factor. *Journal of Clinical Investigation* 76:875–880.

72. Deyton, L.R., J. Kagan, R. Eisenger, I. Robins, and R. Torres. August 30, 1990. Clinical use of hyperthermia in AIDS. In *NIAID Site Visit Report*. Bethesda, MD: NIAID, p. 5.

73. Hilts, P.J. September 5, 1990. Heating blood criticized as treatment of AIDS. *New York Times*.

74. Logan, W.D., Alonso K. 1991. Case report: Total body hyperthermia in the treatment of Kaposi's sarcoma in an HIV positive patient. *Medical Oncology and Tumor Pharmacotherapy* 8:45–47.

75. Anonymous. August 16, 1990. Gay group seeks more data on heat treatment for AIDS. *New York Times*.

76. Steinhart, C.R., S.R. Ash, C. Gingrich, D. Sapir, G.N. Keeling, and M.B. Yatvin. 1996. Effect of whole-body hyperthermia on AIDS patients with Kaposi's sarcoma: A pilot study. *Journal of Acquired Immune Deficiency Syndromes* 11:271–281.

77. Ash, S.R., C.R. Steinhart, M.F. Curfman, et al. 1997. Extracorporeal whole body hyperthermia treatments for HIV infection and AIDS *American Society for Artificial Internal Organs Journal* 43:M830–M838.

78. Fischl, M.S., D.D. Richman, M.H. Grieco, et al. 1987. The efficacy of azidothymidine (AZT) in the treatment of patients with AIDS ad AIDS-related complex. A double-blind, placebo-controlled trial. *New England Journal of Medicine* 317:185–191.

79. Gould, S.J. 1990. AIDS and FDA drug-approval policy: an evolving controversy. *Journal of Health and Social Policy* 2:39–46.

80. Fischl, M.A., D.D. Richman, M.M. Causey et al. 1989. Prolonged zidovudine therapy in patients with AIDS and advanced AIDS-related complex. AZT Collaborative Working Group. *Journal of the American Medical Association* 262:2405–2410.

81. Gail, M.H., P.S. Rosenberg, and J.J. Goedert. 1990. Therapy may explain recent deficits in AIDS incidence. *Journal of Acquired Immune Deficiency Syndromes* 3:296–306.

82. Rosenberg, P.S., M.H. Gail, L.K. Shrager, et al. 1991. National AIDS incidence trends and the extent of zidovudine therapy in selected demographic and transmission groups. *Journal of Acquired Immune Deficiency Syndromes* 4:392–401.

83. Richman, D.D., M.A. Fischl, M.H. Grieco, et al. 1987. The toxicity of azidothymidine (AZT) in the treatment of patients with AIDS and AIDS-related complex. A double-blind, placebo-controlled trial. *New England Journal of Medicine* 317:192–197.

84. Dournon, E., S. Matheron, W. Rozenbaum, et al. 1988. Effects of zidovudine in 365 consecutive patients with AIDS or AIDS-related complex. *Lancet* 2:1297–1302.

85. Altman, L.K. June 6, 1993. At AIDS talks, science faces a daunting maze. *New York Times*.

86. Volberding, P.A., S.W. Lagakos, J.M. Grimes, et al. 1994. The duration of zidovudine benefit in persons with asymptomatic HIV infection. Prolonged evaluation of protocol 019 of the AIDS Clinical Trials Group. *Journal of the American Medical Association* 272:437–442.

87. Graham, N.M.H., S.L. Zeger, L.P. Park et al. 1991. Effect of zidovudine and *Pneumocystis carinii* pneumonia prophylaxis on progression of HIV-1 infection to AIDS. *Lancet* 338:265–269.

88. Graham, N.M.H., S.L. Zeger, L.P. Park, et al. 1992. The effects of survival of early treatment of human immunodeficiency virus infection. *New England Journal of Medicine* 326:1037–1042.

89. Hamilton, J.D., P.M. Hartigan, M.S. Simberkoff, et al. 1992. A controlled trial of early versus late treatment with zidovudine in symptomatic human immunodeficiency virus infection–Results of the Veterans Affairs Cooperative Study. *New England Journal of Medicine* 326:437–443.

90. Hartigan, P.M., J.D. Hamilton, and M.S. Simberkoff. 1992. Early zidovudine and survival in HIV infection [letter]. *New England Journal of Medicine* 327:814–815.

91. Volberding, P.A., and N.M.H. Graham. 1994. Initiation of antiretroviral therapy in HIV infection: a review of interstudy consistencies. *Journal of Acquired Immune Deficiency Syndromes* 7(suppl 2):S12–S23.

92. Hessol, N.A., A.R. Lifson, P.M. O'Malley, L.S. Doll, H.W. Jaffe, and G.W. Rutherford. 1989. Prevalence, incidence, and progression of human immunodeficiency virus infection in homosexual and bisexual men in hepatitis B vaccine trials, 1978–1988. *American Journal of Epidemiology* 130:1167–1175.

93. Stein, D.S., N.M.H. Graham, L.P. Park, et al. 1994. The effect of interaction of acyclovir with zidovudine on progression to AIDS and survival. Analysis of data in the Multicenter AIDS Cohort Study. *Annals of Internal Medicine* 121:100–108.

94. Holmberg, S.D., and R.H. Byers. 1993. Does zidovudine delay development of AIDS? Analysis of data from observational cohorts [letter]. *Lancet* 342:558-559.

95. Aboulker, J.-P., and A.M. Swart. 1993. Preliminary analysis of the Concorde trial [letter]. *Lancet* 341:889–890.

96. Saah, A.J. 1993. Immediate versus deferred zidovudine [letter]. *Lancet* 341:1023.

97. Peto, R., and R. Collins. 1993. Immediate versus deferred zidovudine [letter]. *Lancet* 341:1022–1023.

98. Joint Concorde and Opal Coordinating Committees. 1998. Long-term follow-up of randomized trials of immediate versus deferred zidovudine in symptom-free HIV infection [editorial review]. *AIDS* 12:1259-1265.

99. Collier, A.C. 1994. Early intervention in HIV infection: where are we? *AIDS Research and Human Retroviruses* 10:893–899.

100. McGowan, J.J., J.E. Tomaszewski, J. Cradock, et al. 1990. Overview of the pre-clinical development of an antiretroviral drug, 2'3'-dideoyinosine. *Reviews of Infectious Diseases* 12(suppl 5):S513–S520.

101. Shelton, M.J., A.M. O'Donnell, and G.D. Morse. 1992. Didanosine. *Annals of Pharmacotherapy* 26:660–670.

102. Merigan, T.C., and G. Skowron. 1990. Safety and tolerance of dideoxycyti-dine as a single agent. Results of early-phase studies in patients with acquired im-munodeficiency syndrome (AIDS) or advanced AIDS-related complex. Study Group of the AIDS Clinical Trials Group of the National Institute of Allergy and Infectious Diseases. *American Journal of Medicine* 88:11S–15S.

103. Graham, N.M.H., D.R. Hoover, L.P. Park et al. 1996. Survival in HIV-infected patients who have received zidovudine: Comparison of combination therapy with sequential monotherapy and continued zidovudine monotherapy. *Annals of Internal Medicine* 124:1031–1038.

104. Hirsch, M.S., and P. Yeni. 1996. A bend in the road–Implications of ACTG 175 and Delta trials. *Antiviral Therapy* 1:6–8.

105. Delta Coordinating Committee. 2002. Evidence for prolonged clinical benefit from initial combination antiviral therapy: Delta extended follow-up. *HIV Medicine* 2:181–188.

106. Hammer, S.M., H.A. Kessler, and M.S. Saag. 1994. Issues in combination antiretroviral therapy: A review. *Journal of Acquired Immune Deficiency Syndromes* 7(suppl 2):S24–S37.

107. Hirsch, M.S., and R.T. D'Aquila. 1993. Therapy for human immunodefi-ciency virus infection [review]. *New England Journal of Medicine* 328:1686–1695.

108. Caliendo, A.M., and M.S. Hirsch. 1994. Combination therapy for infection due to human immunodeficiency virus type 1 [commentary]. *Clinical Infectious Diseases* 18:516–524.

109. Altman, L.K. February 18, 1993. Drug mixture curbs H.I.V. in lab, doctors report, but urge caution. *New York Times*.

110. Richman, D.D. 1993. Playing chess with reverse transcriptase. *Nature* 361:588–589.

111. Chow, Y.-K., M.S. Hirsch, D.P. Merrill, et al. 1993. Use of evolutionary limitations of HIV-1 multidrug resistance to optimize therapy. *Nature* 361:650–654.

112. Chow, Y.-K., M.S. Hirsch, J.C. Kaplan, and R.T. D'Aquila. 1993. HIV-1 error revealed [correspondence]. *Nature* 364:679.

113. Larder, B.A., P. Kellam, and S.D. Kemp. 1993. Convergent combination therapy can select viable multidrug-resistant HIV-1 in vitro. *Nature* 365:451–453.

114. Emini, E.A., D.J. Graham, L. Gotlib, J.H. Condra, V.W. Bynes, and W.A. Schleif. 1993. HIV and multidrug resistance [correspondence]. *Nature* 364:679.

115. Anonymous. 1993. Saying sorry quickly: An article on AIDS therapy pub-lished earlier this year turns out not to sustain its hopeful conclusions. *Nature* 364:468.

116. D'Aquila, R.T., M.D. Hughes, V.A. Johnson, et al. 1996. Nevirapine, zidovu-dine, and didanosine compared with zidovudine and didanosine in patients with HIV-1 infection. A randomized, double-blind, placebo-controlled trial. National In-stitute of Allergy and Infectious Diseases AIDS Clinical Trials Group Protocol 241 Investigators. *Annals of Internal Medicine* 124:1019–1030.

117. Zhou, X.J., L.B. Sheiner, R.T. D'Aquila, et al. 1999. Population pharmacokinetics of nevirapine, zidovudine, and didanosine in human immunodeficiency virus-infected patients. The National Institute of Allergy and Infectious Diseases AIDS Clinical Trials Group Protocol 241 Investigators. *Antimicrobial Agents and Chemotherapy* 43:121–128.

CHAPTER EIGHT

The Modern Therapeutic Era (after 1995)

The spirit at the XIth International Conference on AIDS in Vancouver in July 1996 was ebullient. Presentations about HIV health care worker "burn-out," about parsing the differences between sequential vs. combination nucleoside RTI therapy (NRTIs), and about the problems with changing sexual behavior and substance abuse to retard the epidemic were marginalized at this conference by the many HIV clinicians, patients, and others happily comparing favorable treatment notes. These conversations usually contained anecdotes of moribund patients who had almost miraculously recovered CD4+ cells, their weight, and even their jobs after taking protease inhibitor (PI) drugs or non-nucleoside RTIs (NNRTIs). Reports from federally funded AIDS Clinical Treatment Groups (ACTGs) examining the efficacy of these two new classes of drugs were all positive: "This was probably the most optimistic international AIDS conference ever held. It was also atypical in that the grounds for hoping that real progress in the management of disease is being made with advances in direct antiretroviral management rather than, as in previous meetings, with improvements in the prophylaxis and treatment of opportunistic infections."[1]

Not everything is controversial. By the time the first major articles demonstrating the success of highly active antiretroviral therapy (HAART) were published, many if not most patients in the United States were receiving HAART rather than monotherapy or dual therapy with NRTIs only. After publication of an article by Frank Palella and others in the HIV Outpatient Study (HOPS) in 1998, therapy with any regimen other than HAART became untenable.[2] This report has been subsequently referenced thousands of times as indicating the indubitable benefits of the new therapies in the

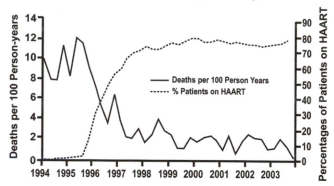

Figure 8.1 Use of highly active antiretroviral therapy (HAART) and mortality rates in the HIV Outpatient Study (HOPS), 1994–2004

real-world setting, specifically of the effectiveness of a PI or NNRTI drug combined with two or more NRTI drugs. As seen in Figure 8.1, that updates mortality rates and HAART usage from the original report, mortality rates in HOPS patients were inversely proportional to the adoption of HAART after 1995. (Many HOPS patients were in experimental trials of these drugs before their FDA approval in 1996 and thereafter.) In a failure-rate analysis, taking combination therapy, especially including a PI drug, was associated with stepwise reductions in mortality and morbidity (opportunistic infections).[2]

Like the HOPS investigators, others reported the same remarkable declines in death and hospitalization rates from elsewhere in the United States and other developed countries.[3–5] By late 1999, the formal recommendations of the International AIDS Society–USA Panel were to initiate therapy for HIV patients with HAART, usually either a PI or an NNRTI drug plus two NRTI drugs.[6] While the Panel did not specify at that time, as they did with later recommendations, exactly which drugs to use, they noted that there were five PI drugs, three NNRTIs and six NRTIs, approved for use in HIV/AIDS from which to select combination therapy (Appendix). This remarkably rapid adoption of HAART followed closely the overwhelming evidence that it was far more potent than earlier mono- or dual therapies with NRTIs: there was essentially no debate as the data were so clear.

However, from the beginning, there have been prominent concerns about toxicity, failure, adherence to, and resistance to the various new therapies and debates about when to start therapy and when, if ever, to end it. These various concerns, considerations, and debates are ongoing, so this chapter mainly recapitulates recent history and indicates trends in thinking.

When to Start Therapy in HIV-Infected People without Symptoms

As there is no cure for HIV/AIDS, the question of at what point in the disease to initiate HIV therapy for the individual patient is a complex consideration of the relative likelihoods of mortality, morbidity, viral drug resistance, adverse events and toxicity, and adherence. While there are questions about when, at what CD4+ cell count, to start therapy for the HIV patient with no symptoms, no one advocates that patients who are late in disease and have developed AIDS not be treated. Thus, the plethora of scientific articles demonstrating that starting therapy before a patient's CD4+ cell count dips below 200 cells/mm^3–itself an AIDS-defining condition–have not been controversial or seriously questioned. The many, many American patients who are not identified or delay treatment when they have a low CD4+ cell count need immediate treatment: that is not debated. The question is when to treat the many HIV patients who have been discovered "early" in infection, for example at CD4+ cells counts above 350 cells/mm^3.

Probably the best approach to this question would be to randomize HIV patients in different CD4+ cell strata to either receive therapy or not and then to follow them over the long term to observe their rates of morbidity, mortality, adverse reactions to drugs, development of drug resistance, etc. A study could start with a group of patients who are observed when they are between 300 and 400 CD4+ cells, randomizing half to receive therapy within that cell stratum and half to receive therapy at the next lowest stratum, say, when they first have a CD4+ cell count between 200 and 300 cells/mm^3. These study-participants would be observed for their rates of "hard outcomes"–for example, mortality rates, percentage developing and maintaining undetectable viral load, numbers and percentage developing drug resistance by a standard assay, etc. Such a study would give some clear indication of the benefit or not of starting earlier vs. later (at the next lower CD4+ cell stratum). Unfortunately, such a study would be prohibitively expensive, probably not yield enough end-events (say, deaths) until years after the study started, and probably be obsolete by the time definitive study results were available, especially given the current rapid rate of development of new and more potent antiretroviral drugs. Further, such a study may not even be ethical: what patient who desires immediate therapy would want to wait to start therapy till the next lower CD4+ cell stratum? Further, such a study would be very hard to "blind," especially if patients receiving a placebo did not do well and HIV clinician and patient want to change to an effective therapy; to deny such therapy would be unethical. Thus, for many good reasons, we are constrained in answering this issue to analyzing observational data from the "real-world" setting

At first, after dramatic declines in morbidity and mortality with HAART, there was enthusiasm for providing these potent new combination therapies as early in the course of infection as possible. However, it quickly became clear that HIV could not be eradicated because of a large pool of latently infected and sequestered cells, and that many patients had toxic or adverse effects from the therapy, were taking many pills each day and frequently nonadherent, and, partly because of inconsistent drug-taking, were developing resistance not just to the drug(s) they were taking but to others in the same class of drugs as well. (For example, resistance to efavirenz results in resistance to the whole first generation of other NNRTIs, such as nevirapine, too.) The duration of sequential drug regimens became shorter, as did options for "salvage" therapy of patients failing initial treatment.[7] All these factors limited treatment options in the first several years after the introduction of HAART, and clinicians became increasingly leery of starting patients who might be able to defer therapy to some later point in their disease process.

Some of these attitudes about delaying therapy until the patient is sick probably had their root in earlier experience with the first antiretroviral therapies such as zidovudine "early" in infection rather than "late," after the onset of AIDS. Immediately following the introduction of zidovudine (AZT) in 1987, the scarcity and cost of the drug, about $10,000 per year,[8] precluded its use except for the sickest patients. In 1987 and 1988 none or very few gay men (less than 17%) with CD4+ cell counts above 200 cells/mm^3 were taking zidovudine; by 1989 about 30–35 percent of gay men in San Francisco who were aware of their HIV infection were taking zidovudine, but still fewer than 20 percent of all known HIV-infected gay men in Denver and Chicago and virtually no injection drug users in New York City were receiving it.[9, 10] By 1990 over 90 percent of gay men with AIDS and 80 percent who had CD4+ cell counts less than 200 cells/mm^3 had used the drug; but because of toxicity and side effects only 68 percent and 63 percent of men with AIDS or low CD4+ cell count, respectively, were able to take the drug for 6 or more months.[9] Thus, by the early 1990s even the largest populations with high rates of HIV and AIDS showed little use of zidovudine in asymptomatic, chronically infected patients; zidovudine and later NRTIs, didanosine and zalcitabine were mainly prescribed for AIDS patients. (Again, a CD4+ cell count less than 200 cells/mm^3 was added to the CDC's definition of AIDS in 1993.)

Another factor influencing the timing of therapy for asymptomatic patients was the preliminary report from the European "Concorde" Study.[11] As described in Chapter 7, Concorde was a randomized double-blind, and placebo-controlled study specifically of immediate vs. deferred zidovudine treatment for HIV patients without symptoms. Analysis of the 1,762 study-subjects showed no significant difference in survival or disease progression for those who took zidovudine "early" or "late" (after AIDS diagnosis). While some questioned this preliminary report, it convinced many that early zidovudine was of transient and modest benefit at best; and that, worse, it might engender resistance not only to zidovudine but also to other drugs of the same NRTI class. The final analyses of Concorde and the similar Opal study data showed limited benefit and no difference between zidovudine started early or late.[12] Thus, by 1994, most clinicians and researchers had concluded that zidovudine provided limited, transient, and even equivocal efficacy in prolonging survival and was frequently associated with adverse effects and toxicities limiting patient adherence.[13]

U.S. guidelines even in July 1998 advocated therapy be considered at any CD4+ cell count, especially for those with a plasma HIV RNA concentration (viral load) more than 5,000–10,000 copies/ml.[14] However, these more lax guidelines started to be reconsidered by the January 2000 guidelines[6] as considerations of adverse effects, adherence to long-term therapy, potential toxicity, and the development of resistance to the new antiretroviral drugs made clinicians more cautious about their earlier use of these drugs. They did not want to repeat perceived mistakes with zidovudine from which many patients got little or modest benefit yet often had adverse effects or developed resistance.

While in 2000 it was thought that treatment could be initiated for asymptomatic HIV patients once their CD4+ cell count had declined to 500 or fewer cells/mm^3,[6] the next few years saw a "pendulum shift" to delaying therapy till patients had "fewer than 350 cells/mm^3,"[15, 16] then even more emphatically till they had "more than 200 cells/mm^3."[17, 18] This trend toward recommendation of later treatment of HIV--that is, near the time but before the patient's CD4+ cell count fell below 200 cells/mm^3--was matched, even anticipated somewhat, by published recommendations from France, Britain, and other European countries.[19–21] It is also likely that clinicians and researchers from those countries, operating under different constraints such as limited availability initially of the "new" drugs compared to the American situation, may have been more conservative and cautious in their use of them.

Because of this shift in attitude, many asymptomatic patients were getting treated later in their disease. For example, in the HOPS--that provided the data for Figure 8.1--the initial CD4+ cell counts of HIV patients who started their therapy while not hospitalized fell from a mean of 317 in 1997, the first year after HAART became available, to 272 cells/mm^3 in 2003[22]; this change occurred despite the fact that many HOPS clinicians described themselves as "early treaters."

What were the data to support this change? The title of an 2003 editorial by NIH's Cliff Lane and Jim Neaton of the University of Minnesota summed up the issue nicely: "When to start therapy for HIV infection: A swinging pendulum in search of data."[23] The data were sparse or nonexistent for recommendations about when to start therapy for an asymptomatic HIV patient. To substantiate their expert opinion, the 2003 U.S. Public Health Service recommendations[18] cited a conference presentation for the recommendation to start therapy at some point greater than 200 cells/mm³ but not for patients with more than 350 cells/mm³. Aside from the fact the presentation did not address the question directly, this[24] and other analyses of mortality of people who started therapy at various CD4+ cell counts were hard to interpret because, while those who start therapy at lower CD4+ cell counts have a greater risk of mortality and morbidity than those who initiate at higher CD4+ cells counts, this is the result of the former group having been infected longer and being later in their HIV disease than the latter. This problem is sometimes called a "lead-time bias."

Several have tried to adjust for lead-time bias by modeling duration of HIV infection before initiation of therapy, finding that earlier therapy did not[25] or, more recently, in collaborative data analysis of the Multicenter AIDS Cohort Study (MACS) and Swiss Cohorts, that it did significantly reduce hazard ratio for AIDS or death (by 35% and 20%, respectively).[26] The interpretation of these is necessarily limited by the fact that varying modeling assumptions can often lead to quite different outcomes.

Thus, the "cleanest" way of looking at this problem is to compare groups of people who have been observed from the time they got infected (a small minority of HIV patients) or from a set "hard" starting time of observation—that is, from a set CD4+ cell count or stratum of CD4+ cells counts—and look at the time to a "hard" outcome, such as death or development of a particular CD4+ cell count (such as 200 cells/mm³ or undetectable plasma HIV RNA [undetectable viral load]). "AIDS" as an outcome is less definitive, as some may develop Kaposi's sarcoma at relatively high CD4+ cell counts (e.g., over 300 cells/mm³) whereas someone may not be seen by a doctor for many months or years and come in with an AIDS diagnosis.

Accordingly, there have been a couple of studies that have tried to avoid such biases of ascertainment by looking at observed HIV progression or mortality from a set CD4+ cell count stratum—that is, in which some study participants started HAART whereas others deferred therapy to a later point. For example, our analysis indicated that for 240 patients who initiated therapy when they were between 350 and 500 CD4+ cells/mm³ (mean, 404 cells/mm³), their mortality rates were roughly 60 percent of 887 patients who were observed from that CD4+ cell stratum but who delayed therapy till some point when their CD4+ cell count was under 350 CD4+ cells/mm^3 (mean, at 258 cells/mm^3).[27] But even with this reasonably large observational cohort analysis, deaths were infrequent, so the study was statistically "underpowered," and the p-value was 0.17. A similar analysis–smaller and shorter term–concluded that, because the 55 percent reduction in mortality rates between those who started therapy at a CD4+ cell count at or above 350 cells/mm^3 and those who delayed or did not start therapy at a lower CD4+ cell count was not statistically significant (log rank test, $p = 0.10$), HAART should not be initiated early, that is, for patients with CD4+ cell counts above 350 cells/mm^3.[28] This conclusion, contradictory to the data presented, seemed designed to "support the [current] recommendation that HAART not be initiated for patients with CD4+ cell counts >350 cells/mm^3."[28] In any case, if one combines the data from the two studies in a meta-analysis, the relative risk of death is 0.46 for those who start therapy above vs. those who start therapy below 350 cells/mm^3, and this result is statistically significant ($p = 0.027$).[22] Other types of analyses have also indicated the benefit of earlier initiation of HAART for chronically infected but asymptomatic patients, [26, 29, 30] but these have had to acknowledge and try to adjust for lead-time bias in their data.

Since 2000, all recommendations have continued to cite the potential for drug toxicity, drug resistance, adverse effects, and other considerations, such as limited "salvage" regimens for those who fail initial and subsequent HAART regimens, as reasons for deferring therapy. Accordingly, we[22] reviewed and summarized data to suggest that those who start therapy at higher CD4+ cell counts (above 350 cells/mm^3) compared to those who start later are much less likely to have adverse effects from therapy, both short-term toxicity and adverse drug reactions[31,32]; and also less likely to have longer term problems such as lipodystrophy (abnormal fat distribution)[33, 34] and peripheral neuropathy.[35, 36]

Another import consideration, early treatment reduces HIV viremia and viral shedding, probably reducing the potential for the treated person to transmit HIV[37, 38] and indicating not just an individual medical benefit but also a potentially substantial public health advantage to getting HIV patients treated early. In addition, cost-effectiveness analysis indicates the economic benefit of starting antiretroviral therapy earlier (above 350 cells/mm^3) rather than later.[39]

Nonetheless, since 2000 there have been no recommendations to start therapy for HIV patients without symptoms who have CD4+ cell counts above 350 cells/mm^3 unless they also have very high viral loads. The most recent recommendations (April 2005 and October 2006) of the U.S. Department of Health and Human Services[40, 41] are also based on expert opinion on this particular subject (obviously, many other issues are covered in this long document) and do not cite data from any study specifically trying to address this issue. These authorities still do not recommend and somewhat discourage, but do not explicitly recommend against, patients' and their physicians' deciding to start HAART at CD4+ cell counts above 350 cells/mm^3.[41] Recommendation for later therapy is mainly predicated on the low risk of development of AIDS or death in those at higher CD4+ cell counts,[42-44] and the thought that they can afford to wait to start therapy. Likewise, the most recent recommendations of the International AIDS Society–USA Panel (August 2006)[45] recognize the tremendous difficulties of performing a randomized controlled trial to address the issue of when-to-start therapy. While at least one study showed the relative benefits and reduced likelihood of toxicity with starting therapy above 350 cells/mm^3,[46] still these recommendations, too, conclude that therapy should normally be started between 200 and 350 CD4+ cells/mm^3 and not at some higher point.[45]

Most expert authorities have not shifted on this point over the past several years, and some have indicated they doubt the likelihood of any study or data to change their recommendations on when to start HIV therapy or require a standard of proof that would not be attainable. However, their opinion has not necessarily been shared by the larger AIDS community. That is, in any cohort data analysis, such as from the NIH's MACS or CDC's HIV Outpatient Study (HOPS) it seems a substantial minority, usually 25–30 percent, of HIV patients have started their antiretroviral therapy before their CD4+ cell counts fell below 350 cells/mm^3.[27] Many patients and their clinicians have decided they would rather start therapy while they are still feeling well rather than waiting till a later point in their disease course.

The pendulum appears to be shifting back toward earlier treatment of HIV in asymptomatic patients. This may have less to do with an objective parsing of unavoidably limited cohort data, but to the ever-increasing number of drugs, combination drugs, and new classes of drugs, such as an approved entry inhibitors (see Appendix) and, as of this writing, an integrase inhibitor. A reduction in both dosage and timing of the drugs and the reduction in toxicity with the newer antiretroviral drugs all make earlier therapy more acceptable for patients. The durability of currently recommended therapies is impressive, as indicated by long-term follow-up data from various cohort studies.[47, 48]

Another major change in the attitudes about when-to-start-therapy has been engendered by the recent results of the Strategies for Management of Antiretroviral Therapy (SMART) study,[49] in which over 5,000 HIV patients in 33 countries were randomly assigned to receive either continuous therapy, starting at some point above 350 cells/mm^3, or to have intermittent therapy at times when their CD4+ cell counts dip below 350 cells/mm^3 (see *Strategic Treatment Interruptions* section). The risk of AIDS-defining conditions and of death were clearly and significantly higher in those who were treated episodically compared with those who were continuously maintained on therapy at a CD4+ cell count great than 350 cells/mm^3. This study did not actually address the issue of whether starting therapy and maintaining it at a CD4+ cell count above 350 cells/mm^3 led to better patient outcomes than starting and maintaining therapy at some point below that CD4+ cell count. However, it did provide enough "circumstantial evidence" to now convince several European experts that HAART therapy should indeed be started for patients above 350 and perhaps even above 500 cells/mm^3.[50]

It is likely that as treatments become ever more easy-to-take, effective, durable, less toxic, and used ever earlier in asymptomatic patients, and as data continue to accrue on the relative benefits of starting earlier, at some point official recommendations will have to address such realities and trends.

Lipodystrophy

After the introduction of HAART in 1996, patients and clinicians increasingly noted the appearance of body distortions caused by fat maldistribution. Broadly termed "lipodystrophy," in fact this syndrome seems to comprise at least two separate phenomena: usually, limb, upper trunk, and facial wasting with or without dorsal fat pad formation (buffalo hump), generally called "lipoatrophy"; or, less commonly, fat accumulation of abdominal fat—"crix belly" as it was originally ascribed to taking "Crixivan" (indinavir, a PI drug)—known as "lipoaccumulation." Lipodystrophy is not only disfiguring, but is often also associated with abnormally high blood lipid levels (cholesterol and triglycerides) and insulin resistance and, so, it may be associated with cardiovascular problems over the long term. A review of patients shows it is quite common: in one survey about 27 percent of all HIV patients had clinician-diagnosed "moderate" or "severe" lipodystrophy, either lipoatrophy or lipoaccumulation[33]; in another, lipoatrophy alone, confirmed by DEXA scan (dual-energy X-ray absorptiometry), was seen in 19 percent.[51] Medical treatment of the condition has not been simple or easy, as discontinuation of drugs that have been suspected of causing the condition have been associated with slow if any improvement.[52] Drug treatment such as with metformin (an oral antidiabetic drug) and the thiazolidinediones (adjunctive therapy for diabetes, introduced in the late 1990s, with effects on lipid hormones such as leptin and adiponectin) such as rosiglitazone have also not been particularly effective.[53-55] Ultimately, because of the disfigurement, patients who can afford it often opt for cosmetic surgery.

Research into the pathogenesis, prevention, and treatment of lipodystrophy is ongoing and beyond the scope of this book, but some early claims about its causes have already been questioned and largely discarded. Specifically, the first researchers to describe lipodystrophy in 1998 and speculate as to its pathogenesis were Andrew Carr and David Cooper of St. Vincent's Hospital in Sydney, Australia.[56] They initially posited two points: one, that lipodystrophy resulted from PI drug use; and two, that mitochondrial toxicity, involving protease-inhibitor-induced inhibition of pathways in the syntheses of ci-9-retioic acid and peroxisome proliferator activator (adipocyte [fat cell]) receptor type gamma, was the postulated mechanism underlying the condition.[57, 58] (Later work by others has focused on inhibition of polymerase gamma [pol gamma], required for replication of mitochondrial DNA, as the pathway by which antiretroviral drugs may be exerting their effect.[59, 60])

Hypothesizing that PI drugs were critical to the pathogenesis of lipodystrophy was attractive for several reasons. HIV-associated lipodystrophy was rarely seen before, but common after, the introduction of PIs in 1996. Also, elevated cholesterol and triglycerides and insulin resistance were recognized complications of the first PI drugs, and as this syndrome clearly involved adipocytes and abnormal fat metabolism it seemed biologically plausible that these drugs could also cause lipodystrophy. However, the association between PI use and lipodystrophy was, in retrospect, confounded by the use of other drugs, especially stavudine, and host factors such as increased age or low CD4+ cell counts.

The first early indication that PIs were not necessary or sufficient to cause lipodystrophy was that many treatment-naïve patients–that is, patients on "protease-inhibitor-sparing regimens"–were also getting the syndrome.[61] When Ken Lichtenstein and collaborators evaluated over 1,000 HIV patients, he found that some with moderate or severe lipodystrophy had taken indinavir (Crixivan), which could be associated with lipoaccumulation, but that many more, especially those with the more common lipoatrophy, had taken the nucleoside RTI stavudine (d4T).[33] Indeed, following this report, several other researchers found that stavudine, zidovudine, and other NRTIs were more likely to be associated with lipodystrophy than the PI drugs.[51, 62–64] All have found that the use of HIV PI drugs are indeed more closely associated with metabolic complications such as dyslipidemia and insulin resistance, but PI drugs have not been convincingly been linked to lipoatrophy.[65] Also, consistent with the clinical and epidemiologic observations, in vitro research showed that stavudine and other NRTIs induced more mitochondrial dysfunction than PI drugs.[59, 66, 67]

The association of any drug–whether PI or NRTI–with lipodystrophy is complicated by the fact that one or more host (nondrug) factors must be present for any therapy to lead to lipodystrophy (lipoatrophy).[34] That is, while stavudine and indinavir were associated with lipodystrophy in the initial HOPS analysis, actually no patient got lipodystrophy who did not also have one or more of the following: older age (greater than 40 years); body mass index loss of 1.0 kg/m or greater; white race; amount and duration of immune (CD4+ cell) recovery with therapy; nadir (lowest) CD4+ cell count less than 100 cells/mm^3; and duration of antiretroviral therapy.[33, 34, 68] There was a dose-response in the sense that the more of these host factors the greater likelihood of developing lipoatrophy. While these host factors do not definitively point to the actual etiology or causative mechanism for lipoatrophy and lipoaccumulation, most researchers have concluded that stavudine and other drugs may exacerbate or initiate the pathogenic process rather than being sole, necessary, and sufficient cause(s).

If non-PI drugs were somehow engendering the syndrome, the originally proposed mechanism, mitochondrial toxicity (from PI drugs), was also questioned. Much recent attention has shifted to adipocyte-derived hormones such as leptin and adiponectin.[69, 70] That is, focus has shifted from mito-chondria to adipocyte differentiation, impairment of adipokine regulation and unopposed production of proinflammatory cytokines.[68] Still, none of these fat hormonal and cytokine mechanisms necessarily eliminate inhibi-tion of mitochondrial RNA transcription, depletion of mitochondrial DNA, and mitochondrial dysfunction as underlying problems, as is still argued by the Australian researchers.[71, 72] There have been some recent data linking mitochondrial and adipocyte dysfunction.[67, 73, 74]

Still, accruing data continue to undercut the "mitochondrial toxicity" hy-pothesis of HIV-associated lipodystrophy, such as that: there is no single or universal toxicity exerted by various antiretroviral drugs within culture models;[75] that mitochondrial DNA changes in tissue may not be reflected in mitochondrial DNA depletion in peripheral blood lymphocytes, as are usu-ally the subject of investigation[76, 77]; and that NNRTI drugs, such as efavirenz and nevirapine, may also show mitochondrial toxicity yet have not been asso-ciated with clinical lipodystrophy.[76, 78] Further complicating the whole field of research is that hepatitis C and its treatment with ribavirin may also be associated with substantial mitochondrial toxicity.[79, 80]

Meanwhile, although the etiology of lipodystrophy is still unknown, "cholesterol-sparing" (favorable effect on blood lipid levels) PI drugs, notably atazanavir,[81] have replaced the older PI drugs, and other nucleoside drugs, such as tenofovir and abacavir, have increasingly replaced stavudine and zidovudine, as well. Switching strategies to improve metabolic and morpho-logic abnormalities[82] putatively prevents future cases of lipodystropy. While not addressing the fundamental issue, continued advances in therapeutics may nonetheless be the most important factor in diminishing the occurrence and controversy (but not the mystery) about the syndrome's pathogenesis.

Protease Inhibitors and Cardiovascular Disease

Shortly after their introduction, it became clear that use of PI drugs, while providing remarkable improvements in morbidity and mortality, also had adverse effects. These drugs increase serum levels of total cholesterol, low-density lipoprotein cholesterol and triglycerides, and increased "insulin resistance," a diabetic diathesis (tendency).[83, 84] Because these metabolic problems can increase the risk of cardiovascular and cerebrovascular disease, a number of investigators were concerned that long-term use of these drugs might increase HIV patients' likelihood of having myocardial infarctions, cerebrovascular events (strokes, transient ischemic attacks, etc.), and other vascular problems. Many if not most U.S. HIV patients are recent or current smokers, and as they survive to later ages other problems including hypertension and frank diabetes often emerge; cardiovascular disease is an ever-increasing cause of death in HIV patients.[85]

Did use of PI drugs predispose to heart attacks, strokes, and other adverse vascular events? By 2002 and 2003, there were preliminary data to suggest this was the case. Analysis of nearly 20,000 HIV-infected patients in the French Hospital Database showed that those who had been treated with a PI had twice the risk of myocardial infarction (54 of these over the period of observation). Further, there was a duration-related effect in that MIs were much higher in those who had taken PI drugs for 18 or more months.[86] Our own analysis of 21 MIs in 5,700 HIV outpatients followed almost 20,000 person-years of observation showed that all but 2 MIs had occurred in patients who had taken PI drugs 6 or more months, with a large strength of association that persisted when the proportional hazards model adjusted for the cardiovascular risk factors of smoking, sex, age, diabetes, hypertension, and hyperlipidemia (hazard ratio, 6.5; $p = 0.06$).[87] A subsequent, expanded analysis of 7,542 of these and other HIV patients showed a clear and statistically significant and "dose response" relationship between PI drug use of 60 or more days and cardiovascular disease (adjusted hazards rate, 1.71; $p = 0.03$).[88] In addition, a review of the claims of 28,000 HIV-infected Medicaid patients in California showed that younger HIV patients (less than 44 years of age for women and less than 34 years of age for men) who had taken antiretroviral agents had twice the risk of coronary heart disease compared with age-matched, but untreated HIV patients.[89] In sum, several different studies indicated that chronic PI drug use might lead to MIs and other cardiovascular and cerebrovascular problems.

However, a prominent article by Sam Bozzette and his colleagues in the Department of Veterans Affairs (VA) in the February 2003 *New England Journal of Medicine* reviewed a retrospective study of almost 37,000 VA HIV patients hospitalized nationally before 2001 and concluded that there was no relation between the use of any category of antiretroviral drug, including and especially PI drugs, and the hazard of cardiovascular or cerebrovascular events.[90] The main analysis was essentially a comparison of rates of mortality from any cause and admissions to the VA hospitals and admission rates for cardio- or cerebrovascular disease and showed both of those declining in the HAART era. It was indicated in the text that "about 1,000" HIV patients had received a PI drug for at least 48 months and "about 1,000" received NNRTI drug recipients for at least 24 months, so there were relatively few patients with substantial PI drug use or comparison non-PI drug takers. Essentially, although this is not easily grasped in the Abstract, the "patient-level" analysis was an ecologic analysis of admission rates for cardiovascular and cerebrovascular disease and rates of PI drug use over the first (mean of) 15 months of exposure to these drugs. Elided over in the text was that while age and sex were known for the persons in the rates being compared, there was only partial information about a host of other important risk factors—such as smoking, diabetes, and hypertension, all very common in the VA population—so the analysis of the rates could not be adequately controlled for these factors. Thus, the paper provided an ecologic argument that since rates of outcome such as myocardial infarction and other vascular events had not increased in the VA hospital population in the first months following introduction of PI drugs, "[f]ear of accelerated vascular disease need not compromise antiretroviral therapy over the short term."[90]

No one seriously disputed this conclusion given the value of PI drugs, but many immediately questioned results based on a relatively crude outcome analysis from only an average of 15 months of observation.[83, 91, 92] These researchers and many others concluded that the weight of data indicated vascular problems with prolonged use of PI drugs; all advocated efforts to reduce modifiable risk factors for cardiovascular disease such as smoking and control of hyperlipidemia, hypertension, and diabetes.

The pressing clinical question was what to prescribe an HIV patient with one or more of these known risk factors for MIs, strokes, and other vascular events; given, for example, that more than 60 percent of HOPS patients are smokers[93] and 43 percent have a body mass index (BMI) greater than 25 (overweight-obese),[94] this was an immediate clinical issue. Should clinicians avoid PI drugs for those many HIV patients with host factors and behaviors that put them at risk of cardiovascular and cerebrovascular disease? Our reanalysis of HOPS data in 2004 showed that both PI drug use and MI incidence were decreasing and that the use of "statin" drugs (such as 'Lipitor' and 'Zocor') and other lipid-lowering drugs were increasing and used by almost 20 percent of HOPS patients.[95]

Recently, the European "D.A.D Study" of adverse effects of antiretroviral drugs has examined 345 HIV patients who had an MI during almost 95,000 person-years of observation: the risk of MI increased by 16 percent per year of PI use,[96, 97] but not with NNRTI use. With such large numbers, and, given that all other clinical studies except the one by Bozzette et al. are consistent with this study, the data will probably convince those who remain previously unconvinced to prescribe PI drugs with caution or not at all for patients at risk of cardio- or cerebrovascular disease or to prescribe "cholesterol-sparing" PI drugs such as atazanavir. The recent availability of not only "lipid-sparing" PI drugs, but also the many other drugs and other classes of antiretroviral drugs should make this ever more easy and possible.

Early Vaccines and Microbicides

It must be noted that some controversial decisions are unavoidable and probably must be made. "AIDSVAX," the first vaccine for HIV, was a notable failure which many predicted before the human trials were undertaken in Thailand and the United States; however, most agreed that these human trials needed to be performed.

While it is well beyond the scope of this book to review past and current HIV vaccinology,[98] the traditional approach for vaccination is to prevent infection by immunization with a killed, neutralized, or nonpathogenic live virus (e.g., vaccinia for smallpox) virus or, in the case of HIV, an engineered part of the viral envelope glycoprotein that, while not infectious, can stimulate immunologic response. These vaccines (antigens) should stimulate protective antibody production, in this case, so-called neutralizing (Neut or NT) antibodies to HIV. However, it has long been understood that HIV envelope glycoprotein evades such NT antibody production.[99–102] AIDSVAX was a preparation of recombinant gp120 (envelope glycoprotein component) from HIV-1 types B and E for use in Thailand, and two HIV-1 B subtypes, so-called "MN" strain and "GNE8" strains, common in North America, for vaccine trial in the United States.

Given the inconsistent neutralizing antibody studies in vitro, many voiced skepticism that these vaccine trials would show AIDSVAX to be efficacious. The vaccine was produced by VaxGen, a subsidiary of Genetech; VaxGen's Director, Dr. Donald Francis, had been made famous as a dedicated AIDS researcher by Randy Shilts' 1987 book, *And the Band Played On*, and the Emmy-winning 1993 HBO movie based on it. Some have accused VaxGen,

Francis, and Dr. Bill Heyward, a former CDC employee who made a deal in 1999 to take a position with VaxGen, of improper political pressure and deal-making. For example, the British investigative reporter Brian Deer had questioned the rationale for such a vaccine trial as early as 1999,[103] and maintains a website following the failures in 2003 of trials both in Thailand and the United States (Available at: http://briandeer.com/vaxgen-aidsvax. htm).

In both trials, the vaccine had been apparently safe and immunogenic in phase I and II trials in 1994 and later,[104] so it was generally thought that AIDSVAX deserved a fair broad trial. Thus, the AIDSVAX B/B (U.S.) and B/E (Thailand) were brought to phase III trials in 1999 but stopped in February (U.S.) and November (Thailand) 2003: vaccinated participants had the same rates of HIV incidence as placebo-vaccinated participants.[105, 106] Does this qualify as an error, or a controversy, that could have been avoided or resolved faster?

Similarly, there is intense interest in finding ways women can protect themselves from getting infected from HIV-infected men. To date, two types of vaginal microbicides have now been tried, and have apparently failed, to protect women in clinical trials of women in developing countries. Nonoxynol-9, which had been shown to inactivate HIV in vitro experiments, did not reduce the incidence rate of HIV and other sexually transmitted diseases in female sex workers in Cameroon.[107] However, even before these trials, some wondered if the local inflammatory effects of nonoxynol-9 might not protect but possibly even lead to easier HIV transmission across the vaginal mucosa;[108, 109] and so this acidic compound was buffered before its use as an applied gel. More recently, phase III trials in India and Africa of an initially promising microbicide, cellulose sulfate,[110] were stopped in early 2007 as women using the vaginal gel actually seemed to have increased risk of HIV infection.[111] Here, too, few would argue that these trials of microbicides that apparently worked in the laboratory should not have been undertaken in human studies.

Strategic Treatment Interruptions

In the first years following the introduction of PIs and NNRTIs in 1996 and 1997, many patients suffered adverse effects from the new drugs or failed therapy and had limited or no new treatment options available to them. Further, therapy was difficult to adhere to (in the mid 1990s, patients too an average 13 or more pills a day for HIV treatment alone[112]). In many settings, especially in the developing world treatment, modern HAART was simply too expensive–about U.S. $ 10,000 per year–and not affordable by the vast majority of HIV patients in the developing world. For these and other reasons, and because some patients who were not fully adherent to their regimens nonetheless could sustain very low or undetectable plasma HIV RNA levels (viral load) and maintain relatively high CD4+ cell counts, some wondered whether it was possible to "cycle" patients on and off therapy in a regimented or structured fashion.

The theory behind such "strategic treatment interruptions" (STI)–or, as he preferred to stress the automatic, non-CD4+ cell- count-driven, "structured intermittent therapy" (SIT)–was explained by Anthony (Tony) Fauci, Director of NIH's National Institute for Allergy and Infectious Diseases (NIAID) at the XIIIth International AIDS Conference in Durban, South Africa in July, 2000, who felt that preliminary data from his laboratory provided a scientific rationale for STIs.[113] Since it was well known that available drugs would not cure HIV infection, or eliminate HIV from a sequestered reservoir of latently infected resting cells,[114] there was eagerness to find an approach that could reduce the long-term pill burden by 30–50 percent. At this and subsequent meetings,[115] Fauci presented data on nine patients receiving intermittent therapy–2 months on and 1 month off–that showed that during periods off therapy, the replication and resurgence of "wild-type virus" (original virus before antiretroviral treatment selected for resistant and other strains) could stimulate CD8+ T cells necessary for the long-term immunologic control of HIV. This stimulation of "killer" T cells by wild type virus was also considered a form of "auto-immunization." However,

> Our previous studies of a single discontinuation of therapy taught us that the virus comes back with a vengeance within four weeks in most patients, but only rarely within the first seven days off therapy ... Therefore, we looked at what would happen if we interrupted therapy every other week. [113]

He then presented preliminary data on five patients receiving HAART on a 7-day-on, then 7-day-off regimen, who, aside from small "blips" of detectable virus, seemed to keep viral load down and CD4+ cells near their treatment baseline (mean, 940 cells/mm^3). In the first 32–68 weeks of therapy, 10 patients on such short-cycle therapy maintained suppression of plasma viremia and no significant change in CD4+ cells.[116]

Fauci is widely respected in the infectious disease community and often asked by print and media journalists for quotes and opinions on virtually any topic in infectious diseases (sometimes to the chagrin of other and specific subject experts who feel slighted). Thus, his suggestion at this meeting, with appropriate caveats about the need for more data, that STIs might decrease total time on antiretroviral medications, improve adherence, and reduce toxicities and cost, was credited more easily and seriously than similar suggestions would have been from many other sources. In turn, the amount of energy, funds, and time spent in scientifically evaluating STIs was accordingly greater than might otherwise be spent on a theory posited by someone else.

There are many scientific problems to evaluating STIs. Drugs must be stopped together, and some drugs, such as the widely used "Sustiva" (liponavir/ritonavir), have long pharmacokinetic half-lives and may persist in the body for days. All STI work until the SMART study (see below) involved few patients, usually less than 20, which made evaluation and extrapolation to the community difficult.

However, the major problem was that in the subsequent years, study after study consistently found that patients taking STIs were at risk of being left with higher viral HIV RNA levels (viral loads) and lower CD4+ cell counts upon restarting therapy after an interruption.[117, 118] Even in 2000 and 2001, well before the results of several studies were available, clinicians were reporting anecdotes of patients who did poorly, even died, when they tried STI.[119, 120] Also, even in the early pilot, nonrandomized studies, CD4+ cells declined, there was an increase in viral load, and a relative shift to drug susceptible wild-type rather than drug-resistant virus; that is, in most studies, "viral failure"—a marked increase in viral load—was the norm, with only a small minority of patients maintaining viral suppression.[121–125] While Spanish[121] and Swiss cohort[124] study researchers indicated that there were modestly encouraged by initial STI data, this was not the impression at most research centers who were discouraged by their own treatment experiences with STIs.[126]

If STI could not be recommended for a majority of patients or it was too difficult to determine who would benefit from STI, the fact that there was a repopulation of wild-type, drug-sensitive virus raised the question whether treatment interruption would be worthwhile for those who were failing drug therapy. That is, while STI might not work on a population basis, would it nonetheless be worthwhile to have heavily treatment-experienced patients have a hiatus between the end of one therapeutic regimen and the start of the next? In this instance, the subsequent therapy would be treating putatively more drug-sensitive virus that replicated after discontinuation of drugs. Thus, investigation of "STI" changed its meaning and direction in the early and mid-2000s.

Unfortunately, here, too, several randomized trials consistently found no benefit and sometimes harm to discontinuing therapy in a heavily pre-treated HIV patient who had had drugs from all (then, three) major classes of antiretroviral drugs (see Appendix). The results of several randomized controlled trials that found no significant benefit to such a strategy were anticipated by the work of Steven Deeks and colleagues at the University of California, San Francisco.[127, 128] These investigators found that despite "virologic failure"—that is, detectable and rising plasma viremia—patients who had exhausted treatment options were nonetheless still suppressing viral replication and maintained or had slowly declining CD4+ cell count levels with continued therapy; this suggested that interrupting for some weeks and restarting with a previous or, more usually, the same therapy plus an additional agent would not substantially improve a relatively stable immunologic and virologic condition. Further, it became clear that once therapy was restarted after treatment interruption of any duration, drug-resistant strains re-emerged:[129] some considered that there was a "library" or "repository" of drug-resistant strains that would not be ablated by allowing wild type virus to predominate during treatment interruption.

Several randomized trials reported at various scientific meetings and conferences between 2001 and 2006 consistently found that treatment-interrupters did worse on several parameters than patients who maintained therapy or who seamlessly changed or added antiretroviral drugs.[130–133] One randomized trial purported to show virologic and immunologic benefit to an STI before "salvage" therapy, but the STI was brief (8 weeks) and the salvage therapy contained 8–9 drugs.[134]: This was not altogether helpful as for reasons of patient adherence, tolerability and cost, few clinicians would put their patients on so many antiviral drugs at one time.

As late as 2004, some researchers continued to try to identify the subset of patients who might benefit from treatment interruption.[135, 136] One consideration was that treatment interruptions had been tried and mainly failed in efficacy when used for patients late in disease, with high viremia and low CD4+ cell counts. Some thought that CD4+ cell count-guided therapy in persons with higher CD4+ cell counts might enable relatively healthy persons relatively early in disease avoid the pill burden and adverse effects, such as multiply drug resistant HIV, attendant to prolonged drug treatment.

Accordingly, a major, multicenter, and multinational cohort study started enrolling patients between 2002 and 2006 in the SMART Study.[49] Almost 5,500 patients were enrolled in the study and randomized to either receive continuous HAART starting at some point before they had a CD4+ cell count above 350 CD4+ cells/mm^3 or to only have such therapy when their CD4+ cell count dipped below 250 cells/mm^3, to be discontinued once they were above 350 cells/mm^3 again. This expensive and extensive study was not without controversy, as many experts were dubious about the likely efficacy of such as strategy given the generally negative findings from the great majority of previous STI studies.

As most patients were enrolled in 2004 and 2005, the mean duration of observation in the SMART was 16 months, but the study was stopped early when data monitoring showed that those having intermittent therapy were at a significantly greater risk of opportunistic disease and death than those in the "drug conservation" (continuous, uninterrupted therapy) group. The gist of the summary article, published in *The New England Journal of Medicine* in November 2006[49] was already known widely in the HIV scientific and treatment community as the SMART investigators promptly reported their results at meetings in early 2006.[137] The conclusion: once antiretroviral therapy is started, it is unwise to stop it. And, as indicated in the previous section (*When to Start Therapy*), some have interpreted the SMART Study results to indicate the advantages of initiating treatment early, before the patient has fewer than 350 CD4+ cells/mm^3.[50]

The situation was well summed up by a clinician colleague:

> Let's hope that the SMART study was the last nail in the coffin for STIs. It was always a bad idea and just about every study on STIs to date have confirmed that ... Denver Health Medical Center was a major center for SMART and many of us in the [HIV treatment] community would not allow our patients to enter it based on previous STI studies ... I feel for those individuals who may have lost ground with their disease by allowing the virus to replicate unabated. I do hope that the concept of STIs finally becomes one of historical interest only as we recount the numerous errors we have made on the way to trying to understand this disease. (Ken Lichtenstein, personal communication, June 10, 2007)

Granting that this concept needed exploration, we may still consider why so much scientific energy and expenditure over several years went into this issue, how much was lost for the patients who underwent STIs, and how considerable investigator effort and study funds might have been more constructively used.

References

1. Radcliffe, K.W., R. Patel, and K.E. Rogstad. 1996. Feedback from the XIth International Conference on AIDS. *International Journal of STD and AIDS* 7:521–524.

2. Palella Jr., F.J., K.M. Delaney, A.C. Moorman, et al. 1998. Declining mortality and morbidity in HIV-infected ambulatory patients. *New England Journal of Medicine* 338:853–860.

3. Hogg, R.S, K.V. Heath, B. Yip, et al. 1998. Improved survival among HIV-infected individuals following initiation of antiretroviral therapy. *Journal of the American Medical Association* 279:450–458.

4. Mocroft, A., S. Vella, T.L. Benfield, et al. 1998. Changing patterns of mortality across Europe in patients infected with HIV-1. EuroSIDA Study Group. *Lancet* 352:1725–1730.

5. Vittinghoff, E., S. Sheer, P.M. O'Malley, G. Colfax, S.D. Holmberg, and S.P. Buchbinder. 1999. Combination antiretroviral therapy and recent declines in AIDS incidence and mortality. *Journal of Infectious Diseases* 179:717–720.

6. Carpenter, C.C.J., D.A. Cooper, M.A. Fischl, et al. 2000. Antiretroviral therapy in adults: Updated recommendations of the International AIDS Society–USA Panel. *Journal of the American Medical Association* 283:381–390.

7. Palella, Jr., F.J., A.C. Moorman, J. Chmiel, C. Chan, S.D. Holmberg, and the HIV Outpatient Study Investigators. 2002. Durability and predictors of success of highly active anti-retroviral therapy (ART) for ambulatory HIV-infected patients. *AIDS* 16:1617–1627.

8. Altman, L.K. July 23, 1992. Cost of treating AIDS patients is soaring. *New York Times.*

9. Holmberg, S.D., L.J. Conley, S.P. Buchbinder, et al. 1993. Use of therapeutic and prophylactic drugs for AIDS by homosexual and bisexual men in three US cities. *AIDS* 7:699–704.

10. Rosenberg, P.S., M.H. Gail, L.K. Schrager, et al. 1991. National AIDS incidence trends and the extent of zidovudine therapy in selected demographic and transmission groups. *Journal of Acquired Immune Deficiency Syndromes* 4:392–401.

11. Aboulker, J.-P., and A.M. Swart. 1993. Preliminary analysis of the Concorde trial [letter]. *Lancet* 341:889–890.

12. Joint Concorde and Opal Coordinating Committees. 1998. Long-term follow-up of randomized trials of immediate versus deferred zidovudine in symptom-free HIV infection [editorial review]. *AIDS* 12:1259–1265.

13. Collier, A.C. 1994. Early intervention in HIV infection: Where are we? *AIDS Research and Human Retroviruses* 10:893–899.

14. Carpenter, C.C.J., M.A. Fischl, S.M. Hammer, et al. 1998. Antiretroviral therapy for HIV infection in 1998: Updated recommendations of the international AIDS Society–USA Panel. *Journal of the American Medical Association* 280:78–86.

15. CDC. 2002. Guidelines for using antiretroviral agents among HIV-infected adults and adolescents: Recommendations of the Panel on Clinical Practices for Treatment of HIV. *Morbidity and Mortality Weekly Report* 51(RR-7):1–55.

16. Dybul, M., A.S. Fauci, J.G. Bartlett, J.E. Kaplan, and A.K. Pau. 2002. Guidelines for using antiretroviral agents among HIV-infected adults and adolescents. The Panel on Clinical Practices for Treatment of HIV. *Annals of Internal Medicine* 137:381–433.

17. Yeni, P.G., S.M. Hammer, C.C.J. Carpenter, et al. 2002. Antiretroviral treatment for using adult HIV infection in 2002: updated recommendations of the International AIDS Society–USA Panel. *Journal of the American Medical Association* 288:222–235.

18. U.S. Department of Health and Human Services (DHHS). November 10, 2003. Guidelines for the use of antiretroviral agents in HIV-1-infected adults and adolescents. Available at http://www.hivcommission-la.info/2003_guidelines.pdf.

19. Delfraissy, J.F. 1999. *Rapport 1999-Prise en charge thérapeutique des personnes infectees par le VIH.* Médicine-Sciences, Flammarion, Paris, 1999.

20. Murphy, R., and B. Gazzard. 2003. Antiretroviral treatment guidelines. *AIDS* 17(suppl 2):S1.

21. British HIV Association (BHIVA). 2003. BHIVA guidelines for the treatment of HIV-infected adults with antiretroviral therapy. *HIV Medicine* 4(suppl 1):1–41.

22. Holmberg, S.D., F.J. Palella Jr., K.A. Lichtenstein, and D.V. Havlir. 2004. The case for earlier treatment of HIV infection. *Clinical Infectious Diseases* 39:1699–1704.

23. Lane, H.C., and J.D. Neaton. 2003. When to start therapy for HIV infection: A swinging pendulum in search of data [editorial]. *Annals of Internal Medicine* 138:680–681.

24. Kaplan, J., D. Hanson, J. Karon, et al. 2001. Late initiation of antiretroviral therapy (at CD4+ lymphocyte count <200 cells/μL) is associated with increased risk of death [abstract 520]. In *Program and Abstracts of the 8th Conference on Retroviruses and Opportunistic Infections,* Chicago, February 4–8, 2001.

25. Ahdieh-Grant, L., T.E. Yamshita, J.E. Phair, et al. 2003. When to initiate highly active antiretroviral therapy: A cohort approach. *American Journal of Epidemiology* 157:738–746.

26. Sterne, J., M. May, D. Costagliola, et al. 2006. Estimating the optimum CD4 threshold for starting HAART in antiretroviral-naïve HIV-infected individuals [abstract 525]. In *Program and Abstracts of the 13th Conference on Retroviruses and Opportunistic Infections,* Denver, February 5–8, 2006.

27. Palella Jr., F.J., M.D. Knoll, J.S. Chmiel, et al. 2003. Survival benefit of initiating antiretroviral therapy in HIV-infected patients in different CD4+ cell strata. *Annals of Internal Medicine* 138:620–626.

28. Sterling, T.R., R.E. Chaisson, and R.D. Moore. 2003. Initiation of highly active antiretroviral therapy at CD4+ T lymphocyte counts of 350 cells/mm^3: disease progression, treatment durability, and drug toxicity. *Clinical Infectious Diseases* 36:812–815.

29. Wang, C., D. Vlahov, M. Galai, et al. 2004. Mortality in HIV-seropositive versus-seronegative persons in the era of highly active antiretroviral therapy: Implications for when to initiate therapy. *Journal of Infectious Diseases* 190:1046–1054.

30. Opravil, M., B. Ledergerber, H. Furrer, et al. 2002. Clinical efficacy of early initiation of HAART in patients with asymptomatic HIV infection and CD4 cell count > 350 X 10^6/l. *AIDS* 16:1371–1381.

31. Staszewski, S., J. Gallant, A.L. Pozniak, et al. 2003. Efficacy and safety of tenofovir DF (TDF) versus stavudine (d4T) when used in combination with lamivudine and efavirenz in antiretroviral naïve patients: 96-week preliminary results [abstract 564b]. In: *Program and Abstracts of the 10th Conference on Retroviruses and Opportunistic Infections,* Boston, February 10–14, 2003.

32. Lucas, G.M., R.E. Chaisson, and R.D. Moore. 1999. Highly active antiretroviral therapy in a large urban clinic: Risk factors for virologic failure and adverse drug reactions. *Annals of Internal Medicine* 131:81–87.

33. Lichtenstein, K.A., D.J. Ward, A.C. Moorman, et al. 2001. Clinical assessment of HIV-associated lipodystrophy in an ambulatory population. *AIDS* 15:1389–1398.

34. Lichtenstein, K.A. K.M. Delaney, C. Armon, et al. 2003. Incidence of and risk factors for lipoatrophy (abnormal fat loss) in ambulatory HIV-1 infected patients. *Journal of Acquired Immune Deficiency Syndromes* 32:48–56.

35. Kelleher, T., A. Cross, L. Dunkle. 1999. Relation of peripheral neuropathy to HIV treatment in four randomized clinical trials involving didanosine. *Clinical Therapeutics* 21:1182–1192.

36. Simpson, D.M., A-B Haidich, G. Schifitto, et al. 2002. Severity of HIV-associated neuropathy is associated with plasma HIV-1 RNA levels. *AIDS* 16:407–412.

37. Quinn, T.C., M.J. Wawer, N. Sewankambo, et al. 2000. Viral load and heterosexual transmission of human immunodeficiency virus type 1. Rakai Project Study Group. *New England Journal of Medicine* 342:921–929.

38. Cohen, M.S., C. Gay, A.D. Kashuba, S. Blower, and L. Paxton. 2007. Narrative review: antiretroviral therapy to prevent the sexual transmission of HIV-1. *Annals of Internal Medicine* 146:591–601.

39. Schackman, B.R., K.A. Freedberg, M.C. Weinstein, et al. 2002. Cost-effective implications of the timing of antiretroviral therapy in HIV-infected adults. *Archives of Internal Medicine* 162:2478–2486.

40. U.S. Department of Health and Human Services (DHHS). April 7, 2005. Guidelines for the use of antiretroviral agents in HIV-1-infected adults and adolescents. Available at http://aidsinfo.nih.gov/ContentFiles/AdultandAdolescentGL04072005001.pdf.

41. U.S. Department of Health and Human Services (DHHS).October 10, 2006. Guidelines for the use of antiretroviral agents in HIV-1-infected adults and adolescents. Available at http://aidsinfo.nih.gov/contentfiles/AdultandAdolescentGL.pdf.

42. Mellors, J.W., A. Muñoz, J.V. Giorgi, et al. 1997. Plasma viral load and CD4+ lymphocytes as prognostic markers of HIV-1 infection. *Annals of Internal Medicine* 126: 946–954.

43. Egger, M., M. May, G. Chene, et al. 2002. Prognosis of HIV-1-infected patients starting highly active antiretroviral therapy: A collaborative analysis of prospective studies. *Lancet* 360:119–129.

44. Phillips, A., and CASCADE Collaboration. 2004. Short-term risk of AIDS according to current CD4 cell count and viral load in antiretroviral drug-naïve individuals and those treated in the monotherapy era. *AIDS* 18:51–58.

45. Hammer, S.M., M.S. Saag, M. Schechter, et al. 2006. Treatment for Adult HIV Infection. 2006. Recommendations of the International AIDS Society- USA Panel. *Journal of American Medical Association* 296:827–843.

46. Lichtenstein, K., C. Armon, K. Buchacz, et al. 2006. Early, uninterrupted ART is associated with improved outcomes and fewer toxicities in the HIV Outpatient Study (HOPS) [abstract 769]. In *Program and Abstracts of the 13th Conference on Retroviruses and Opportunistic Infections,* Denver, February 5–8, 2006.

47. Landay, A., B.A. da Silva, M.S. King, et al. 2007. Evidence of ongoing immune reconstitution in subjects with sustained viral suppression following 6 years of lopinavir-ritonovir treatment. *Clinical Infectious Diseases* 44:749–54.

48. Gallant, J.E., S. Staszewski, A.L. Pozniak, et al. 2004. Efficacy and safety of tenofovir DF vs stavudine in combination therapy in antiretroviral-naïve patients: A 3-year randomized trial *Journal of the American Medical Association* 292:191–201.

49. SMART Study Group. 2006. CD4+ count-guided interruption of antiretroviral treatment. *New England Journal of Medicine* 355:2283–2296.

50. Phillips, A.N., B.G. Gazzard, N. Clumeck, M.H. Losso, and J.D. Lundgren. 2007. When should antiretroviral therapy for HIV be started? *British Medical Journal* 334:76–78.

51. Carter, V.M., J.F. Hoy, M. Bailey, P.G. Colman, I. Nyulasi, and A.M. Mijch. 2001. The prevalence of lipoatrophy in an ambulant HIV-infected population: it all depends on the definition. *HIV Medicine* 2:174–180.

52. Tavassoli, N., H. Baghieri, A. Sommet, et al. 2006. Effects of discontinuing stavudine or protease inhibitor therapy on human immunodeficiency virus-related

fat redistribution evaluated by dual-energy X-ray absorptiometry. *Pharmacotherapy* 26:154–161.

53. Benavides, S., and M.C. Nahata. 2004. Pharmacologic therapy for HIV-associated lipodystrophy. *Annals of Pharmacotherapy* 38:448–457.

54. Kovacic, J.C., A. Martin, D. Carey, et al. 2005. Influence of rosiglitazone on flow-mediated dilation and other markers of cardiovascular risk in HIV-infected patients with lipoatrophy. *Antiviral Therapy* 10:135–143.

55. Cavalcanti, R.B., J. Raboud, S. Shen, K.C. Kain, A. Cheung, and S. Walmsley. 2007. A randomized, placebo-controlled trial of rosiglitazone for HIV-related lipoatrophy. *Journal of Infectious Diseases* 195:1754–1761.

56. Carr, A., K. Samaras, S. Burton, et al. 1998. A syndrome of peripheral lipodystrophy, hyperlipidaemia and insulin resistance in patients receiving protease inhibitors. *AIDS* 12:F51–F58.

57. Carr, A., K. Samaras, D.J. Chisholm, and D.A. Cooper. 1998. Pathogenesis of HIV-1-protease inhibitor-associated peripheral lipodystrophy, hyperlipidaemia, and insulin resistance. *Lancet* 351:1881–1883.

58. Carr, A., K. Samaras, A. Thorisdottir, G.R. Kaufmann, D.J. Chisholm, and D.A. Cooper. 1999. Diagnosis, prediction, and natural course of HIV-1 protease-inhibitor-associated lipodystrophy, hyperlipidaemia, and diabetes mellitus: A cohort study. *Lancet* 353:2093–2099.

59. Miro, O., S. Lopez, F. Cardellach, and J. Casademont. 2005. Mitochondrial studies in HAART-related lipodystrophy: From experimental hypothesis to clinical findings. *Antiviral Therapy* 10(suppl 2):M73–M81.

60. Yamanaka, H., H. Gatanaga, P. Kosalaraksa, et al. 2007. Novel mutation of human DNA polymerase gamma associated with mitochondrial toxicity induced by anti-HIV treatment. *Journal of Infectious Diseases* 195:1419–1425.

61. Brinkman, K., J.A. Smeitink, J.A. Romijn, and P. Reiss. 1999. Mitochondrial toxicity induced by nucleoside-analogue reverse-transcriptase inhibitors is a key factor in the pathogenesis of antiretroviral-therapy-related lipodystrophy. *Lancet* 354:112–115.

62. Young, J., M. Rickenbach, R. Weber, et al. 2005. Body fat changes among antiretroviral-naïve patients on PI- and NNRTI-based HAART in the Swiss HIV cohort study. *Antiviral Therapy* 10:73–81.

63. Martin, A., D. Smith, A. Carr, et al. 2004. Progression of lipodystrophy (LD) with continued thymidine analogue usage: Long-term follow-up from a randomized clinical trial (the PILR study). *HIV Clinical Trials* 5:192–200.

64. Ergun-Longmire, B., K. Lin-Siu, A.M. Dunn, et al. 2006. Effects of protease inhibitors on glucose tolerance, lipid metabolism, and body composition in children and adolescents infected with human immunodeficiency virus. *Endocrine Practice* 12:514–521.

65. Nolan, D. and S. Mallal. 2005. Antiretroviral-therapy-associated lipoatrophy: Current status and future directions. *Sexual Health* 2:153–163.

66. Dagan, T., C. Sable, J. Bray, and M. Gerschenson. 2002. Mitochondrial dysfunction and the antiretroviral nucleoside analog toxicities: What is the evidence? *Mitochondrion* 1:397–412.

67. Nolan, D., E. Hammond, A. Marti, et al. 2003. Mitochondrial DNA depletion and morphologic changes in adipocytes associated with nucleoside reverse transcriptase inhibitor therapy. *AIDS* 17:1329–1338.

68. Lichtenstein, K.A. 2005. Redefining lipodystrophy syndrome: Risks and impact on clinical decision making. *Journal of Acquired Immune Deficiency Syndromes* 39:395–400.

69. Sweeney, L.L., A.M. Brennan, and C.S. Mantzoros. 2007. The role of adipokines in relation to HIV lipodystrophy [editorial review]. *AIDS* 21:895–904.

70. Kosmiski, L., D. Kuritzkes, K. Lichtenstein, and R. Eckel. 2003. Adipocyte-derived hormone levels in HIV lipodystrophy. *Antiviral Therapy* 8:9–15.

71. Mallon, P.W. 2007. Pathogenesis of lipodystrophy and lipid abnormalities in patients taking antiretroviral therapy. *AIDS Review* 9:3–15.

72. Carr, A. 2003. HIV lipodystrophy: risk factors, pathogenesis, diagnosis and management. *AIDS* 17(suppl 1):S141–S18.

73. Jones, S.P., N. Ozaki, J. Morelese, et al. 2005. Assessment of adipokine expression and mitochondrial toxicity in patients with lipoatrophy on stavudine- and zidovudine-containing regimens. *Journal of Acquired Immune Deficiency Syndromes* 40:565–572.

74. Galluzzi, L., M. Pinti, G. Guaraldi, et al. 2005. Altered mitochondrial RNA production in adipocytes from HIV-infected individuals with lipodystrophy. *Antiviral Therapy* 10(suppl 2):M91–M99.

75. Lund, K.C., L.L. Peterson, and K.B. Wallace. 2007. The absence of a universal mechanism of mitochondrial toxicity by nucleoside analogs. *Antimicrobial Agents and Chemotherapy* 51:2531–2539.

76. Casula, M., G.J. Weverling, F.W. Wit, et al. 2005. Mitochondrial DNA and RNA increase in peripheral blood mononuclear cells from HIV-1 patients randomized to receive stavudine-containing or stavudine sparing combination therapy. *Journal of Infectious Diseases* 192:1794–1800.

77. Maagaard, A., M. Holberg-Petersen, G. Kollberg, A. Oldfors, L. Sandvik, and J.N. Bruun. 2006. Mitochondrial (mt)DNA changes in tissue may not be reflected by depletion of mtDNA in peripheral blood mononuclear cells in HIV-infected patients. *Antiviral Therapy* 11:601–608.

78. Nolan D. 2005. Do non-nucleoside reverse transcriptase inhibitors contribute to lipodystrophy? *Drug Safety* 28:1069–1074.

79. Sulkowski, M.S., and Y. Benhamou. 2007. Therapeutic issues in HIV/HCV-coinfected patients. *Journal of Viral Hepatitis* 14:371–386.

80. Laguno, M., A. Milinkovic, E. de Lazzari, et al. 2005. Incidence and risk factors for mitochondrial toxicity in treated HIV/HCV-coinfected patients. *Antiviral Therapy* 10:423–429.

81. Swainston Harrison, T., and L.J. Scott. 2005. Atazanavir: A review of its use in the management of HIV infection. *Drugs* 65:2309–2336.

82. Barragan, P. C. Fisac, and D. Podzamczer. 2006. Switching strategies to improve lipid profile and morphologic changes. *AIDS Review* 8:191–203.

83. Kuritzkes, D.R., and J. Currier. 2003. Cardiovascular risk factors and antiretroviral therapy [perspective]. *New England Journal of Medicine* 348:679–680.

84. Rhew, D.C., M. Bernal, D. Aguilar, U. Iloeje, and M.B. Goetz. 2003. Association between protease inhibitor use and increased cardiovascular risk in patients infected with human immunodeficiency virus: A systematic review. *Clinical Infectious Diseases* 37:959–972.

85. Palella, F.J., R.K. Baker, A.C. Moorman, et al. 2006. Mortality in the highly active antiretroviral era: changing causes of death and disease in the HIV Outpatient Study. *Journal of Acquired Immune Deficiency Syndromes* 43:27–34.

86. Mary-Krause, M., L. Cotte, A. Simon, et al. 2003. Increased risk of myocardial infarction with duration of protease inhibitor therapy in HIV-infected men. *AIDS* 17:2479–2486.

87. Holmberg, S.D, A.C. Moorman, J.M. Williamson, et al. 2002. Protease inhibitors and cardiovascular outcomes in patients with HIV-1. *Lancet* 360:1747–1748.

88. Iloeje, U.H., Y. Yuan, G. L'Italien, et al. 2005. Protease inhibitor exposure and increased risk of cardiovascular disease in HIV-infected patients. *HIV Medicine* 6:37–44.

89. Currier, J.S., A. Taylor, F. Boyd, et al. 2003. Coronary heart disease in HIV-infected individuals. *Journal of Acquired Immune Deficiency Syndromes* 33:506–512.

90. Bozzette, S.A., C.F. Ake, H.K. Tam, S.W. Chang, and T.A. Louis. 2003. Cardiovascular and cerebrovascular events in patients treated for human immunodeficiency virus infection. *New England Journal of Medicine* 348:702–710.

91. Sklar, P., and H. Masur. 2003. HIV infection and cardiovascular disease–Is there really a link [editorial]? *New England Journal of Medicine* 349:2065–2067.

92. Klein, D., L.B. Hurley, and S. Sidney. 2003. Cardiovascular disease and HIV infection [correspondence]. *New England Journal of Medicine* 349:1869–1870.

93. Moorman, A.C., S.D. Holmberg, S.I. Marlowe, et al. 1999. Changing conditions and treatments in a dynamic cohort of ambulatory HIV patients: the HIV Outpatient Study (HOPS). *Annals of Epidemiology* 9:349–357.

94. Tedaldi, E.M., J.T. Brooks, P.J. Weidle, et al. 2006. Increased body mass index does not alter response to initial highly active antiretroviral therapy in HIV-1-infected patients. *Journal of Acquired Immune Deficiency Syndromes* 43:35–41.

95. Holmberg, S.D., A.C. Moorman, and A.E. Greenberg. 2004. Trends in rates of myocardial infarction among patients with HIV [correspondence]. *New England Journal of Medicine* 350:730–732.

96. The Data Collection on Adverse Events of Anti-HIV Drugs (DAD) Study Group. 2007. Class of antiretroviral drugs and the risk of myocardial infarction. *New England Journal of Medicine* 356:1723–1735.

97. The Data Collection on Adverse Events of Anti-HIV Drugs (DAD) Study Group. 2003. Combination antiretroviral therapy and the risk of myocardial infarction. *New England Journal of Medicine* 349:1993–2003.

98. Catanzaro, A.T., and B.S. Graham. 2006. Rationale for current HIV vaccine clinical trials. In *Recent Advances in HIV Infection Research*. M. Sanchez and G. Buela-Casal (eds.). Hauppauge, NY: Nova Science Publishers, Inc, pp. 261–291.

99. Moore, J.P., Y. Cao, L. Qing, et al. 1995. Primary isolates of human immunodeficiency virus type 1 are relatively resistant to neutralization by monoclonal antibodies to gp120, and their neutralization is not predicted by studies with monomeric gp120. *Journal of Virology* 69:101–109.

100. Koch, M., M. Pancera, P.D. Kwong, et al. 2003. Structure-based, targeted deglycosylation of HIV-1 gp120 and effects on neutralization sensitivity and antibody recognition. *Virology* 313:387–400.

101. Kwong, P.D., M.L. Doyle, D.J. Casper, et al. 2002. HIV-1 evades antibody-mediated neutralization through conformational masking of receptor-binding sites. *Nature* 420:678–682.

102. Burton, D.R., R.C. Desrosiers, R. Doms, et al. 2004. HIV vaccine design and the neutralizing antibody problem. *Nature Immunology* 5:233–236.

103. Deer, B. October 3, 1999. The VaxGen experiment. *The Sunday Times Magazine (London)*.

104. Pitisuttithum, P., P.W. Berman, B. Phonrat, et al. 2004. Phase I/II study of a candidate vaccine designed against the B and E subtypes of HIV-1. *Journal of the Acquired Immune Deficiency Syndromes* 37:1160–1165.

105. Pitisuttithum, P. 2005. HIV-1 prophylactic vaccine trials in Thailand. *Current HIV Research* 3:17–30.

106. Flynn, N.M., D.N Forthal, C.D. Harro, et al. 2005. Placebo-controlled phase 3 trial of a recombinant glycoprotein 120 vaccine to prevent HIV-1 infection. *Journal of Infectious Diseases* 191:654–655.

107. Roddy, R.E., L. Zekeng, K.A. Ryan, U. Tamoufé, S.S. Weir, and E.L. Wong. 1998. A controlled trial of nonoxynol 9 film to reduce male-to-female transmission of sexually transmitted diseases. *New England Journal of Medicine* 339:504–510.

108. Anonymous. 1998. Trial shows Nonoxynol 9 efficacy is questionable. *AIDS Alert* 13:117–120.

109. Doncel, G.F., N. Chandra, R.N Fichorova. 2004. Preclinical assessment of the proinflammatory potential of microbicide candidates. *Journal of Acquired Immune Deficiency Syndromes* 37(suppl 3):S174–S180.

110. El-Sadr, W.M., K.H. Mayer, L. Maslankowski, et al. 2006. Safety and acceptability of cellulose sulfate as a vaginal microbicide in HIV-infected women. *AIDS* 20:1109–1116.

111. World Health Organization (WHO). January 31, 2007. Cellulose sulfate microbicide trial stopped. Available at http://www.who.int/hiv/mediacentre/news65/en/.

112. Von Bargen, J., A. Moorman, and S. Holmberg. 1998. How many pills do patients with HIV infection take [letter]? *Journal of the American Medical Association* 280:29.

113. Fauci, A.S. July 11, 2000. Plenary Address. XIIIth International Conference on AIDS, held in Durban, South Africa.

114. Chun, T.W., J.S. Justement, S. Moir, et al. 2007. Decay of the HIV reservoir in patients receiving antiretroviral therapy for extended periods: Implications for eradication of virus. *Journal of Infectious Diseases* 195:1762–1764.

115. Fauci, A.S. 2001. Host factors in the pathogenesis of HIV disease: Implications for therapeutic strategies [abstract S16]. In *Program and Abstracts of the 8th Conference on Retroviruses and Opportunistic Infections*, Chicago, February 4–8, 2001.

116. Dybul, M., T.-W. Chun, C. Yoder, et al. 2001. Short-cycle structured intermittent treatment of chronic HIV infection with highly active antiretroviral therapy: Effects on virologic, immunologic, and toxicity parameters. *Proceedings of the National Academy of Science USA* 98:15161–15166.

117. Garcia, F., M. Plana, C. Vidal, et al. 1999. Dynamics of viral load rebound and immunological changes after stopping effective antiretroviral therapy. *AIDS* 13:F79–F86.

118. Davey, R.T., N. Bhat, C. Yoder, et al. 1999. HIV-1 and T cell dynamics after interruption of highly active antiretroviral therapy (HAART) in patients with a history of sustained viral suppression. *Proceedings of the National Academy of Sciences USA* 96:15109–15114.

119. Mirken, B. 2000. Treatment interruption: Experts sound cautious note at San Francisco Forum; meeting proceeds despite disruption. The Body: The complete HIV/AIDS resource. Available at http://www.thebody.com/content/art32155.html.

120. Anonymous (Reuters). July 20, 2001. Experts caution against an AIDS therapy. *New York Times.*

121. Ruiz, L., G. Carcelain, J. Martinez-Picado, et al. 2001. HIV dynamics and T-cell immunity after three structured treatment interruptions in chronic HIV-1 infection. *AIDS* 15:F19–F27.

122. Ruiz, L., E. Esteban, A. Bonjoch, et al. 2003. Role of structured treatment interruption before a 5-drug salvage antiretroviral regimen: The Retrogene Study. *Journal of Infectious Diseases* 188:977–985.

123. Oxenius, A., D.A. Price, H.F. Güthard, et al. 2002. Stimulation of HIV-specific cellular immunity by structured treatment interruption fails to enhance viral control in chronic HIV infection. *Proceedings of the National Academy of Sciences USA* 99:13747–13752.

124. Fagard, C., A. Oxenius, H. Günthard, et al. 2003. A prospective trial of structured treatment interruptions in human immunodeficiency virus infection. *Archives of Internal Medicine* 163:1220–1226.

125. Ananworanich, J., R. Nuesch, M. Le Braz, et al. 2003. Failures of 1 week on, 1 week off antiretroviral therapies in a randomized trial. *AIDS* 17:F33–F37.

126. Achenbach, C.J., M. Till, F.J. Palella, et al. 2005. Extended antiretroviral treatment interruption in HIV-infected patients with long-term suppression of plasma HIV RNA. *HIV Medicine* 6:7–12.

127. Deeks, S.G., T. Wrin, T. Liegler, et al. 2001. Virologic and immunologic consequences of discontinuing combination antiretroviral-drug therapy in HIV-infected patients with detectable viremia. *New England Journal of Medicine* 344:472–480.

128. Deeks, S.G., J.D. Barbour, R.M. Grant, and J.N. Martin. 2002. Duration and predictors of CD4 T-cell gains in patients who continue combination therapy despite detectable plasma viremia. *AIDS* 16:201–207.

129. Izopet, J., C. Souyris, A. Hance, et al. 2002. Evolution of human immunodeficiency virus type 1 populations after resumption of therapy following treatment interruption and shift in resistance genotype. *Journal of Infectious Diseases* 185:1506–1510.

130. Beatty, G., P. Hunt, A. Smith, et al. 2006. A randomized pilot study comparing combination therapy plus enfuvirtide versus a treatment interruption followed by combination therapy plus enfuvirtide. *Antiviral Therapy* 11:315–319.

131. Lawrence, J., K.H. Hullsiek, L.M Thackery, et al. 2006. Disadvantages of structured treatment interruption persist in patients with multidrug-resistant HIV-1: Final results of the CPCRA 064 study. *Journal of Acquired Immune Deficiency Syndromes* 43:169–178.

132. Benson, C.A., F. Vaida, D.V. Havlir, et al. 2006. A randomized trial of treatment interruption before optimized antiretroviral therapy for persons with drug-resistant HIV: 48-week virologic results of ACTG A5086. *Journal of Infectious Diseases* 194:1309–1318.

133. Ananworanich, J., A. Gayet-Ageron, M. Le Braz, et al. 2006. CD4-guided scheduled treatment interruptions compared with continuous therapy for patients infected with HIV-1: Results of the Staccato randomised trial. *Lancet* 368:459–465.

134. Delaguerre, C., G. Peytavin, S. Dominguez, et al. 2005. Virological and pharmacological factors associated with virological response to salvage therapy after

an 8-week of treatment interruption in a context of a very advanced HIV disease (GigHAART ANRS 097). *Journal of Medical Virology* 77:345–350.

135. Tarwater, P.M., M. Parish, and J.E. Gallant. 2003. Prolonged treatment interruption after immunologic response to highly active antiretroviral therapy. *Clinical Infectious Diseases* 37:1541–1548.

136. Florence, E., F. Garcia, P. Montserrat, et al. 2004. Long-term clinical follow-up, without antiretroviral therapy of patients with chronic HIV-1 infection with good virological response to structured treatment interruption. *Clinical Infectious Diseases* 39:569–574.

137. El-Sadr, W., J. Neaton, for the SMART Study Investigators. 2006. Episodic CD4-guided use of ART is inferior to continuous therapy: results of the SMART Study [abstract 106LB]. In *Program and Abstracts of the 13th Conference on Retroviruses and Opportunistic Infections*, Denver, February 5–8, 2006.

CHAPTER NINE

Errors, Their Consequences, and Their Management

Scientific error and controversy spring from biases and flourish in the absence of data. Biases, which underlay errors and controversies, are probably unavoidable. There seems to be a natural bias to notice and analyze data that shows what one expects to find, while minimizing or dismissing contrary evidence. Also, it is probably natural to defer to the wisdom of received authority, which is why, for example, blood-letting survived as a medical practice into the twentieth century. Intellectual laziness, wishful thinking, fear of reporting something different from expectations of colleagues or teachers, desire to be original, and sometimes even financial motivations all influence our ability to see things clearly. Perhaps there is an irreducible minimum of biased thinking that leads HIV scientists to err. As experience in the HIV/AIDS epidemic shows, all scientists, including some who are infrequently wrong, can make errors. Only training, experience, and dedication to honest and frequent evaluation of data can hedge against bias.

Controversies will always occur, and, indeed, it is understood that they are fundamental to the scientific process; given incomplete or inadequate data and each person's innate tendency to believe or disbelieve selected information, sincere disagreements are inevitable. Controversies in HIV/AIDS often spur broader research and are usually resolved with more data. Errors, however, are rarely helpful and must be avoided.

This chapter reviews considerations of the types and consequences of scientific error in HIV/AIDS; how errors and controversies may best be resolved by hastening the process by which studies are funded, executed, and their data reviewed and reported; and, more difficult to achieve and requiring better education and real-world practice, preventing errors by learning critical evaluation of one's own and others' work.

This book has attempted to review some of the most egregious scientific errors, missteps, and controversies in the first 25 years of the U.S. HIV/AIDS epidemic. It does not review the much larger body of HIV scientific data that has been reproduced and widely accepted. Also, many controversies that have had less impact on scientific and public thinking about HIV and AIDS could not be covered in this book. These have been errors in articles that appeared in less influential medical and scientific journals, that were not duplicated or developed, or have had relatively little currency in the AIDS community or research time expended by HIV scientists. Also, reflecting the author's bias, most of the controversies covered here reflect epidemiologic, medical, and preventive health issues, and mainly treat adult and adolescent infection.

Further, with the exception of some recent controversies (Chapter 8), the errors and controversies subjected to "autopsy" were selected from those now widely accepted as dead issues. Some other controversies have not yet been resolved and so cannot offer insights regarding how error and controversy influence scientific, medical, and epidemiologic thinking and progress. For example, two biologic mysteries continue to elude us: why most people exposed by sexual contact to HIV-infected partners, sometimes repeatedly, do not get infected (Chapter 4, *Issues in Sexual Transmission* section); and why some people once infected rapidly develop AIDS, whereas others go on without symptoms many more than the average 10 years between HIV and an AIDS-defining disease or condition. Associations have been reported, such as the longer survival of patients who preserve numbers and function of CD8+ cells specifically or cytotoxic T lymphocytes generally.[1-3] In this instance, the researchers reporting long-term infection without symptoms and persistence of certain types of white blood cells recognize that this association is confounded by biologic phenomena not yet understood. However, knowing the association may help in evaluating the efficacy of experimental HIV vaccines. In any case, such areas of ongoing research and murkiness do not provide good case studies (yet) of how incorrect data, its analysis, or conclusions drawn from it may divert our attentions.

Types of Errors and Their Consequences

Some errors can be considered "classic" epidemiologic or analytic errors. For example, *biases of ascertainment* occurred in reports throughout the epidemic, especially early, when people were not able to distinguish adequately between stages of HIV infection. A classic case of such a bias occurred when some investigators reported that women had shorter incubation periods—from HIV infection to AIDS—or shorter survival after HIV infection than men;[4] however, because in the mid-1980s, HIV was considered a "gay disease," women were tested later, often when they were already ill or in hospital. That is, these women were diagnosed or "ascertained" later in their disease course, so "progressed" more rapidly to disability and death. In fact, numerous later studies found that women actually had lower viral loads (plasma HIV RNA levels) than men at the same stage of HIV disease progression (CD4+ cell count). Put another way, women consistently have higher CD4+ cell counts than men at the same stage of disease progression as measured by their having the same levels of plasma viremia (viral load).[5–8] It appears that uninfected women start with higher normal CD4+ cell counts than uninfected men,[9] and even in early stages of HIV infection, then tend toward the same CD4+ cell counts as HIV infection progresses to late stages.[5, 6] Thus, conclusions drawn from measurements of CD4+ counts during HIV infection need to be interpreted with these trends in mind. Although differences in natural progression of HIV disease in men and women may exist, gender differences other than in genital diseases do not seem to affect the overall course of this chronic infection[10, 11] and probably only have import if they affect timing of treatment of women.[12]

However, this (erroneous) tendency to report the supposedly more rapid disease progression in women may have had the salutary effect of highlighting the growing problem in them; from a few percent in the 1980s and 1990s, women currently comprise over 20 percent and an increasing percentage of reported AIDS cases.

The term *confounding* has been used to refer to a few different concepts, but in epidemiology usually refers to bias in estimating causal effects, an unmeasured or unanalyzed factor that significantly affects a purported association. (For example, associations between coffee drinking and cancer may be confounded if one does not control for usually greater cigarette-smoking in coffee- vs. non-coffee drinkers.) Certainly errors of confounding have occurred several times in the brief history of the HIV/AIDS epidemic. The reported association between the use of protease inhibitor (PI) drugs and lipoatrophy (fat wasting of limbs) [13, 14] was, in retrospect, probably confounded by the concurrent use of stavudine (d4T), a nucleotide reverse transcriptase inhibitor (Chapter 8, *Lipodystrophy* section). Stavudine was FDA-approved in June 1994, and was widely used when PI drugs (saquinivir, ritonavir, and indinavir) were being introduced as "highly effective antiretroviral therapy" (HAART) in 1995 and 1996 (Appendix). The PI drugs do induce many of the metabolic effects purportedly associated with lipodystrophy, such as hyperlipidemia and diabetes (insulin resistance). However, it turned out that these effects of PIs were separate from clinical lipodystrophy (lipoatrophy), which subsequent researchers repeatedly found was actually most closely associated with the use of stavudine, zidovudine, and some other NRTI, not PI, drugs.[15-17]

This error engendered some reluctance for physicians to prescribe and patients to want to take protease inhibitors and distracted from the real problem; further, because the original researchers who reported the association with PI use also advocated mitochondrial toxicity as the underlying pathogenesis, much research has been focused on this pathogenic mechanism. However, increasingly more researchers are now beginning to wonder if mitochondrial toxicity is the real or sole biologic factor underlying lipodystrophy (Chapter 8, *Lipodystrophy* section).[18]

Similarly, the early reported association of inhaled nitrites (poppers) and Kaposi's sarcoma (KS) in gay men in the United States distracted some researchers (Chapter 2, *"Poppers" and Kaposi's sarcoma* section).[19, 20] Before the AIDS epidemic, KS, a rare tumor of proliferating blood vessels, was found mainly in elderly men in Italy and elsewhere in the Mediterranean; after the AIDS epidemic began, KS was widely seen in African patients. Thus, as these non-Americans were not exposed to "poppers" or other evident sources of nitrites, many thought the association was confounded by the sexual activity of gay men (i.e., many partners, unprotected sex). With hindsight, it is now clear that KS represents the dual effects of HIV-induced immunodeficiency and underlying infection with human herpesvirus 8 (HHV-8). It took over a decade before the isolation of this virus from KS tissue;[21] given that there were not effective treatments for HIV or KS in the 1980s, this error and controversy about the KS agent probably led to more wasted laboratory time (and ink) than adverse clinical ramifications.

Another example of a potentially important confounder in HIV epidemiologic and clinical research is current or history of smoking cigarettes. As seen in gay men and injection drug users generally, about 60 percent of HIV patients currently in care are past or current smokers,[22] and some populations such as patients at Veterans Affairs (VA) are almost 80 percent current or former smokers.[23] These are rates two-, three- or more times the rates of smoking seen in the general public. Thus, for example, any analysis of cancer or of cardiovascular disease in HIV patients should control or adjust analysis for cigarette smoking in the HIV-infected population, although some have not been able to do so adequately[24] or at all.[25] High rates of smoking-related diseases may be attributed to immunodeficiency from HIV infection—which certainly may affect the occurrence of some cancers, lung disease, and cardiovascular disease—but would normally be expected to occur in proportion to the increased rates of smoking in the HIV patient population anyway.

Ironically, the opposite problem–that is, inflating smoking's influence–can also occur, a bias to think that this exposure must be associated with all bad HIV-related outcomes. Cigarette smoking is firmly associated with heart, lung, and vascular disease, and over 20 cancers. However, does this also translate to a negative effect on HIV/AIDS disease progression? Early in the epidemic, public service announcements and brochures warned HIV-patients that continuing to smoke cigarettes could accelerate HIV disease. In fact, though, the few studies that have purported to show this were either small, for example 84 HIV-infected smokers who were reported to have more rapid progression to AIDS,[26] or reflected questionable ascertainment, as in 521 HIV-infected patients admitted to a tertiary care hospital[27] who were more likely to have *Pneumocystis carinii* pneumonia (PCP) or community-acquired pneumonia. Except for the association with community-acquired pneumonia, almost all other studies, including the largest ones, have actually not been able to find any association between cigarette smoking and HIV disease progression or even, contrary to expectations, with the lung condition PCP.[28–30] Thus, while it is important to the health of HIV patients, especially as they live longer, to discontinue cigarette smoking, it appears this personal health measure is more important to their avoiding cardiovascular, pulmonary and malignant diseases than to influencing the progression of AIDS or avoiding opportunistic infections associated with HIV.

Analytic errors or weaknesses can easily be hidden in arcane statistical procedures that nonstatistical readers may not be able to discern. Mathematical modeling is especially prone to these as many simplifying assumptions may need to be made, and such assumptions may be based on poor, lacking, or incorrect data. For example, few readers would be able to discern that a model predicting that zidovudine would decrease the incidence of AIDS cases (Chapter 7, *Zidovudine* section) would know that this represented assumptions both of widespread use of zidovudine in 1988 and 1989 by people who did not yet have AIDS and of long-term efficacy of zidovudine,[31] or that modeling the numbers of AIDS cases in the United States (Chapter 3, *Estimating the Impact of AIDS* section) were substantially derived from an estimated 6,000 HIV infections in a survey of child-bearing women in 1989,[32] an estimate not provided in the report;[33] or that my and others' estimates of numbers of injection drug users in the United States or HIV incidence in them were skewed because of somewhat inflated "expert opinion" (Chapter 3, *Estimating the Impact of AIDS* section).[34, 35]

Ecologic fallacies may be hidden in masses of extraneous data, as that there was an overlap in the sites where oral polio vaccination was administered and where early African HIV cases were purportedly found (Chapter 2, *The*

River section);[36] or in statistical procedures that obscure that essentially two trend lines are being compared between the use of PI drugs and cardiovascular disease, for a very brief period (mean, 15 months, not long enough to see chronic effects)(Chapter 8, *Protease Inhibitors and Cardiovascular Disease* section).[24] In the former case, this increases public mistrust of scientific and medical authorities, especially those authorities funded or paid by the government.[37] In the latter case, dismissing the association between PI drugs and adverse cardiovascular events may have distracted some clinicians and patients from the need to avoid such drugs when the patient had underlying risk factors for cardiovascular disease. Indeed, some modify their risk factors–such as stopping smoking, and controlling their hypertension or diabetes–but many will not: should such patients receive or continue to receive PI drugs?

The ability to recognize such epidemiologic, statistical, and analytic errors should be honed in graduate schools of medicine, science, and public health, but there are categories of errors that are harder to recognize and may have more profound and detrimental effects. In particular, *laboratory errors* can substantially bollix up the research direction and activities of many other laboratories. The contamination that led Robert Gallo and his laboratory to conclude that HTLV-III was the cause of AIDS,[38] when a human T-lymphotropic virus was not the AIDS agent, serve as an illustration of how such a "simple" lab error may have large consequences (Chapter 2, *HTLV-III* section). The prominent backing of the then U.S. Department of Health, Education and Welfare of the Gallo lab's claim meant that all American researchers had to refer to HIV as HTLV-III or HTLV-III/LAV (to acknowledge the French "lymphadenopathy-associated virus"). This annoying circumlocution distracted some basic research to a virus that was not the cause of AIDS. Most important, it putatively resulted in some lives lost as the United States and France wrangled about patent rights on a serum test that could have been available 6–12 months earlier to screen the U.S. blood supply for HIV.

Unrecognized contamination also led to the reports of HTLV-IV,[39] which was ultimately found to be a simian immunodeficiency virus (SIV) laboratory contaminant (Chapter 2, *HIV-2, HTLV-IV* section).[40] Scores of research articles about this nonexistent virus attest to the research distraction such a contamination can engender. Once HTLV-IV was debunked, the discoverers of this nonexistent virus tried unsuccessfully to convince the AIDS scientific community that previous infection with HIV-2 protected against HIV-1.[41] As these researchers came from a prestigious institution (Harvard), had received prestigious awards (Lasker Award), and reported in a prestigious journal

(*Science*), their suggestions had to be taken seriously and required further research on the part of others who pointed out—along with data of the many people coinfected with both HIV-1 and HIV-2—errors in their epidemiologic reasoning.[42]

Another kind of laboratory error, other than contamination, involves the misapplication or poor laboratory technique of a newly introduced test. For example, in the U.S. HIV/AIDS epidemic, much public confusion was created by use of the newly introduced polymerase chain reaction (PCR) to report that people could be long-term HIV-serum-test "negative" (seronegative) yet actually HIV-infected, as detected by PCR (Chapter 4, "*Silent Sequences*" section).[43] This prominent report in the *New England Journal of Medicine* certainly rattled many who had tested "HIV negative," yet now wondered if they were HIV-infected nonetheless. Others could not detect such seronegative but HIV-infected persons in several other investigations of test-negative persons and wondered if contamination, clerical errors, or inappropriate PCR technique (e.g., too many cycles of replication) could explain this error.[44] Indeed, the authors of the original report could not duplicate their original results.[45] Similar concerns attached to a report, also in 1989, that raised false hopes that some HIV-infected persons could lose their HIV antibody and perhaps their HIV infection as well (Chapter 4, "*Silent Sequences*" section).[46] Here, too, further research was never able to substantiate this remarkable finding.[47] Similarly, no research unit has duplicated the finding of HIV in insect cells[48] as reported at AIDS conferences in the mid-1980s (Chapter 5, *Belle Glade* section); nor has any other researcher reported finding (by in situ PCR) inside (not attached) to human sperm cells.[49] Each of these findings were widely reported and both created public anxiety and also required research by many other teams to try to (unsuccessfully) replicate these incorrect findings.

Human Bias

To the extent it can be differentiated from errors, human bias is the underlying force behind skewed analyses and conclusions rather than a problem of methodology or analysis alone. For example, there was an underlying desire on the part of many researchers to justify the benefits of the first antiretroviral drug, zidovudine (Chapter 7, *Zidovudine* section). Thus, analyses that did not seem to be inherently wrong were nonetheless viewed by some as not according with their experience. In retrospect, for example, zidovudine, with or without acyclovir,[50] is not a particularly effective treatment; its therapeutic benefits can usually be measured in months.

In reference to financial factors that bias researchers, many worry about the role of pharmaceutical companies who may influence physicians' attitudes to their products by providing sometimes substantial honoraria for doctors' service on speaking panels or for enrolling their (the clinicians') patients in studies of the company's drugs and therapies. One form of effective influence by drug companies is to analyze data from a clinical study, ghost-write it as a journal manuscript, and to make a participating clinician the lead author: what doctor does not want to be the prime author of a published paper that burnishes his or her reputation and, perhaps, chances of academic advancement? That this can be provided with relatively modest input and time on the doctor's part further sweetens financial compensation for enrolling one's patients in drug company-financed studies.

Journal editors and conference organizers have made many strides in recent years to make the commercial, usually pharmaceutical company, backing of speakers and journal authors more transparent to the audience or the readers. Typically, a list of the pharmaceutical companies compensating each author or speaker is appended to the article or made clear in the meeting program. These are good and necessary disclosures, but the most prominent writers and speakers often have received honoraria or research support from a host of companies, including the few major pharmaceutical companies producing most antiretroviral drugs. How does the reader or audience member know whether some support is much greater and, thus, more likely to bias a presentation or article than other listed sources of support? There is a big difference between receiving major research grants and receiving, say, a single modest honorarium for a one-time educational activity. Perhaps there is some way that major support can be somehow distinguished from more minor support in disclosures.

On the other hand, sources or amount of funding do not necessarily match up with bias: to a greater or lesser extent, almost all researchers try to eliminate bias from their research results and interpretations (or, at least try to convince themselves they are not being biased). Ultimately, as indicated at the start of this book, scientists need to examine their own biases, if only for enlightened self-interest: ultimately, it does not help anyone to report results that others cannot reproduce.

Sometimes even data and reason will not suffice, and public mischief can be created from misrepresenting risk to the public. People have difficulty estimating risk, so that if it is reported that a chance of something is "one in hundred," or even "one in a million," one tends to think he or she will be the "one," not part of the "million." Our focus is on the numerator, not the denominator. This human tendency also makes bracketing risk difficult, so that even though the likelihood getting HIV from the sweat or exhaled air from another person must be infinitesimally small, if it occurs at all, still some think will read that "one in a million risk" as that it can occur rather than the reality, which is that it doesn't.

As discussed in Chapter 2, ever since the discovery of HIV and its role in the pathogenesis of AIDS, there have been vociferous "AIDS deniers" and conspiracy theorists. Peter Duesberg, a molecular and cell biologist at University of California at Berkeley started by insisting that HIV does not cause AIDS,[51] and, when it was widely accepted that HIV infection leads to AIDS, elided to the view that HIV *alone* does not cause AIDS.[52] Lorraine Day, an orthopedic surgeon who relinquished her practice because she charged that CDC was downplaying the risk to her of operating on HIV patients (Chapter 5, *Health Care Workers* section), has not changed her views despite the rare occupational infections in surgeons and other health care workers over the past two decades[53]; she now promotes alternative therapies for AIDS and for cancer. And there have been other, less public conspiracy theories or skewing of facts to bolster bias: for example, water fluoridation opponents thought that, since such treatment occurred in New York City, San Francisco and Miami—from which cities the first AIDS cases were reported—fluoridation was damaging the immune system and predisposing to AIDS,[54] a classic example of an ecological fallacy driven by serious personal bias.

If these attitudes were just confined to persons who, for whatever reason, stubbornly refuse to face facts, their effects would be minimal. The net effect of critics such as Day or Duesberg—even though they are advocating somewhat contradictory points—is directly negative to the extent that HIV patients (or potential patients) believe them and avoid appropriate behaviors or treatments. In the case of Peter Duesberg, his discredited argument that HIV does not cause AIDS was seized upon by Thabo Mbeki, the South African President since 1999 who has resisted federally funding treatment and prevention programs in his country: he argues that AIDS is caused by poverty, not by HIV, and repeatedly cites Duesberg's theoretic objections.

In the United States, it is the overall indirect effect that may be most destructive as unreasonable yet highly visible critics increase the difficulty of getting official or expert health messages to some of the people who need it most. Iconoclasts reinforce the general distrust of the federal government and other authorities among African Americans who cite the Tuskegee syphilis experiments of the 1960s and other valid examples of racial prejudice. The net result is that 27 percent of respondents in a door-to-door survey of black adults in San Bernardino, California, recently agreed with the belief that "HIV/AIDS is a man-made virus that the federal government made to kill and wipe out black people."[55] It is hard to measure this indirect but large negative effect of public skepticism and its effect on HIV prevention efforts[56, 57]; but it is especially frustrating as HIV infection and AIDS are spreading rapidly through young African Americans living in the South.

Bureaucracy, the "Killer Bees," and Other Considerations about Retarding Research

Again, scientific controversies flourish and errors persist in an absence of data. However, there are practical or systematic as well as theoretic reasons why errors can persist. Many controversies are decided and errors corrected in direct proportion to the length of time for more data and more accurate data to become available. The faster that better data can be presented, the faster errors can be recognized, controversies resolved, or essentially correct observations improved.

For example, there was wide public, medical, and scientific concern with the potential development of another epidemic of "AIDS" caused by something other than HIV, called "idiopathic CD4 lymphocytopenia" (ICL, low CD4 cells in the absence of HIV infection or other clear cause)(see Chapter 3, *Idiopathic CD4-lymphocytopenia* section). ICL lasted as an issue almost exactly from the time of the Eighth International Conference on AIDS in Amsterdam in July 1992, when it was first raised on the floor of the Conference as an issue, till the publication of the national study in the *New England Journal of Medicine* in February 1993.[58] The result of rapid identification, interview, and examination of 47 persons across the United States who met the ICL case definition showed no evidence of a new transmissible agent causing lymphopenia (low CD4+ cell counts).

Some issues, however, will continue to need evolving data and continuous re-thinking. The controversy about when—that is, at what CD4+ cell count or viral load—to start therapy for persons who are still without symptoms has been ongoing for over a decade (Chapter 8, *When to Start Therapy* section). In the unavoidable absence of a definitive, timely, yet long-term study of what happens to patients who start therapy at different CD4+ cell counts, official guidelines for the recommendations about the use of antiretroviral drugs rely on "expert opinion." A definitive study would take a long period and probably be obsolete by the time it was completed, as evolving and improving therapy now continuously shifts clinicians' attitudes on when to recommend their patients start therapy. Normally, however, many controversies fall between these two extremes and can be resolved and errors corrected if the process is not too drawn out and misinformation does not become solidified in people's minds.

If resolving controversies and errors depends on the rapidity with which correct data becomes available, we should ask what speeds the process of scientific enquiry or how we can resolve obstacles to science. The example of the ICL investigation is illustrative in this regard. This was undertaken and completed rapidly because the federal government allows an exception to normal procedures in the face of an outbreak or suspected outbreak of disease with public health implications. The ICL investigation took about 4 months from start to finish (publication of results); if it had undergone usual governmental procedures it would have taken well over 4 years. The whole process is referred to by a colleague as a bureaucratic "Chutes and Ladders."

First, the idea of investigating cases of our example, ICL, under a Cooperative Agreement, a type of Grant that would draw on the strengths both of federal and non-governmental (e.g., academic or hospital) investigators, would have required convincing every supervisory level at the Agency of the need for funding such an investigation. Other means of funding studies, by Grant or by Contract, have their own problems. Grants, as the name suggests, allow most freedom to the individual or institution receiving the grant: the federal scientist mainly reviews and tries to manage bureaucratic issues–not what most people come to NIH or CDC to do–and, in fact, have limited ability to make sure that research dollars are spent well. If a Contract, the federal researchers get to specify all aspects of the research, but every change to the protocol–and these are inevitable as situations change over the years of a contract–must be reviewed and approved by the federal government, often very slowly. Depending upon how the relationship is structured, the contracting institution may have difficulties with the research and other constraints. No matter what the relationship–Grant, Cooperative Agreement, or Contract–Agency delays to issuing a Request for Applications (RFA) or Request for Proposals (RFP) are considerable.

At CDC and other Agencies recent trends to put more power and decision-making in the hands of successively higher levels of administration removes such priority setting for research and service from the hands of subject-experts. At CDC, the construction of a power pyramid and the addition of layers of bureaucracy were epitomized by the 2003 decision to delete the job title and supervisory authority of "Section Chief" (the first rung of supervisory authority) but to add another level, "Coordinating Centers," above the level of the several CDC Centers, just below the CDC Director's office. Funding decisions and research directions are now decided at increasing higher levels of the bureaucracy, and less by those closest to the subject. The time it takes now to explain, "lobby," and get a funding commitment up the chain of command, many of whom are already busy, burdened, traveling, and not necessarily knowledgeable about the issue, can be considerable.

Once past this internal approval process, an RFP or an RFA is issued, asking interested parties to apply to participate in a multicenter investigation. Of course, writing the RFP often takes many weeks, as this is a long and complicated document. Then, posting in the Federal Register and collecting applications takes many more.

Then, grant and cooperative agreement applications must be reviewed by an External Review Committee, comprised mainly or entirely of persons outside the funding unit. Previously, the Section, Branch, or Division that issued the RFP would also provide Technical Reviews of the proposals received; this was an opportunity to point out for the Review Committee the evident strengths and weaknesses of each proposal as perceived by the researchers trying to do the study. Also, at least one third of the reviewers on the External Review Committee could be comprised of officials working within the Center or Institute funding the research. In recent years, however, no Technical Review or other input from the RFA- or RFP-issuing unit can be provided; and external reviewers must mainly or entirely come from outside the Center and some from outside the Agency.

This sounds like it would provide objective review, until one has read these reviews, many of which are neither objective nor informed. External reviewers who may have never done nor have any idea what the specific research entails are asked to evaluate it. Often, too, persons with hidden agendas or axes to grind end up on these committees: so, both good and bad proposals may easily get unfair or prejudicial evaluation, positive or negative. There is no appeal process, and the unit issuing the RFP (or at NIH, the RFA) may receive a priority ranking from the External Committee that have several poor proposals getting higher scores than much better ones. The unit funding and managing the research may only take the top-scored applications; in some cases, the resulting list of highly scored applications is so unacceptable that the Agency decides not to fund any sites, nullifying the RFA or RFP.

If this important hurdle can be overcome—that is, good sites are available and selected after External Review—the always difficult process begins of hammering out a common protocol describing study-participants to be recruited, timing, and the timing and types of examinations and interview all agree should form the guide for the multisite investigation of, in our example, ICL. This is often useful and necessary, as it may crystallize the many researchers' thoughts about what can or can not be accomplished. Still, it is always a time-consuming process, even when the federal unit tries to outline a skeleton or draft protocol ahead of time. Now, though, comes some of the most painful delay.

At this point, in the argot of federal researchers, the "Killer Bees"–the various Institutional Review Boards (IRBs) and the federal Office of Management and Budget (OMB)–come into play. IRBs, rightly, became the sine qua non after the disastrous Tuskegee syphilis study, and were designed to prevent such unethical research. Thus, all human research needs to be approved by the federal Agency's IRB and the IRBs of every participating institution in the study (e.g. hospital or university, state or local health departments, etc.). Technically, each IRB should focus on issues of ethical review–specifically, that the research will entail no undue or inappropriate risk to the study-subjects, and that the Consent Form a study-participant signs is clear, complete, and comprehensible. Many IRBs, such as those at CDC, now require that Consent Forms are at no higher than an eighth-grade reading level. Unfortunately, many IRBs overstep this boundary and refuse to sign off on research unless it includes some methodologic or material changes to the research protocol. Sometimes such suggestions are helpful, often they are not, and rarely are they requested or wanted. Thus, some have recently argued that "mission creep" in IRBs have led to simultaneous overregulation of researchers and under protection of study-participants.[59]

Even if the several IRBs focus mainly on ethical conduct of the proposed study, different IRBs may have markedly different evaluation standards. Sometimes, the federal and external investigators who wish to do a study are caught between "ping-pong" IRBs; for example, one IRB insists on a particular wording of the Consent form, often at the behest of their institution's lawyers, whereas a separately reviewing IRB also insists on a very different wording, also often at the behest of their lawyers. Hapless investigators then have to appeal to one, the other, or several IRBs to compromise, as without all IRBs agreeing to the research, it cannot move forward.

A review of almost 5,000 hours of staff time over a 19-month period in Veterans Affairs primary care clinic IRBs[60] showed that long turnaround times, lost paperwork, difficulty obtaining necessary forms and unavailability of key staff were frequent process problems: the median time to obtain IRB approval was 286 days (range, 52–708 days). These reviewers of IRB reviewers concluded that "the IRB system as currently configured impose costly burdens of administrative activity and delay on observational health services research studies, and paradoxically decreases protection of human subjects."[60]

Certainly, it occurs to every intelligent analyst of the IRB system, especially its researcher "victims," that there must be a better, more expeditious way to ensure ethical research. For example, one may ask why there is not some standard Consent Form or Consent Form outline that lists the necessary components of consent and even the specific language agreed upon by a nationally constituted body of ethicists. (Currently the federal Office of Human Research Protections [OHRP] credentials the many IRBs, but does not provide such guidance.) Better yet would be standard, sitting, and centralized IRBs–IRBs are currently composed of rotating membership from the institution and the community–that could serve as nationally recognized review panels, such that any proposed research could be submitted and be rapidly reviewed by one standard, central and "expert" IRB. This single IRB would suggest improvements; however, hopefully, the membership of an objective, separate IRB would be more informed and less adversarial, delayed, and anarchic as many local institutional IRBs can be.

Yet even when one is past the IRB process, the proposal–if it intends to ask questions of study-participants–must be approved by the federal OMB. Under the amendments to the ironically titled Paperwork Reduction Act sponsored by then North Carolina U.S. Senator Jesse Helms in 1995 (44 USC Sec. 3506), all information collected from ten or more citizens, such as questionnaires administered as part of a study, need to be approved by the Director of OMB. Helms had become staunchly opposed to all AIDS research and service in 1987 after being shocked by the contents of a prevention brochure released by the Gay Men's Health Crisis. Although this brochure was not funded by any public dollars, Helms wanted all material produced with public funds containing sensitive questions, particularly about sex behaviors, reviewed first by OMB as a sort of "power of the purse-string." Sociologist Edward Laumann, of the University of Chicago, described[61] how Helms' and others 6-year obstruction of two NIH-funded and review process-approved grants to perform a much-needed national sex survey. (There is currently no authoritative and representative national survey of American sexual behaviors.) After repeated review and even approval, this survey was eventually scotched in 1991 by the administrative action of Wendy Baldwin, a newly appointed Director of the National Institute of Child Health and Human Development who may have been under pressure to do so.[61]

Two years before his retirement from the Senate, Helms himself regretted his many years' opposition to AIDS funding after a deeply religious conversation with the Irish Rock star Bono in 2000, and, in that year, actually sponsored $600 million in funding for AIDS relief for Africa. However, the OMB regulations and requirements from his earlier time have remained in place.

At the time of this writing, all questionnaires in AIDS need to be reviewed by a small and inexpert staff at OMB: the process now takes at least nine months, longer if the proposing researchers are not then asked to provide more details for OMB re-review. It would be difficult to find a scientific justification for this delay, especially given that there are already internal Agency,

External Committee, and usually several IRB reviews of the proposed project.

After the governmental bureaucratic delays, there are inevitably non-governmental institutions' difficulties. Hiring and training those to perform the study, making sure the physical space and research infrastructure are adequate, programming computerized data entry, collection, storage and analytic capacity, and many other details and unforeseen snags usually delay any study several months. Then, actual performance of the study, collection and analysis of data, depending upon the project—even with, say, only a few hundred potential ICL subjects to screen and examine—can still take many months or, usually, years. Finally, the resulting multiauthored conference presentations or journal articles must be written and undergo an Agency review process even before submission to a conference committee or journal review.

Thus, returning to the hypothetical example, if concerned persons had first published their description of ICL patients in a major journal, rather than verbally and spontaneously presented them at an AIDS conference, and if CDC did not have an option to investigate this putative outbreak as a so-called "Epi-aid," the normal process could easily have taken several years to provide confirmation or refutation of the original reports. Meanwhile, if indeed there were another virus or other agent causing immunodeficiency was being transmitted in the public, especially if like HIV this were a chronic infection without symptoms for several years, this information like that for the early stages of the AIDS epidemic would be too late for effective prevention efforts.

Journals

Many of the examples in this book of erroneous or controversial research in HIV/AIDS over the first 25 years of the epidemic were published in the most respected journals—*New England Journal of Medicine, Science, Journal of the American Medical Association (JAMA), Lancet,* to name just a few. Are these journals more prone to accepting erroneous research, or is this simply an artifact, a bias of ascertainment, that the deepest scientific controversies are engendered by original publication in these prominent journals? It would be interesting to somehow measure the rate of "correct"—meaning largely reproducible—research and the rate of "incorrect"—meaning not reproducible or otherwise discredited—research reported in several journals. The results might be surprising. In any case, timely revisiting and "autopsy" of previous articles would be helpful to those journals improve their rate of publishing correct, reproducible science.

Many misunderstand the journal review process as mainly a means of elim-inating fraudulent or commercial research. In fact, wrong or poor research that is not fraudulent or commercially biased can still be quite misleading when published in a prominent journal and can spark controversy requiring much research time and dollars to confirm or refute the original report. Many times, subsequent, more correct data and analyses by others are published in lesser read journals, so the public and even many members of the sci-entific AIDS community may be left with misinformed opinions based on an original, highly visible, and incorrect journal article. It takes a while for true, reproducible information to percolate through the research and then the larger community.

The journal review process of submitted manuscripts can be flawed and time-consuming. Peer-reviewers for journals are often selected from re-searchers who can be envious, competitive, or otherwise negatively disposed to the research of another institution or researcher. Peer-reviewers may also be selected by their prominence in a field, but may not understand the need for observational studies (as opposed to randomized clinical trials), may be dazzled by big numbers, or by arcane statistical or laboratory techniques they themselves cannot do, or otherwise distracted by any number of issues. Also, senior specialists are busy, and they may delay reviewing for many weeks. Often they will forward manuscripts they have been asked to review to a junior staff member, who may be eager to show the senior expert how in-sightful, analytic, and critical he or she can be. No paper can withstand such scrutiny: there are always problems in doing and reporting studies in the real world as circumstances cannot be controlled. (Most scientific papers include a discussion of various usually unavoidable limitations to the research.) For many reasons, journal peer reviews that are inappropriate in substance or tone are not uncommon.

Many have questioned the peer-review process, and journals often try to improve it.[62] There seems to be no background training or experience that predicts which peer reviewers will provide a quality review.[63] One solution, of course, would be dedicated peer review by panels of experts who have a proven track record of objectivity, fairness, knowledge of the specialty, and a history of providing appropriate review. The idea of fixed, professional peer review committees (similar to the suggestion for central IRBs) seems to have occurred to many.[64] However, many important journals and probably all smaller journals, would not be able to afford to empanel such full- or part-time review committees. Thus, the larger ones review the reviewers for the value, thoroughness, and punctuality of the critique and rate them as to the quality of their reviews. They have to trust the ability of associate editors to fairly chose and consider the reviewers of submitted manuscripts and to detect bias or unfairness, both positive and negative, in reviews when they receive them.

Higher Education

In addition to facilitating or speeding up the process by which studies and projects are funded, completed and reported, and the ongoing efforts of journals to do an ever better job of making sure peer review is timely, insightful and reasonably unbiased, errors will nonetheless be made and prominently reported. There are ways the scientific process can be improved and hastened such that errors get detected and corrected more promptly. Better yet, but also more difficult, is the recognition, the prevention, of error before it becomes embedded in the literature and imaginations of medical and public health scientists. As there are some scientists who seem to maintain objectivity and to be less prone to bias and error (are "right" more often), recognizing error may be something that can be learned, even taught.

We can do a better job of educating medical, biology, and public health students about how to fairly evaluate reports in the literature, information upon which many will be designing and executing their own research or clinical practice. Can they recognize common biases and confounded associations? Are they trained to evaluate Methods and Results critically and with a "common sense" viewpoint, and to interpret authors' conclusions within the context of what the research actually shows? How much practical training do they receive such that they understand that it is the development of an accurate and complete-as-possible database that is the hard, essential work, not the computer application of complicated statistical tests to that data? In the real world, no one will be providing a "clean" dataset to practice on. Can they recognize that information reported based on new laboratory techniques need to be interpreted cautiously and with an open mind, that a new technique in the hands of still-inexperienced researchers might be unreliable?

Students of medicine, the natural sciences, and public health have ever more to learn during their course of study. Many learn several practical considerations about human research as they write and defend a thesis or as part of a residency program. Many, however, will never do research and will base their medical and public health practice based on the opinions of persons they respect and their reading of the scientific literature. A critical sense needs to be developed in evaluating both written and oral scientific opinion, even if one's career only involves reviewing the scientific work and publications of others and not original research on one's own part. So, as institutional bureaucracies and journals may benefit from re-thinking and revising their review and approval processes, graduate schools of medicine, science, and public health, too, would probably benefit from re-evaluating their courses of instruction: how well are they preparing their graduates to recognize and avoid error?

References

1. Lifson, A.R., S.P. Buchbinder, H.W. Sheppard, et al. 1991. Long-term human immunodeficiency virus infection in asymptomatic homosexual and bisexual men with normal CD4+ lymphocyte counts: Immunologic and virologic characteristics. *Journal of Infectious Diseases* 163:959–965.

2. Harrer, T., E. Harrer, S.A. Kalams, et al. 1996. Cytotoxic T lymphocytes in asymptomatic long-term nonprogressing HIV-1 infection, Breadth and specificity of the response and isolation of the response and relation to in vivo viral quasispecies in a person with prolonged infection and low viral load. *Journal of Immunology* 156:2616–2623.

3. Giorgi, J.V., H.N. Ho, K. Hirji, et al. 1994. CD8+ lymphocyte activation at human immunodeficiency virus type 1 seroconversion: Development of HLA-DR+ CD38- CD8+ cells is associated with subsequent stable CD4+ cell levels. The Multicenter AIDS Cohort Study Group. *Journal of Infectious Diseases* 170:775–781.

4. Rothenberg, R., M. Woelfel, R. Stoneburner, J. Milberg, R. Parker, and B. Truman. 1987. Survival with the acquired immunodeficiency syndrome. Experience with 5833 cases in New York City. *New England Journal of Medicine* 317:1297–1302.

5. Bush, C.E., R.M. Donovan, N. Makowitz, D. Baxa, P. Kvale, and L.D. Saravolatz. 1996. Gender is not a factor in serum human immunodeficiency virus type 1 RNA levels in patients with viremia. *Journal of Clinical Microbiology* 34:970–972.

6. Farzadegan, H., D.R. Hoover, J. Astemborski, et al. 1998. Sex differences in HIV-1 viral load and progression to AIDS. *Lancet* 352:1510–1514.

7. Rompalo, A.M., J. Astemborski, E. Schoenbaum et al. 1999. Comparison of clinical manifestations of HIV infection among women by risk group, CD4+ cell count, and HIV-1 plasma viral load. HER Study Group. HIV Epidemiology Research Study. *Journal of the Acquired Immune Deficiency Syndrome and Human Retrovirology* 20:448–454.

8. Lyles, C.M., D. Vlahov, H. Farzadegan, et al. 1998. Comparison of two measures of human immunodeficiency virus (HIV) type 1 load in HIV risk groups. *Journal of Clinical Microbiology* 36:3647–3652.

9. Maini, M.K., R.J. Gilson, N. Chavda, et al. 1996. Reference ranges and sources of variability of CD4 counts in HIV-seronegative women and men. *Genitourinary Medicine* 72:27–31.

10. Melnick, S..L, R. Sherer, T.A. Louis, et al. 1994. Survival and disease progression according to gender of patients with HIV infection. The Terry Beirn Community Programs for Clinical Research on AIDS. *Journal of the American Medical Association* 272:1915–1921.

11. Hader, S.L., D.K. Smith, J.S. Moore, and S.D. Holmberg. 2001. HIV infection in women in the United States: Status at the Millenium. *Journal of the American Medical Association* 285:1186–1192.

12. Prins, M., J.R. Robertson, R.P. Brettle, et al. 1999. Do gender differences in CD4 cell counts matter? *AIDS* 13:2361–2364.

13. Carr, A., K. Samaras, S. Burton, et al. 1998. A syndrome of peripheral lipodystrophy, hyperlipidaemia and insulin resistance in patients receiving protease inhibitors. *AIDS* 12:F51–F58.

14. Carr, A., K. Samaras, D.J. Chisholm, and D.A. Cooper. 1998. Pathogenesis of HIV-1-protease inhibitor-associated peripheral lipodystrophy, hyperlipidaemia, and insulin resistance. *Lancet* 351:1881–1883.

15. Lichtenstein, K.A., D.J. Ward, A.C. Moorman, et al. 2001. Clinical assessment of HIV-associated lipodystrophy in an ambulatory population. *AIDS* 15:1389–1398.

16. Carter, V.M., J.F. Hoy, M. Bailey, P.G. Colman, I. Nyulasi, and A.M. Mijch. 2001. The prevalence of lipoatrophy in an ambulant HIV-infected population: It all depends on the definition. *HIV Medicine* 2:174–180.

17. Martin, A., D. Smith, A. Carr, et al. 2004. Progression of lipodystrophy (LD) with continued thymidine analogue usage: long-term follow-up from a randomized clinical trial (the PILR study). *HIV Clinical Trials* 5:192–200.

18. Lund, K.C., L.L. Peterson, and K.B. Wallace. 2007. The absence of a universal mechanism of mitochondrial toxicity by nucleoside analogs. *Antimicrobial Agents and Chemotherapy* 51:2531–2539.

19. Marmor, M., A.E. Friedman-Kien, L. Laubenstein, et al. 1982. Risk factors for Kaposi's sarcoma in homosexual men. *Lancet* 1:1083-1086.

20. Goedert, J.J., C.Y. Neuland, W.C. Wallen, et al. 1982. Amyl nitrate may alter T lymphocytes in homosexual men. *Lancet* 1:411–416.

21. Chang, Y., E. Cesarman, M.S. Pessin, F. Lee, J. Culpepper, D.M. Knowles, and P.S. Moore. 1994. Identification of herpesvirus-like DNA sequences in AIDS-associated Kaposi's sarcoma. *Science* 266:1865–1869.

22. Holmberg, S.D., A.C. Moorman, J.M. Williamson, et al. 2002. Protease inhibitors and cardiovascular outcomes in patients with HIV-1. *Lancet* 360:1747–1748.

23. Joseph, A.M., N.J. Arikian, L.C. An, et al. 2004. Results of a randomized controlled trial of intervention to implement smoking guidelines in Veterans Affairs medical centers: increased use of medications without cessation benefit. *Medical Care* 42:1100–1110.

24. Bozzette, S.A., C.F. Ake, H.K. Tam, S.W. Chang, and T.A. Louis. 2003. Cardiovascular and cerebrovascular events in patients treated for human immunodeficiency virus infection. *New England Journal of Medicine* 348:702–710.

25. Obel, N., H.F. Thomsen, G. Kronborg, et al. 2007. Ischemic heart disease in HIV-infected and HIV-uninfected individuals: A population-based cohort study. *Clinical Infectious Diseases* 44:1625–1631.

26. Nieman, R.B., J. Fleming, R.J. Coker, J.R. Harris, and D.M. Mitchell. 1993. The effect of cigarette smoking on the development of AIDS in HIV-1-seropositive individuals. *AIDS* 7:705–710.

27. Miguez-Burbano, M.J., D. Ashkin, A. Rodriguez, et al. 2005. Increased risk of Pneumocystis carinii and community-acquired pneumonia with tobacco use in HIV disease. *International Journal of Infectious Diseases* 9:208–217.

28. Conley, L.J., T.J. Bush, S.P. Buchbinder, K.A. Penley, F.N. Judson, and S.D. Holmberg. 1996. The association between cigarette smoking and selected HIV-related medical conditions. *AIDS* 10:1121–1126.

29. Burns, D.N., D. Hillman, J.D. Neaton, et al. 1996. Cigarette smoking, bacterial pneumonia, and other clinical outcomes in HIV-1 infection. Terry Beirn Community Programs for Clinical Research on AIDS (CPCRA). *Journal of Acquired Immune*

Deficiency Syndromes and Human Retrovirology 13:374–383.

30. Galai, N., L.P. Park, J. Wesch, B. Visscher, S. Riddler, and J.B. Margolick. 1997. Effect of smoking on the clinical progression of HIV-1 infection. *Journal of Acquired Immune Deficiency Syndromes and Human Retrovirology* 14:451–458.

31. Gail, M.H., P.S. Rosenberg, and J.J. Goedert. 1990b. Therapy may explain recent deficits in AIDS incidence. *Journal of Acquired Immune Deficiency Syndromes* 3:296–306.

32. Gwinn, M., M. Pappaioanau, J.R. George, et al. 1991. Prevalence of HIV infection in childbearing women in the United States: Surveillance using newborn blood samples. *Journal of the American Medical Association* 265:1704–1708.

33. Karon, J.M., P.S. Rosenberg, G. McQuillan, M. Khare, M. Gwinn, and L.R. Petersen. 1996. Prevalence of HIV infection in the United States, 1984 to 1992. *Journal of the American Medical Association* 276:126–131.

34. Hahn, R.A., I.M. Onorato, T.S. Jones, and J. Dougherty. 1989. Prevalence of HIV infection among intravenous drug users in the United States. *Journal of the American Medical Association* 261:2677–2684.

35. Holmberg, S.D. 1996. The estimated prevalence and incidence of HIV in 96 large US metropolitan areas. *American Journal of Public Health* 86:642–654.

36. Hooper, E. 1999. *The River: A Journey to the Source of HIV and AIDS*. Boston: Little, Brown and Company.

37. Buchbinder, S.P., B. Metch, S.E. Holte, S. Scheer, A. Coletti, and E. Vittinghoff. 2004. Determinants of enrollment in a preventive HIV vaccine trial: Hypothetical versus actual willingness and barriers to participation. *Journal of Acquired Immune Deficiency Syndromes* 36:604–612.

38. Popovic, M., M.G. Sarngadharan, E. Read, and R.C. Gallo. 1984. Detection, isolation, and continuous production of cytopathic retroviruses (HTLV-III) from patients with AIDS and pre-AIDS." *Science* 224:497–500.

39. Kanki, P.J., F. Barin, S. M'Boup, et al. 1986. New human T-lymphotropic retrovirus related to simian T-lymphotropic virus III (STLV-IIIAGM). *Science* 232:238–242.

40. Kestler 3rd, H.W., Y. Li, Y.M. Naidu, et al. 1988. Comparison of simian immunodeficiency virus isolates. *Nature* 331:619–622.

41. Kanki, P.J., G. Eisen, K.U. Travers, et al. 1996. HIV-2 and natural protection against HIV-1 infection [letter]. *Science* 272:1960.

42. Greenberg, A.E., S.F. Wiktor, K.M. DeCock, P. Smith, H.W. Jaffe, and T.J. Dondero Jr. 1996. HIV-2 and natural protection against HIV-1 infection [technical comments]. *Science* 272:1959.

43. Imagawa, D.T., M.H. Lee, S.M Wolinsky et al. 1989. Human immunodeficiency virus type 1 infection in homosexual men who remain seronegative for prolonged periods. *New England Journal of Medicine* 320:1458–1462.

44. Horsburgh Jr., C.R., C.-Y. Ou, S.D. Holmberg, et al. 1989. Human immunodeficiency virus type infections in homosexual men who remain seronegative for prolonged periods [letter]. *New England Journal of Medicine* 321:1679–1680.

45. Imagawa, D., and R. Detels. 1991. HIV-1 in seronegative homosexual men [letter]. *New England Journal of Medicine* 325:1250–1251.

46. Farzadegan, H., M.A. Polis, S.M. Wolinsky, et al. 1988. Loss of human immunodeficiency virus type 1 (HIV-1) antibodies with evidence of viral infection in asymptomatic homosexual men. A report from the Multicenter AIDS Cohort Study. *Annals of Internal Medicine* 108:785–790.

47. Holmberg, S.D., C.R. Horsburgh Jr., R.H. Byers, et al. 1988. Errors in reporting seropositivity for infection with human immunodeficiency virus (HIV)[letter]. *Annals of Internal Medicine* 109:679–680.

48. Becker, J.T., U. Hazan, M.Y. Nguyere, et al. Infection of cultured insect cells with HIV, the causative agent of AIDS, and demonstration of infection in African insects with this virus (French). 1986. *Comptes rendus de l'Académie des sciences. Série III, Sciences de la vie* 303:303–306

49. Bagasra, O., H. Farzadegan, T. Seshamma, J.W. Oakes, A. Saah, and R.J. Pomerantz. 1994. Detection of HIV-1 proviral DNA in sperm from HIV-1-infected men. *AIDS* 8:1669–1674.

50. Stein, D.S., N.M.H. Graham, L.P. Park, et al. 1994. The effect of interaction of acyclovir with zidovudine on progression to AIDS and survival. Analysis of data in the Multicenter AIDS Cohort Study. *Annals of Internal Medicine* 121:100–108.

51. Duesberg, P. 1988. HIV is not the cause of AIDS [policy forum]. *Science* 241:514, 517.

52. Duesberg, P. 1994. Infectious AIDS–Stretching the germ theory beyond its limits. *International Archives of Allergy and Immunology* 103:118–127.

53. Day, L. 1991. *AIDS: What the Government Isn't Telling You.* Palm Desert, CA: Rockford Press.

54. Culbert, M. 1989. *AIDS: Hope, Hoax and Hoopla.* Chula Vista, CA: Robert W. Bradford Foundation.

55. Klonoff, E.A., and H. Landrine. 1999. Do blacks believe that HIV/AIDS is a government conspiracy against them? *Preventive Medicine* 28:451–457.

56. Bird, S.T., and L.M. Bogart. 2005. Conspiracy beliefs about HIV/AIDS and birth control among African Americans: Implications for the prevention of HIV, other STIs and unintended pregnancy. *Journal of Social Issues* 62:109–126.

57. Bogart, L.M., and S. Thorburn. 2005. Are HIV/AIDS conspiracy beliefs a barrier to HIV prevention among African Americans? *Journal of the Acquired Immune Deficiency Syndromes* 38:213–218.

58. Smith, D.K., J.J. Neal, and S.D. Holmberg. 1993. Unexplained opportunistic infections and CD4+ T-lymphocytopenia without HIV infection. The Centers for Disease Control Idiopathic CD4+ T-lymphocytopenia Task Force. *New England Journal of Medicine* 328:429–431.

59. Gunsalus, C.K., E.M. Bruner, N.C. Burbules, et al. 2006. Mission creep in the IRB world [editorial]. *Science* 312:1441

60. Green, L.A., J.C. Lowery, C.P. Kowalski, and L. Wyszewianski. 2006. Impact of institutional review board practice variation on observational health services research. *Health Services Research* 41:214–230.

61. Laumann, E.O., R.T. Michael, and J.H. Gagnon. 1994. A political history of the national sex survey of adults. *Family Planning Perspectives* 26:34–38.

62. Laine, C., S.N. Goodman, M.E. Griswold, and H.C. Sox. 2007. Reproducible research: Moving toward research the public can really trust. *Annals of Internal Medicine* 146:450–453.

63. Callaham, M.L., and J. Tercier. 2007. The relationship of previous training and experience of journal peer reviewers to subsequent review quality. *Public Library of Science (PloS) Medicine.* 4 (online):e40. Available at http://www.pubmedcentral.nih.gov/articlerender.fcgi?tool=pubmed&pubmedid=17411314

64. Agee, C. 2007. Improving the peer review process: Develop a professional review committee for better and quicker results. *Healthcare Executive* 22:72–73.

Appendix: Antiretroviral Drugs Approved by the U.S. Food and Drug Administration, 2007

Generic name (trade name)	Current adult dosage (pills/day)	Manufacturer	Approval date (time to approval, months)
Nucleos(t)ide Reverse Transcriptase Inhibitors (NRTIs)			
zidovudine, AZT (Retrovir)	2	GlaxoSmithKline	March 1987 (3.5)
didanosine, ddI (Videx)	1–4	Bristol-Myers Squibb	October 1991 (6.0)
zalcitabine, ddC (Hivid)	3	Hoffman-La Roche	June 1992 (7.6)
stavudine, d4T (Zerit)	2	Bristol-Myers Squibb	June 1994 (5.9)
lamivudine, 3TC (Epivir)	2	GlaxoSmithKline	November 1995 (4.4)
AZT/3TC (Combivir)	2	GlaxoSmithKline	September 1997 (3.9)
abacavir, ABC (Ziagen)	2	GlaxoSmithKline	December 1998 (5.8)
abacavir/AZT/3TC (Trizivir)	2	GlaxoSmithKline	November 2000 (10.9)
tenofovir, TDF (Viread)	1	Gilead Sciences, Inc.	October 2001 (5.9)
emtricitabine, FTC (Emtriva)	1	Gilead Sciences, Inc.	July 2003 (10.0)
abacavir/lamivudine (Epzicom)	1	GlaxoSmithKline	August 2004 (10.0)
tenofovir/emtricitabine (Truvada)	1	Gilead Sciences, Inc.	August 2004 (5.0)

Generic name (trade name)	Current adult dosage (pills/day)	Manufacturer	Approval date (time to approval, months)
Protease Inhibitors (PIs)			
saquinavir (Invirase)	6	Hoffman-La Roche	December 1995 (3.2)
ritonavir (Norvir)[a]	2–12	Abbott Laboratories	March 1996 (2.3)
indinavir (Crixivan)[b]	6	Merck & Co., Inc.	March 1996 (1.4)
nelfinavir (Viracept)	9–10	Agouron Pharmaceuticals	September 1998 (2.6)
lopinavir and ritonavir (Kaletra)[b]	4	Abbott Laboratories	September 2000 (3.5)
atazanavir (Reyataz)[b]	2	Bristol-Myers Squibb	June 2003 (6.0)
fosamprenavir (Lexiva)[b]	4	GlaxoSmithKline	October 2003 (10.0)
tipranavir, TPV (Aptivus)[b]	8	Boehringer Ingelheim	June 2005 (6.0)
darunavir (Prezista)[b]	6	Tibotec, Inc.	June 2006 (6.0)
Non-Nucleoside Reverse Transcriptase Inhibitors (NNRTIs)			
nevirapine (Viramune)	2	Boehringer Ingelheim	June 1996 (3.9)
delavirdine, DLV (Rescriptor)	6	Pfizer	April 1997 (8.7)
efavirenz (Sustiva)	1	Bristol Myers-Squibb	September 1998 (3.2)
Fusion Inhibitor efuvirtide, T-20 (Fuzeon)	2[c]	Hoffman-LaRoche/Trimeris	March 2003 (6.0)
Multiclass Combination Product efavirenz/emtricitabine/ tenofovir (Atripla)	1	Bristol-Myers Squibb/Gilead	July 2006 (2.5)

[a] Now rarely used at full dose (12 pills/day), but as a 50–100 mg pill twice per day to "boost" efficacy of other protease inhibitor drugs.

[b] "Boosted" with low-dose ritonavir; pills per day includes ritonavir dosage.

[c] Two subcutaneous injections per day.

Source: Adapted from U.S. Food and Drug Administration (FDA), "Drugs Used in the Treatment of HIV Infection," May 2007. Available at http://www.fda.gov/oashi/aids/virals.html

Index

About the Author

SCOTT D. HOLMBERG, M.D., joined the Centers for Disease Control in 1982. As a Peace Corps Volunteer working in smallpox eradication in Ethiopia, he had become dedicated to a professional life of investigating and controlling epidemics. He then returned to the United States, and, after premedical courses, medical school, and residency, joined the CDC. The history of scientific errors and controversies in this book is based on his experience as Chief of Epidemiology for the CDC's Division of HIV/AIDS Prevention from 1986 to 2005. Holmberg has authored or co-authored more than 150 scientific articles about HIV/AIDS, and has received many awards from the CDC, the Department of Health and Human Services, and the U.S. Public Health Service, in which he served as a Commissioned Officer. He is a graduate of Columbia University College of Physicians and Surgeons and Emory University.